# Dysphagia Assessment and Treatment Planning

## A TEAM APPROACH

*Second Edition*

# Dysphagia Assessment and Treatment Planning

## A TEAM APPROACH

*Second Edition*

Rebecca Leonard, Ph.D.
Katherine Kendall, M.D.

PLURAL
PUBLISHING
INC.

SAN DIEGO
OXFORD
BRISBANE

5521 Ruffin Road
San Diego, CA 92123

e-mail: info@pluralpublishing.com
Web site: http://www.pluralpublishing.com

49 Bath Street
Abingdon, Oxfordshire OX14 1EA
United Kingdom

Typeset in 10½ × 13 Palatino by Flanagan's Publishing Services, Inc.
Printed in Hong Kong by Paramont Printing

**Library of Congress Cataloging-in-Publication Data:**

Dysphagia assessment and treatment planning : a team approach / [edited by]
Rebecca Leonard and Katherine Kendall. — 2nd ed.
     p. ; cm.
  Includes bibliographical references and indexes.
  ISBN-13: 978-1-59756-153-2 (pbk.)
  ISBN-10: 1-59756-153-3 (pbk.)
  1. Deglutition disorders. I. Leonard, Rebecca. II. Kendall, Katherine, M.D.
  [DNLM: 1. Deglutition Disorders—diagnosis. 2. Deglutition Disorders—
therapy. 3. Patient Care Planning. 4. Patient Care Team. WI 250 D9976 2007]
  RC815.2.D86 2007
  616.3'23—dc22
                                         2007018791

# Contents

# Introduction

In the 10 years since the publication of the first edition of this text, many changes have occurred in the assessment and treatment of dysphagic patients. New emphasis on the relationship between pharyngeal and esophageal function has driven clinicians to be more knowledgeable about the role of each, and the instrumentation for assessing each, in understanding dysphagia. New information regarding the possible benefits of exercise therapies in selected dysphagic patients is just beginning to emerge, and will hopefully encourage therapists to tap into and utilize knowledge banks previously unfamiliar to them, such as exercise physiology and kinesiology. Surgical techniques, particularly reconstructive procedures in head and neck cancer, are increasingly incorporating principles of retaining or restoring function of critical oral and pharyngeal structures and, as a consequence, creating new hope for post-treatment swallowing capabilities in patients.

Many of these changes are considered in this second edition. Entire chapters are devoted, respectively, to esophageal phase dysphagia and to the role of reflux in dysphagia. In another chapter, emerging technologies in dysphagia assessment are reviewed, with succinct and clear discussions of the kinds of data they provide, and how these are interpreted. Behavioral, medical, and surgical treatments for dysphagia are critically reviewed not only in terms of their demonstrated effectiveness, but also with respect to questions that need to be answered regarding their appropriate uses. In other chapters, extensive revisions by the authors have contemporized material pertinent to nursing evaluations and concerns in dysphagia management, clinical evaluation of adult and pediatric populations, and endoscopic and radiographic assessment practices. The revised chapter on nutrition incorporates, among other things, new information about the National Dysphagia Diet, and how this can be translated into the realities of both hospital and home practice. Chapters concerned with dysphagia specific to neurogenic and head and neck surgery populations, respectively, have been updated to reflect our current understanding of swallowing impairment associated with these types of disorders, as well as treatment considerations in the management of patients who experience them.

Four chapters in the revised text are devoted to the dynamic fluoroscopic swallow study (DSS). This emphasis reflects our great interest in the topic, and our view that the study represents a powerful diagnostic tool. Our sense is that most clinicians just "scratch the surface" of its capabilities, using it primarily to make determinations about aspiration or recommendations for diet, and possibly, to probe strategies that facilitate safe and effective swallowing. Alhough these are of course important considerations, the use of a standard protocol in performing the exam, and the extraction of objective measurements from it, adds significantly to the power of the DSS. Our approach to it as a standardized test pemits us to compare our patients to normal, to other patient populations, and across time and treatments, in an objective manner. Over the last several years, we have collected fluoroscopic data for a relatively large number of normal subjects, and for several thousand dysphagic patients. We have learned a great deal about normal swallow function, and how it varies according to age and gender. In addition, we have acquired useful insights into characteristics of swallowing in a wide variety of patient populations. As we review this information, we are also finding that some measures are particularly useful in assessing risk and potential in patients. A number of these measures, and how they allow us to anticipate patient performance beyond the context of the fluoro study, are discussed in the text. An animated tutorial that describes how those measures are made, DSS TUTOR, is included on the DVA accompanying the text. In addition, an entire chapter has been devoted to interpretation of the dynamic swallow study. The author of this chapter, as well as the chapter on conduct of the DSS, is a clinician who has spent many years not only directing fluoro studies, but also making objective measures and forming subjective impressions from them. Readers who are already involved in directing these studies, as well as clinicians who are just beginning, will undoubtedly learn from and appreciate her excellent insights.

The measurement chapter includes instructions, materials, and even programs required to extract objective measures from fluoroscopy studies. In addition, several normal and patient studies are included with our measurement data. Readers can make measurements, themselves, and compare them to our findings. Attempting to measure various biomechanical aspects of swallowing, i.e. timing and displacement, is an excellent way to learn about swallow function, and it is in the spirit of learning and having fun that this material is offered.

Another addition to the revised text is an entire chapter on the anatomy and physiology of deglutition. Information presented provides the groundwork for understanding all other discussions of anatomy and physiology that appear in the text, and we think it's an extremely valuable addition. The other major inclusion in the revised text are numerous video clips of fluoroscopic and endoscopic swallow studies demonstrating both normal and disordered swallow function. Other videos are used to illustrate new technologies, for example, fluoromanometry and guided observation of swallowing in the esophagus (GOOSE). Videos of endoscopic studies are utilized to model structures of the upper airway during swallowing as a series of valves and chambers. The model presented provides a useful perspective for understanding swallowing physiology, and for assessing its adequacy for swallowing via fluoroscopy and endoscopy. Other clips illustrate the implementation and use of various strategies that facilitate safe and effective swallow in particular patients.

One thing that has not changed since the first edition of the text is our belief in the value of a team approach in the management of dysphagic patients. Dysphagia can be defined as the impaired transfer of nutrition/hydration from the lips to the stomach. The symptoms associated with this impairment may be subtle or dramatic, immediate or delayed, and perceived or not by an individual swallower. Many different diseases and conditions can produce dysphagia, in both pediatric and adult populations. The broad scope of these disorders exceeds the expertise of any one specialist, and the content area of any one discipline. Consequently, the ideal approach to assessment and treatment planning is from the perspective of a team. A group of specialists, each with a unique background and particular skills, is likely to identify, understand, and treat a given disorder more comprehensively, and more effectively, than an individual caregiver.

This has been our belief since we began to evaluate and treat dysphagic patients, and our conviction has only become stronger in the intervening years. A "team" may take different forms, be comprised of different specialists, and operate in different ways. But, whatever the form, we are convinced that patients are best served by a group of specialists who recognize how multifaceted and complex dysphagia can be, and who appreciate an approach to patient care that incorporates this recognition, seeks ongoing input from pertinent sources, and attempts to translate this into the best treatment plan possible. This edition of *Dysphagia Assessment and Treatment Planning: A Team Approach* provides a comprehensive view of the interdisciplinary approach practiced in our own setting. We hope it will encourage those who seek to develop similar groups in their own settings, and offer an additional perspective to those who already practice in the context of a "team."

# Acknowledgments

The authors gratefully acknowledge the significant contributions of the members of the U.C. Davis Dysphagia Team to this project. Their enthusiasm, skill, knowledge, and insights, apparent weekly in their function as members of our team, are no less apparent in this text. We are extremely fortunate to have developed and maintained a strong interdisciplinary and collegial approach to the management of our patients, and we firmly believe that it represents an excellent model for professionals involved in the management of dysphagia. We would also like to thank those patients and volunteer subjects who have shared their time and efforts willingly and generously to our collection of normative and other data. Finally, the U.C. Davis staff who make our work more pleasant, and more possible, are also high on our thank you list. These include Chitra Rao and Linsey Jordan, for their assistance in retrieving, compiling, and editing, and Geoff Chan, for resolving computer glitches on a daily basis. Their support is greatly appreciated.

# Contributors

**Peter C. Belafsky, M.D., Ph.D., M.P.H**
Assistant Professor
Department of Otolaryngology
University of California Davis
Sacramento, California
*Chapters 5, 6, and 13*

**Margie Crandall, R.N., R.S.N., Ph.D.**
Center for Nursing Research
University of California Davis,
Children's Hospital
Sacramento, California
*Chapter 9*

**Susan J. Goodrich, M.S.**
Senior Speech Pathologist
Voice and Swallowing Center
Sacramento, California
*Chapters 8, 9, and 18*

**E. Ralph Johnson, M.D.**
Cameryn Park, California
*Chapter 4*

**Katherine Kendall, M.D.**
Department of Otolaryngology
Veterans Administration Medical Center
Minneapolis, Minnesota
*Chapters 1, 2, 3, 16, and 18*

**Rebecca Leonard, Ph.D.**
Adjunct Professor
Department of Otolaryngology
University of California Davis
Sacramento, California
*Chapters 11, 14, 16, 17, and 18*

**Beverly Lorens**
Clinical Dietician
Food and Nutrition Service
University of California Davis Medical
    Center
Sacramento, California
*Chapter 10*

**Susan McKenzie, M.S.**
Senior Speech Pathologist
Voice and Swallowing Center
Univesity of California Davis
Sacramento, California
*Chapters 14, 15, 16, 17, and 18*

**Janet Pitcher, R.N., M.S., P.N.P.**
Child Neurology Nurse Practioner
University of California Davis Medical
    Center
Sacramento, California
*Chapter 9*

**Catherine J. Rees, M.D.**
Center for Voice and Swallowing
    Disorders
Assistant Professor of Otoloryngology
Wake Forest University School of
    Medicine
Winston-Salem, North Carolina
*Chapters 5, 6, and 13*

**C. John Rosenquist, M.D.**
Professor of Radiology
University of California Davis
Sacramento, California
*Chapter 12*

**Ann E. F. Sievers, R.N., M.A.,
C.O.R.L.N.**
Department of Otolaryngology
University of California Davis
Sacramento, California
*Chapter 7*

**Alice Walker, M.S.**
Sr. Speech Pathologist
Voice and Swallowing Center
University of California Davis
Sacramento, California
*Chapter 8*

# 1

# *Anatomy and Physiology of Deglutition*

## Katherine Kendall

Familiarity with the anatomy and physiology of normal deglutition enables a more focused approach to the evaluation of patients with disordered swallowing. This chapter will discuss those head and neck structures involved in swallowing and review the sequence of events resulting in a successful swallow.

The oral cavity, oropharynx, and esophagus can be thought of as a series of expanding and contracting chambers, divided by muscular sphincters. Propulsion of a bolus through this part of the alimentary tract is the result of forces or positive pressure developed behind the bolus, as well as a vacuum or negative pressure developed in front of the bolus. The creation of propulsion pressures depends upon the sequential contraction and expansion of the chambers of the upper aerodigestive tract and the competency of the sphincters dividing the chambers. Any distur-bance in the functional elements or coordination of this system is likely to result in less efficient transfer of a bolus from the oral cavity to the stom-ach, resulting in dysphagia. Swallow-ing involves coordination of the sequence of activation and inhibition for more than 25 pairs of muscles in the mouth, pharynx, larynx, and esopha-gus (Appendix 1A). An understanding of how the structures of the head and neck interact and coordinate to bring about the propulsion pressures required for normal swallowing is vital for the clinician involved in the evaluation and treatment of patients with swal-lowing complaints.

For simplicity, the act of deglutition is traditionally divided into four parts: the preparatory phase, the oral phase, the pharyngeal phase, and the esoph-ageal phase (Dodds, Stewart, & Loge-mann, 1990; Miller, 1982).

## PREPARATORY PHASE

The preparatory phase of swallowing includes mastication of the bolus, mixing it with saliva, and dividing the food for transport through the pharynx and esophagus. The preparatory phase takes place in the oral cavity, the first chamber in the swallowing system. This oral preparatory phase of swallowing is almost entirely voluntary and can be interrupted at any time.

During bolus preparation, facial muscles play a role in maintaining the bolus on the tongue and between the teeth for chewing. Specifically, the obicularis oris muscle, the circular muscle of the lips, maintains oral competence and can be considered as the first sphincter of the swallowing system.

The buccinator muscle of the cheek contracts to keep the bolus from pooling in the pockets formed by the gingival buccal sulcii. These muscles receive neural input from the facial nerve or cranial nerve VII (Figures 1–1A, 1–1B, and 1–1C).

Most of the movement and positioning of the bolus is carried out by the tongue muscles. In addition to four intrinsic muscles, the tongue has four extrinsic muscles: the genioglossus, palatoglossus, styloglossus, and hyoglossus muscles (Figure 1–2). Along with the genioglossus muscle, the intrinsic muscles act primarily to alter the shape and tone of the tongue while the other three extrinsic muscles aid in the positioning of the tongue relative to other oral cavity and pharyngeal

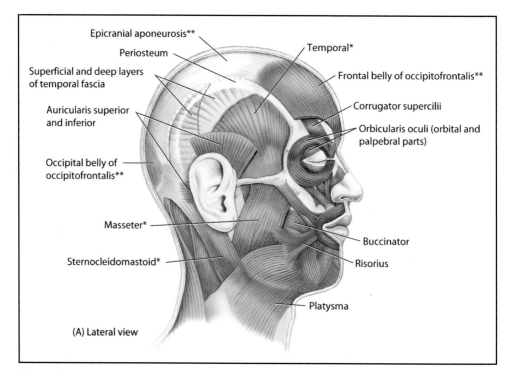

**Figure 1-1. A.** Facial musculature shown in relationship to muscles of head and neck. *(continues)*

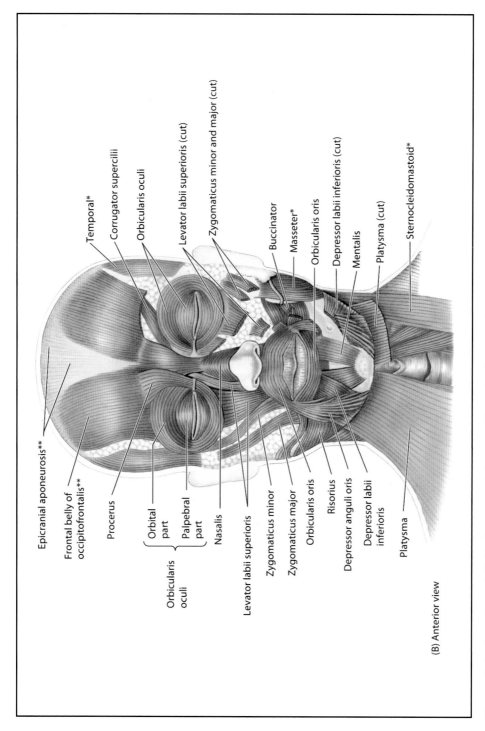

Epicranial aponeurosis**

Frontal belly of occipitofrontalis**

Procerus

Orbicularis oculi { Orbital part / Palpebral part }

Nasalis

Levator labii superioris

Zygomaticus minor

Zygomaticus major

Orbicularis oris

Risorius

Depressor anguli oris

Depressor labii inferioris

Platysma

Temporal*

Corrugator supercilii

Orbicularis oculi

Levator labii superioris (cut)

Zygomaticus minor and major (cut)

Buccinator

Masseter*

Orbicularis oris

Depressor labii inferioris (cut)

Mentalis

Platysma (cut)

Sternocleidomastoid*

(B) Anterior view

**Figure 1–1.** *(continued)* **B.** Facial musculature and buccinator muscle, anterior view. *(continues)*

3

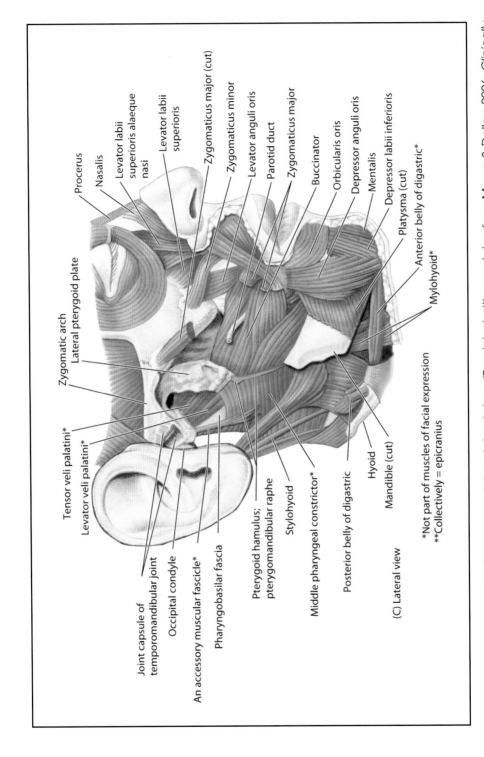

**Figure 1-1.** *(continued)* **C.** Facial musculature, lateral view. (Reprinted with permission from Moore & Dalley, 2006, *Clinically Oriented Anatomy* (5th ed., pp. 934, 935). Copyright 2006 Williams and Wilkins, Figures 7–4a, 7–4b, and 7–4c, respectively.)

Zygomaticus major (cut)

Levator labii superioris alaeque nasi

Levator labii superioris

Procerus

Nasalis

Zygomaticus minor

Levator anguli oris

Parotid duct

Zygomaticus major

Buccinator

Orbicularis oris

Depressor anguli oris

Mentalis

Depressor labii inferioris

Platysma (cut)

Anterior belly of digastric*

Mylohyoid*

Zygomatic arch

Lateral pterygoid plate

Tensor veli palatini*

Levator veli palatini*

Joint capsule of temporomandibular joint

Occipital condyle

An accessory muscular fascicle*

Pharyngobasilar fascia

Pterygoid hamulus; pterygomandibular raphe

Stylohyoid

Middle pharyngeal constrictor*

Posterior belly of digastric

Hyoid

Mandible (cut)

(C) Lateral view

*Not part of muscles of facial expression
**Collectively = epicranius

4

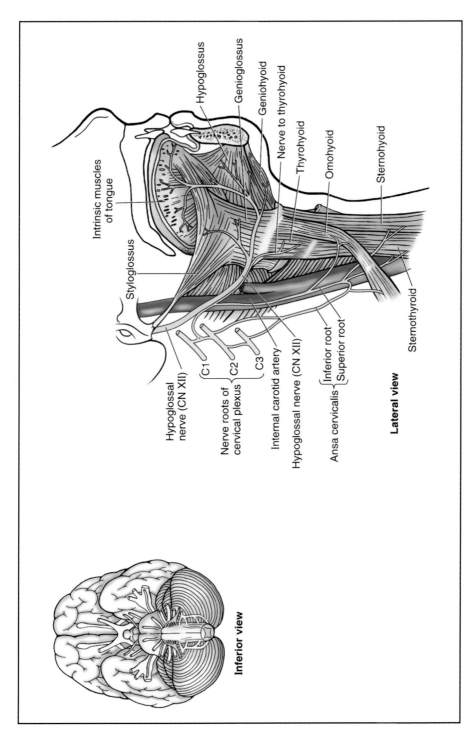

**Figure 1-2.** Distribution of the hypoglossal nerve. (Reprinted with permission from Moore & Dalley, 2006, *Clinically Oriented Anatomy* (5th ed., p. 1154). Copyright 2006 Williams and Wilkins, Baltimore, Figure 9–15.)

5

structures. Cranial nerve XII, the hypoglossal nerve, carries the motor nerve fibers that innervate both the intrinsic and extrinsic tongue muscles, except for the palatoglossus muscle (see Figure 1–2). A branch of the pharyngeal plexus from the vagus nerve (X) sends motor fibers to innervate the palatoglossus muscle. A high density of mechanoreceptors within and on the surface of the tongue indicates that the tongue is an important sensory region for determining the size of the bolus. Sensory information from the anterior two thirds of the tongue is carried back to central swallowing control centers via the lingual nerve, a branch of the trigeminal nerve, or cranial nerve V. Sensory information from the posterior one third of the tongue is carried centrally by the glossopharyngeal nerve, or cranial nerve IX (Figures 1–3A and 1–3B). During the bolus preparatory phase of deglutition, the posterior part of the tongue elevates against the soft palate, which pushes downward to keep the bolus from escaping prematurely into the pharynx. The palate is the second sphincter in the swallowing system. Contraction of the palatoglossus muscles approximates the palate and posterior tongue, effectively closing the back of the oral cavity (Figures 1–4 and 1–5) (Reprinted from Moore & Dalley, 2002, 2006).

Mastication of the bolus involves the masseter muscles, the temporalis muscles, and the medial and lateral pterygoid muscles. This muscle group is known collectively as the muscles of mastication. Motor fibers controlling the contraction of these muscles are carried in branches of the trigeminal nerve (V) (Figure 1–6, A–E) (Moore & Dalley, 2006, 1992).

## Salivation

Successful transfer of a food bolus from the oral cavity into the esophagus requires the mixing of the bolus with saliva. Saliva lubricates and dilutes the bolus to a consistency proper for swallowing. Saliva contains two major types of protein secretion: an enzyme for digesting starches, and mucus for lubricating purposes. Normal salivary secretion ranges from 1.0 to 1.5 liters per day. Saliva also plays an important role in maintaining healthy oral tissues. It is bacteriostatic and controls the pathogenic bacteria normally present in the oral cavity that are largely responsible for dental caries. The secretion of saliva is controlled by the salivatory nucleus in the brainstem. The nerve fibers of the parasympathetic nervous system carry signals from the salivatory nucleus to the salivary glands (Guyton, 1981).

## ORAL PHASE

The bolus is propelled from the oral cavity to the pharynx during the oral phase of swallowing. The top of the tongue is placed on the superior alveolar ridge behind the maxillary central incisors. Voluntary opening of the pharynx then begins with elevation of the soft palate and depression of the posterior tongue (see videoclip of straw drinking in the materials folder for Chapter 1). In this way, there is expansion of the posterior oral cavity and a chute forms down which the bolus moves into the pharynx. Elevation of the palate occurs as a result of contraction of the levator palati muscle.

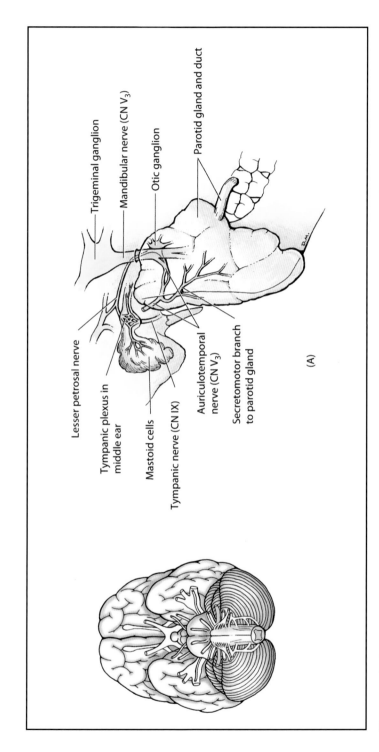

**Figure 1–3.** Distribution of the glossopharyngeal nerve (A and B). (Reprinted with permission from Moore & Dalley, 2006, *Clinically Oriented Anatomy* (5th ed., p. 1148). Copyright 2006 Williams and Wilkins, Baltimore, Figure 9–10B.) *(continues)*

7

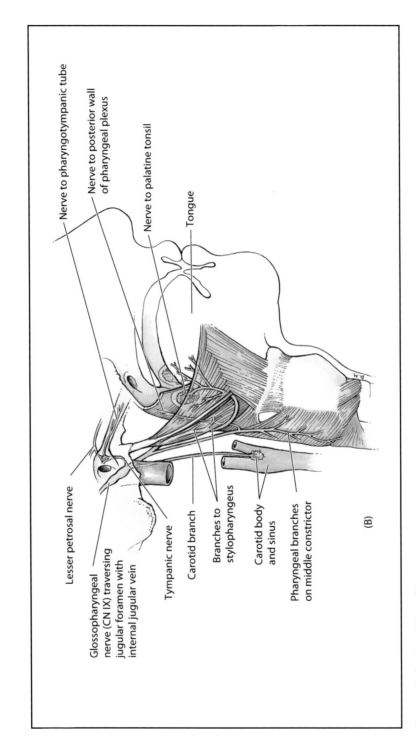

Nerve to pharyngotympanic tube

Nerve to posterior wall of pharyngeal plexus

Nerve to palatine tonsil

Tongue

Lesser petrosal nerve

Glossopharyngeal nerve (CN IX) traversing jugular foramen with internal jugular vein

Tympanic nerve

Carotid branch

Branches to stylopharyngeus

Carotid body and sinus

Pharyngeal branches on middle constrictor

(B)

**Figure 1–3.** *(continue6)*

**Figure 1-4.** Lateral view from video-fluorscopic swallowing study: Oral phase. Note bolus in the oral cavity on the superior surface of the tongue. Palate closes against tongue base to close posterior oral cavity from oropharynx.

The levator palati muscle receives motor innervation from the vagus nerve (X) via the pharyngeal plexus. The hyoglossus muscle (XII), and to a lesser extent the styloglossus muscle (XII), are active in posterior tongue depression. The anterior half of the tongue is then pressed against the maxillary alveolar ridge and the anterior half of the hard palate in rapid sequence, moving the bolus posteriorly on the dorsum of the tongue. Contraction of the obicularis oris and buccinator muscles prevents pressure escape forward, out of the mouth, or laterally (Moore & Dalley, 2002, 2006).

Soft palate elevation allows the bolus to pass through the tonsillar pillars. Once the soft palate is fully elevated, it contacts the adjacent pharyn-geal walls in a valving action that acts to prevent penetration of the bolus or pressure into the nasopharynx. The side walls of the nasopharynx, consisting of the superior pharyngeal constrictor muscle, also appose one another to make a more forceful closure of the nasopharynx (Figure 1–7). Motor nerve fibers from the vagus nerve (X) via the pharyngeal plexus innervate the superior pharyngeal constrictor and palatal musculature. The hyoid bone is then moderately elevated in preparation for the pharyngeal phase of swallowing. Early hyoid bone elevation occurs primarily as a result of mylohyoid muscle contraction. Motor innervation of the mylohyoid muscle comes from a branch of the trigeminal nerve (V) (Moore & Dalley, 2002, 2006).

The muscles involved in the oral phase of swallowing represent three anatomical regions: the suprahyoid suspensory muscles (which affect the position of the posterior tongue and thus, the hyoid bone), the muscles surrounding the tonsillar pillars, and the muscles involved in the closure of the nasopharynx. Muscles that discharge during the oral phase of swallowing include the muscles of the face, (specifically, those within the lips and cheeks), the tongue muscles, the superior pharyngeal constrictor, the styloglossus, stylohyoid, geniohyoid, and mylohyoid muscles with the palatoglossus and palatopharyngeus muscles demonstrating their maximal activity later. The anterior and posterior bellies of the digastric muscle participate in the subsequent elevation of the hyoid and larynx (see Figures 1–1A, 1–1B, and 1–6E).

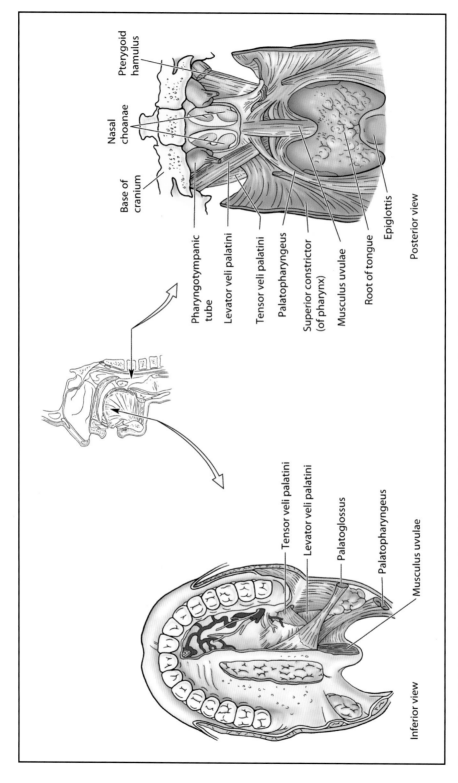

**Figure 1-5.** Palate and oral cavity (posterior view) showing tensor veli palatine and levator veli palatini muscles. (Reprinted with permission from Moore & Dalley, 2006, *Clinically Oriented Anatomy* (5th ed., p. 829). Copyright 2006 Williams and Wilkins, Baltimore, Figure 8–45.)

Pterygoid hamulus

Nasal choanae

Base of cranium

Pharyngotympanic tube

Levator veli palatini

Tensor veli palatini

Palatopharyngeus

Superior constrictor (of pharynx)

Musculus uvulae

Root of tongue

Epiglottis

Posterior view

Tensor veli palatini

Levator veli palatini

Palatoglossus

Palatopharyngeus

Musculus uvulae

Inferior view

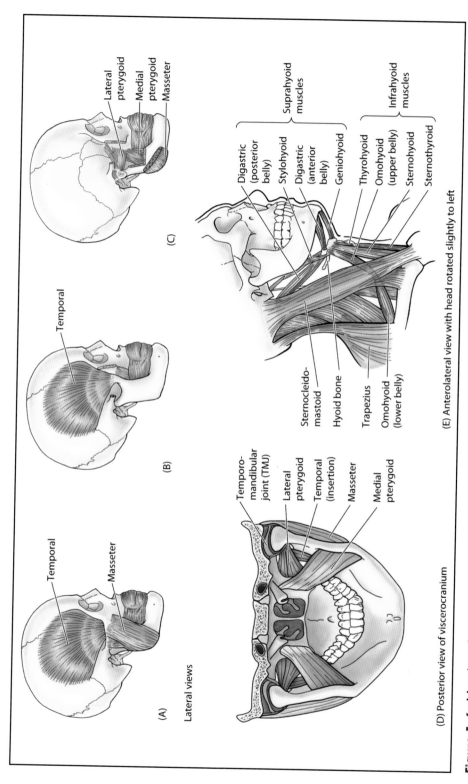

**Figure 1-6.** Muscles of mastication (A–E). (Reprinted with permission from Moore & Dalley, 2006, *Clinically Oriented Anatomy* (5th ed., p. 988). Copyright 2006 Williams and Wilkins, Baltimore, Figure 7–12.)

11

**Figure 1–7.** Lateral view from videofluoroscopic swallowing study: Oropharyngeal phase. Note elevation of palate and contact with posterior pharyngeal wall.

## PHARYNGEAL PHASE

Passage of food through the pharynx and into the esophagus occurs during the pharyngeal phase of swallowing. Respiration and swallowing must be coordinated during this portion of the swallow, since both functions occur through the common portal of the pharynx. Because respiration must cease during the pharyngeal phase of deglutition, the central control of pharyngeal swallowing must involve an efficient, automatic mechanism. The pharyngeal phase of swallowing is also involuntary and, once initiated, the pharyngeal phase is an irreversible motor event.

At the onset of the pharyngeal phase of swallowing, the tongue carries the bolus into the oropharynx as the entire posterior mass of the tongue is rolled backward on the hyoid bone, while maintaining the bolus on the tongue surface. The mandibular muscles (medial and lateral pterygoid muscles, masseter, and temporalis muscles [CN V]) contribute to stabilization of the tongue

base during the development of the tongue's piston-like movements, and this stabilization of the tongue is more critical with boluses of thicker consistency. The mandible is held in a closed position during swallowing.

As the bolus is propelled posteriorly by the piston-like movement of the tongue, the pharynx, as a whole, elevates and then contracts to create a descending peristaltic wave. Elevation of the pharynx occurs when the paired palatopharyngeus muscles contract (X). The walls of the pharyngeal chamber stiffen because of the sequential contraction of its three constrictors (CN X) (Figure 1–8 and Figures 1–9A and 1–9B). Because the oropharynx is a closed cavity at the time of bolus passage, the pressure generated by the tongue and pharyngeal walls provides a force that drives the bolus inferiorly. Simultaneously, the hyoid and larynx rise and are pulled forward under the root of the tongue by the contraction of the suprahyoid muscles. The larynx moves with the hyoid bone because it is attached to the hyoid bone by the thyrohyoid membrane and paired thyrohyoid muscles. This anterior movement of the larynx simultaneously protects the larynx from penetration by the bolus and expands the hypopharyngeal chamber causing a decrease of pressure in the pharyngoesophageal (PE) segment. This decrease in pressure in front of the bolus, along with the piston action of the tongue base against the pharyngeal constrictors, drives bolus through the pharynx and into the upper esophagus (Figure 1–10).

As the bolus is driven inferiorly and the larynx begins to move forward, the epiglottis folds down over the laryngeal opening. The epiglottis moves

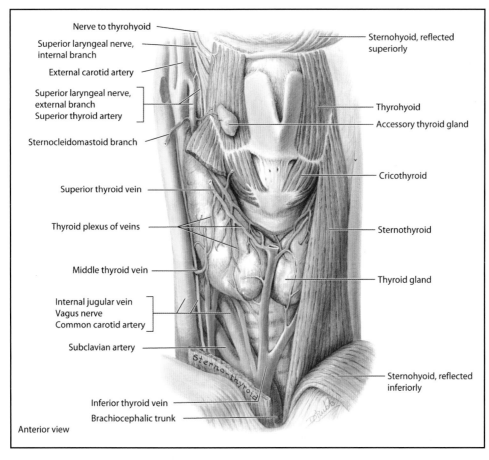

**Figure 1–8.** Anterior view of larynx and neck. (Reprinted with permission from Moore & Dalley, 2006, *Clinically Oriented Anatomy* (5th ed., p. 1085). Copyright 2006 Williams and Wilkins, Baltimore, Figure 8–23.)

from an upright to a horizontal position and then tips downward. This positional change of the epiglottis is caused mainly by elevation of the hyoid and larynx as well as by contraction of the paired thyrohyoid muscles followed by contraction of the intrinsic laryngeal muscles to close the vocal folds. The abductors of the vocal folds, the posterior cricoarytenoid muscles, are inhibited during this phase, ensuring closure of the vocal folds. The true and ventricular vocal folds play a major role in protecting the laryngeal vestibule by constricting the laryngeal aperture. The larynx closes anatomically from below upward: first, the vocal folds, then the vestibular folds, then the lower vestibule (approximation and forward movement of the arytenoids), and then the upper vestibule (horizontal position of the epiglottis that contacts the closed arytenoids). Opening of the larynx proceeds from above downward. Many of the mechanisms that contribute to airway protection also contribute to bolus transportation as closure of the larynx creates pressures

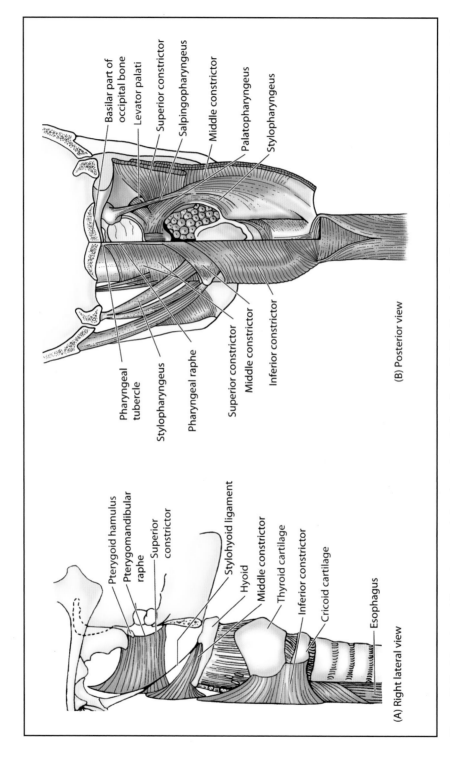

**Figure 1-9.** Muscles of the pharynx: lateral and posterior views (A, B). (Reprinted with permission from Moore & Dalley, 2006, *Clinically Oriented Anatomy* (5th ed., p. 1107). Copyright 2006 Williams and Wilkins, Baltimore, Figure 8–6.)

**Figure 1-10.** Lateral view from videofluoroscopic swallowing study: Pharyngeal phase. Note anterior displacement of hyoid and larynx with expansion of the hypopharynx. The tongue base contacts the posterior pharyngeal wall. Subject has a cricopharyngeal bar at cervical vertebra 5.

that promote movement of the bolus away from the larynx and into the upper esophagus (Figures 1–10 and 1–11) (Doty & Bosma, 1956; Kidder, 1995).

The upper esophageal sphincter, also known as the PE segment, is the third and final sphincter involved in the oropharyngeal phase of deglutition. At rest, the sphincter is closed by the tonic contraction of the cricopharyngeus muscle. Inhibition of the tonic contraction, which results in relaxation and allows for opening of the sphincter, starts at the onset of the oropharyngeal phase of swallowing and lasts until the cricopharyngeus muscle becomes active and propels the bolus into the esophagus. Both laryngeal elevation (which pulls the cricoid lamina away from the

posterior pharyngeal wall) and cricopharyngeal relaxation are essential for normal opening of the pharyngoesophageal segment for bolus passage (see Figures 1–8, 1–10, and 1–11). Manometric studies have shown that a successful swallow depends on the tongue driving pressure and the negative pressure developed in the PE segment more than the peristaltic-like pressure of the constrictors (McConnel, 1988a, 1988b).

Once the bolus passes into the pharyngoesophageal segment, the force of the pharyngeal contraction eliminates the bolus from the level of the glottic opening. If pharyngeal contractions do not fully clear the bolus from the pharynx while the laryngeal aperture is closed, then a portion of the residual bolus will be aspirated upon reopening the airway and inhaling. The pharyngeal phase of swallowing is completed when the soft palate returns to its original position and the larynx is reopened for respiration.

The oropharyngeal phase of swallowing is a complex sequence of not only excitatory but also inhibitory events that take place generally in less than one second. It involves a set of striated muscles that always participate in the fundamental motor pattern. Electromyographic studies of the muscles involved in the pharyngeal phase of swallowing have delineated that the onset of swallowing begins with a contraction of the mylohyoid muscle. At the same time or very shortly thereafter, the anterior digastric and the pterygoid muscles begin to contract (innervation from the trigeminal nerve V) followed by the geniohyoid (XII), stylohyoid (VII), styloglossus (XII), posterior tongue, superior constrictor (X),

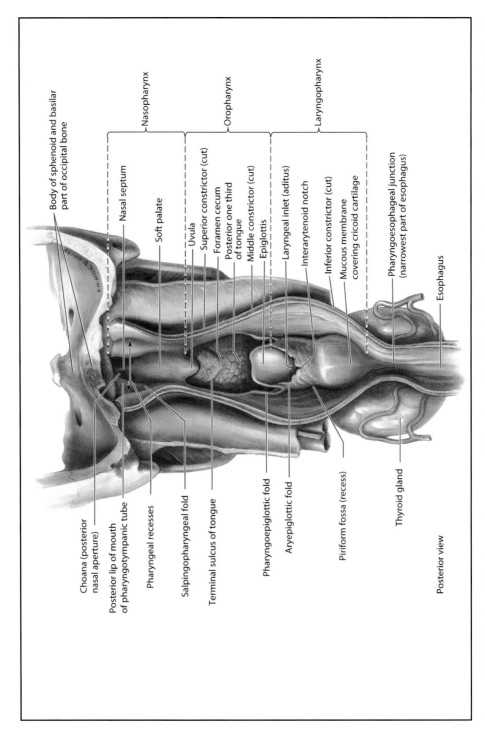

**Figure 1–11.** Muscles of the hypopharynx, posterior view. (Reprinted with permission from Moore & Dalley, 2006, *Clinically Oriented Anatomy* (5th ed., p. 1102). Copyright 2006 Williams and Wilkins, Baltimore, Figure 8–36.)

Body of sphenoid and basilar part of occipital bone

Nasopharynx

Nasal septum

Soft palate

Uvula

Superior constrictor (cut)

Foramen cecum

Posterior one third of tongue

Middle constrictor (cut)

Epiglottis

Oropharynx

Laryngeal inlet (aditus)

Interarytenoid notch

Inferior constrictor (cut)

Mucous membrane covering cricoid cartilage

Laryngopharynx

Pharyngoesophageal junction (narrowest part of esophagus)

Esophagus

Choana (posterior nasal aperture)

Posterior lip of mouth of pharyngotympanic tube

Pharyngeal recesses

Salpingopharyngeal fold

Terminal sulcus of tongue

Pharyngoepiglottic fold

Aryepiglottic fold

Piriform fossa (recess)

Thyroid gland

Posterior view

palatoglossus (X), and paltopharyngeus muscles (innervation from pharyngeal plexus: X). This group of muscles is called the "leading complex." The middle and inferior constrictor muscles then contract in an overlapping sequence. The oropharyngeal sequence ends when the wave of contraction reaches the upper esophageal sphincter. Electrophysiologic studies have shown that any background electrical activity in the swallowing muscles is inhibited with the onset of electrical activity in the leading complex and that inhibition is also found in the muscles of the leading complex just before they contract during swallowing (Doty, 1968; Doty & Bosma, 1956; Hrycyshyn & Basmajian, 1972; Miller, 1982; Moore & Dalley, 2002, 2006).

## NEURAL CONTROL OF THE PHARYNGEAL PHASE OF SWALLOWING

The complex oropharyngeal muscle contraction and relaxation sequence that results in a successful swallow is triggered and controlled by a group of neurons within the reticular formation of the brainstem. These neurons are collectively referred to as a central pattern generator because they drive a sequence of complex but repetitive movements. The neurons of the central pattern generator directly stimulate several pools of motor neurons located in various brainstem cranial motor nuclei responsible for excitatory and inhibitory signals to the muscles of the oropharynx involved in swallowing. Peripheral feedback from sensory receptors in the muscles and mucosa of the pharynx is thought to modify the swallow sequence via direct input to the neurons of the central pattern generator. The central pattern generator can therefore be subdivided into three systems: an afferent input system from peripheral sensory mechanisms to the center, an efferent system corresponding to the motor outputs from the center to the muscles of the pharynx, and an organizing system corresponding to the interneuronal network within the brainstem that programs the motor pattern. Within the central pattern generator, some neurons may participate in activities other than swallowing such as respiration, mastication, and vocalization. Respiration is also likely controlled via a central pattern generator that coordinates with the swallowing pattern generator to integrate swallowing and respiratory functions (Altschuler, Bao, Bieger, Hopkins, & Miselis, 1989; Broussard, 2000; Doty & Bosma, 1956; Jean, 1990; Jean, Car, & Roman, 1975).

### Afferent Input to the Central Pattern Generator

Branches from three cranial nerves: the trigeminal (V), the glossopharyngeal (IX), and the vagus (X) provide peripheral sensory feedback to the central pattern generator. The most sensitive oropharyngeal mucosal receptor regions for the stimulation of the swallowing sequence are innervated by fibers of the glossopharyngeal nerve via the pharyngeal plexus and by the superior laryngeal nerve (SLN) via the vagus nerve. Stimulation of the SLN induces pure swallowing with a short latency, and this finding has led to the belief that the fibers of the SLN constitute the main afferent pathway involved in the initiation of swallowing. Stimulation of the glossopharyngeal nerve facilitates swallowing, but alone, does not trigger the pure motor pattern of oropharyngeal swallowing (Doty & Bosma, 1956; Jean, 1990, 2001; Kessler & Jean, 1985; Miller, 1982; Ootani, Umezaki, Shin, & Murata, 1995).

Both the glossopharyngeal and the SLN send fibers to the nucleus tractus solitarius (NTS) in the brainstem. The NTS is the principal sensory nucleus of the pharynx and esophagus and all the afferent fibers involved in initiating or facilitating swallowing converge in the NTS, mainly in the interstitial subdivision. Almost all of the NTS neurons that are involved in swallowing are activated with stimulation of the SLN. Most of the same NTS neurons can be activated by stimulation of the glossopharyngeal nerve. During swallowing, stimulation of sensory receptors in the pharynx by the posterior projection of the bolus is thought to initiate the involuntary pharyngeal phase of swallowing coordinated by the central pattern generator via the SLN (Altschuler, 2001; Jean, 2001).

Although the oropharyngeal swallowing motor sequence is centrally organized, it can change in response to peripheral afferent information. The same irreversible muscle sequence is exhibited during swallowing of food, liquids, or saliva but sensory information received from peripheral receptors can modulate the central network activity to adapt the swallowing motor sequence according to bolus consistency and size. Oropharyngeal muscle contraction timing, duration, and likely intensity, change with changes in bolus size and consistency. Sensory feedback

likely modifies the central program, by adjusting the motor outputs depending on the contents of the oropharyngeal tract. In other words, continuous sensory feedback from the pharynx may influence the neurons of the central pattern generator and thus modulate the central program. Considerable variability in the sequence of events that occurs during the pharyngeal phase of swallowing can be appreciated on videofluoroscopic studies of swallowing in normal individuals. Ablation of sensory feedback does not, however, disrupt sequential discharge of the cranial motor nerve fibers that occurs during swallowing (Hamdy et al., 1997, 1999; Jean, 2001; Kendall, 2002; Kendall, McKenzie, Leonard, Goncalves, & Walker, 2000; Kendall, Leonard, & McKenzie, 2003).

## Higher Cortical Input to the Central Pattern Generator

Higher cortical input is also thought to influence the coordination of swallowing by the central pattern generator. Many of the neurological disorders that result in dysphagia do not involve the brainstem but rather affect a wide range of supramedullary central neural regions. In addition, the fact that swallowing can be initiated voluntarily without stimulation of the pharynx by a bolus, such as in a "dry" swallow, indicates that input from cerebral cortex can trigger swallowing.

The mechanism by which higher cortical centers impact swallowing function is poorly understood, but it appears that a widespread network of brain regions participate in the control of swallowing. It is hypothesized that speech movements and perhaps the oral phase of swallowing rely on the lateral regions of the primary motor cortex and the premotor areas that are mapped somatotopically to the anterior vocal tract. There are a number of subcortical sites, including the corticofugal swallowing pathway, which can trigger or modify swallowing, in particular the internal capsule, subthalamus, amygdala, hypothalamus, substantia nigra, mesencephalic reticular formation, and monoaminergic brain stem nuclei. Many studies of central swallowing control emphasize the importance of the inferior precentral gyrus. The anterior insula/claustrum and the cerebellum are also likely active in the initiation of voluntary swallowing (Barlow & Burton, 1990; Hamdy et al., 1999; Kendall et al., 2003; Mosier & Bereznaya, 2001; Zald & Pardo, 1999).

## Motor Output from the Central Pattern Generator

The main motor nuclei of the brainstem involved in deglutition are the hypoglossal (XII) motor nucleus and the nucleus ambiguus (X) (Figure 1–12). The cell bodies of the hypoglossal nucleus are organized myotopically, related to the different tongue muscles innervated by the hypoglossal motor neurons. The nucleus ambiguus is organized in a rostrocaudal pattern with respect to the motor neurons innervating the esophagus, pharynx, and larynx. The esophageal motor neurons are localized in the rostral compact formation of the nucleus, the pharyngeal and soft palate motor neurons are in the intermediate semicompact formation and most of the laryngeal motor

neurons are in the caudal loose formation of the nucleus. The organization scheme results in sequential firing of the motor neurons within the nucleus ambiguus during swallowing. Because the neurons in the nucleus fire sequentially during swallowing, each group of neurons in this chain may control more and more distal regions of the swallowing chain and be responsible for the successive firing behavior. In addition to excitatory drive, these motor neurons may also receive inhibitory inputs or have complex intrinsic properties that are activated by the swallowing sequence.

The motor neurons also exhibit extensive dendritic extensions into the adjacent reticular formation with a distinct pattern for each muscle group. Because the reticular formation is the location of the neuronal network that is the central pattern generator, these dendrites provide an anatomical basis for the interaction of the swallowing motor neurons and the neurons of the central pattern generator (Bieger & Hopkins, 1987; Doty & Bosma, 1956; Gestreau, Dutschmann, Obled, & Bianchi, 2005; Lawn, 1966, 1988; Tomomune & Takata, 1988; Zoungrana, Amri, Car, & Roman, 1997).

It has been reported that when the motor neurons responsible for the beginning of the swallowing sequence fire, the neurons controlling the more distal parts of the tract are inhibited and their activity is delayed. In some cases, the activity of distal neurons is inhibited before the motor activity of proximal muscle groups is initiated. These inhibitory mechanisms may contribute directly to the sequential excitation of the motor neurons. Via mechanisms such as disinhibition or

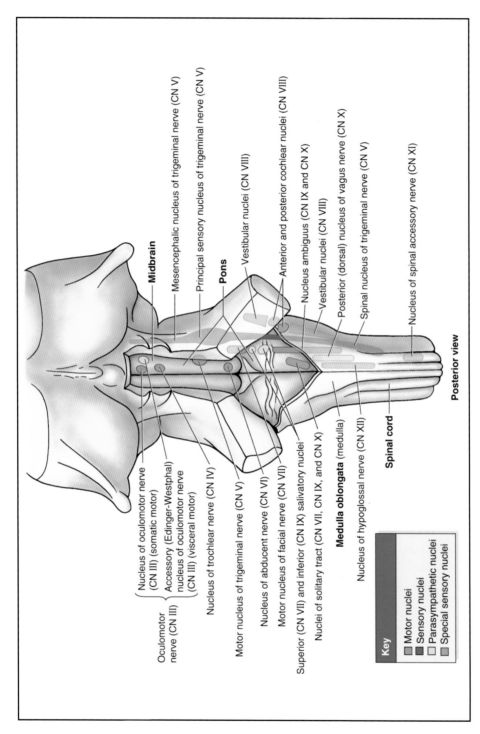

**Figure 1-12.** Brainstem motor nuclei. (Reprinted with permission from Moore & Dalley, 2006, *Clinically Oriented Anatomy* (5th ed., p. 1085). Copyright 2006 Williams and Wilkins, Baltimore, Figure 8–23.)

postinhibitory rebounds, the inhibitory connections may be at least partly responsible for the progression of the contraction wave (Jean, 2001).

## Brainstem Interneurons Responsible for the Programming and Coordination of the Swallowing Sequence

The network of brainstem neurons thought to be responsible for the coordination of the pharyngeal swallowing motor sequence is called interneurons or premotor neurons. In general, central nervous system interneurons are identified by their connectivity with multiple areas of the brainstem and other areas of the central nervous system. Specifically, the physical connections of the central swallowing pattern generator interneurons provide an anatomic substrate for the integration of swallowing-related activities with airway-protective reflexes. The interneurons of the central swallowing pattern generator are thought to be located in two main brainstem areas, although some controversy exists regarding their exact locations. The dorsal swallowing group (DSG) of interneurons is located in the dorsal medulla within the NTS and adjacent reticular formation. The neurons of the NTS receive and integrate sensory information. The ventral swallowing group (VSG) of interneurons is located in the ventrolateral medulla just above the nucleus ambiguus. The motor nuclei of the nucleus ambiguus control the pharyngeal muscles (Amirali, Tsai, Weisz, Schrader, & Sanders, 2001; Chiao, Larson, Yajima, Ko, & Kahrilas, 1994; Ezure, Oku, & Tanaka, 1993;

Gestreau et al., 2005; Kessler & Jean, 1985; Larson, Yajima, & Ko, 1994).

DSG interneurons are thought to be involved in triggering, shaping, and timing the sequential swallowing motor pattern. These interneurons exhibit a sequential firing pattern that parallels the sequential motor pattern typical of deglutition, with considerable overlap between the sequential firing of the various neurons. The neurons in this part of the reticular formation have been shown to have direct connections with the motor neurons that drive the musculature of the pharynx involved in swallowing. Each DSG neuron may be directly activated by signals from peripheral afferent fibers originating in the corresponding part of the oropharynx that is under its control.

Stimulation of the SLN results in initial activity, producing a single spike, in all of the DSG interneurons (see Figure 1–12). Some of the neurons in the DSG exhibit activity before the onset of the swallowing motor sequence, which is continuous and is called "preswallowing activity." Those DSG interneurons that display preswallowing activity can be activated by stimulation of both the SLN and the glossopharyngeal nerve. This pattern of activity observed in the DSG interneurons suggests that these neurons are involved in the initiation of swallowing. Cortical input into the swallowing central pattern generator has been found to involve the neurons of the DSG. The DSG neurons, therefore, receive convergent information from both cortical and peripheral inputs that trigger swallowing. Finally, the two hemi-central pattern generators located in each half of the medulla are tightly synchronized and it is thought that this connection occurs within the DSG of interneurons (Cunningham & Sawchenko, 2000; Jean, 2001; Kessler & Jean, 1985).

The interneurons of the VSG are thought to be "switching" neurons that distribute and coordinate the swallowing drive to the various pools of motor neurons involved in swallowing. The firing behavior of these neurons also exhibits a sequential pattern, but with more overlap, longer latency, greater duration variability, and lower frequency than the interneurons of the DSG. This type of firing behavior indicates that the connections between the VSG interneurons and their afferent fibers are likely to be polysynaptic. The VSG interneurons are probably activated by the interneurons of the DSG. They, in turn, are connected to all the various groups of motor neurons involved in swallowing and, within the VSG interneurons, each neuron can project to more than one motor nucleus. The trigeminal and hypoglossal motor nuclei are connected only to the VSG interneurons and not to the DSG. Swallowing motor neurons only receive input from the ipsilateral efferent fibers of the ventral swallowing interneurons (Amri, Car, & Roman, 1990; Jean, 2001; Kessler & Jean, 1985; Larson et al., 1994).

In addition to the interneurons of the ventral and DSGs, swallowing interneurons have been identified within the trigeminal and hypoglossal motor nuclei, or in close proximity. They may play the role of premotor neurons or be involved in the organization of the swallowing drive to the various motor neurons involved in swallowing within a single motor nucleus. They might

also be involved in the bilateral coordination of the motor neuron pools (Car & Amri, 1987; Jean, 2001; Kessler & Jean, 1985; Ono, Ishiwata, Kuroda, & Nakamura, 1998).

There is also a population of interneurons, identified more rostrally in the pons, that fire during the oropharyngeal phase of swallowing. These interneurons have been classified as sensory relay neurons and are thought to provide information from the oropharyngeal receptors to the higher nervous centers (Jean, Kessler, & Tell, 1994).

In conclusion, the DSG interneurons are involved in initiating the swallowing sequence. They stimulate the interneurons of the VSG which then modulate and coordinate the stimulation of the various motor neurons involved in the swallowing sequence (Bieger, 2001; Roda, Gestreau, & Biachi, 2002).

## ESOPHAGEAL PHASE

The bolus is transported down the esophagus into the stomach. The esophageal phase is quite simple and consists of a peristaltic wave of contraction that propagates down the esophagus. There is considerable variability in the speed and strength of the esophageal contractile wave. Once initiated, it is not an all-or-none phenomenon, but may dissipate before reaching the lower esophageal sphincter. Sensory feedback likely plays a role in regulating the speed and intensity of the esophageal peristaltic wave, depending on the characteristics of the bolus. The lower esophageal sphincter is a site of high pressure, resulting from tonic contraction of the smooth muscle making up the sphincter. Increased pressure within the sphincter prevents reflux of stomach contents into the esophagus. During swallowing, the lower esophageal sphincter tone is inhibited, relaxing the sphincter for bolus passage into the stomach (Jean, 2001).

Secondary esophageal peristalsis is defined as peristalsis without a preceding oropharyngeal phase of swallowing. Secondary peristalsis occurs in response to stimulation of esophageal sensory receptors by distension of the esophageal lumen, and is otherwise similar in character, with regard to strength and speed of contraction, to primary esophageal peristalsis. Tertiary peristalsis of the esophagus refers to peristalsis of the smooth muscle portion of the esophagus, unrelated to extrinsic innervation (Jean, 2001).

The esophageal phase of swallowing requires both excitatory and inhibitory input to the muscles of the esophagus. At rest, the esophagus is electromyographically silent. All of the esophageal motor neurons are strongly inhibited during the oropharyngeal phase of swallowing and the contractile wave of the esophagus during the esophageal phase is preceded by inhibitory input. Once the bolus enters the esophagus, bolus movement involves the coordinated contraction of the smooth and striated muscles of the esophagus. Contraction of esophageal striated muscle is controlled by the motor nuclei of the brainstem (nucleus ambiguus) whereas smooth muscle contraction is controlled by the autonomic nervous system. Smooth muscle of the esophagus is innervated by preganglionic fibers originating in the vagal motor nucleus. As are the muscles of the oropharynx,

the muscles of the esophagus are inhibited and stimulated by motor neurons under the control of interneurons associated with the swallowing central pattern generator. Less information is available regarding the location of the central pattern generator interneurons. They regulate the esophagus and coordinate the oropharyngeal and esophageal phases of swallowing. Similarly, little is known regarding the interaction of these interneurons with the esophageal motor neurons. It is believed that fewer interneurons are involved in regulating the esophageal phase of deglutition, and that central control may be more dependent on afferent input than during oropharyngeal swallowing (Jean, 2001).

## STUDY QUESTIONS

1. What are the four phases of deglutition and which are under voluntary control and which are primarily involuntary or "reflexive" in nature?
2. What are the three sphincters in the upper aerodigestive tract? Which chambers do they divide? How do they open and close?
3. What muscles are involved in bolus propulsion through the pharynx?
4. What sensory nerves are important in triggering the pharyngeal phase of swallowing and what areas of the mucosa do they supply?
5. Describe in general terms what is known about the central control of pharyngeal swallowing. What is the central pattern generator? What are the inputs to the central pattern generator? How does the central pattern generator control swallowing?

## REFERENCES

Altschuler, S. M. (2001). Laryngeal and respiratory protective reflexes. *American Journal of Medicine, 111,* 90S–94S.

Altschuler, S. M., Bao, X., Bieger, D., Hopkins, D. A., & Miselis, R. R. (1989). Viscerotopic representation of the upper alimentary tract in the rat: Sensory ganglia and nuclei of the solitary and spinal trigeminal tracts. *Journal of Comparative Neurology, 283,* 248–268.

Amirali, A., Tsai, G., Weisz, D., Schrader, N., & Sanders, I. (2001). Mapping of brain stem neuronal circuitry active during swallowing. *Annals of Otology, Rhinology and Laryngology, 110,* 502–513.

Amri, M., Car, A., & Roman, C. (1990). Axonal branching of medullary swallowing neurons projecting on the trigeminal and hypoglossal motor nuclei: Demonstration by electrophysiological and fluorescent double labeling techniques. *Experimental Brain Research, 81,* 384–390.

Barlow, S.M., & Burton, M. K. (1990). Ramp-and-hold force control in the upper and lower lips: Developing new neuromotor assessment applications in traumatically brain injured adults. *Journal of Speech and Hearing, 33,* 660–675.

Bieger, D. (2001). Rhombencephalic pathways and neurotransmitter controlling deglutition, *American Journal of Medicine, 111,* 85S–89S.

Bieger, D., & Hopkins, D. A. (1987). Viscerotopic representation of the upper alimentary tract in the medulla oblongata in the rat: The nucleus ambiguus. *Journal of Comparative Neurology, 262,* 546–562.

Broussard, D. L., & Altschuler S. M. (2000). Central integration of swallow and airway-protective reflexes, *American Journal of Medicine, 108,* 62S–67S.

Car, A., & Amri, M. (1987). Activity of neurons located in the region of the hypoglossal motor nucleus during swallowing in sheep. *Experimental Brain Research, 69,* 175–182.

Chiao, G. Z., Larson, C. R., Yajima, Y., Ko, P., & Kahrilas, P. J. (1994). Neuronal activity in nucleus ambiguus during deglutition and vocalization in conscious monkeys. *Experimental Brain Research, 100,* 29–38.

Cunningham, E. T., & Sawchenko, P. E. (2000). Dorsal medullary pathways subserving oromotor reflexes in the rat: implications from the central neural control of swallowing. *Journal of Comparative Neurology, 417,* 448–466.

Dodds, W. J., Stewart, E. J., & Logemann, J. A. (1990). Physiology and radiology of the normal and pharyngeal phases of swallowing. *American Journal of Roentgenology, 154,* 953-963.

Doty, R. W. (1968). Neural organization of deglutition. In: *Handbook of physiology. The alimentary canal* (pp. 1861–1902), Washington, DC: American Physiology Society, sect. VI.

Doty, R. W., & Bosma, J. F. (1956). An electromyographic analysis of reflex deglutition. *Journal of Neurophysiology, 19,* 44–60.

Ezure, K., Oku, Y., & Tanaka, I., (1993). Location and axonal projection of one type of swallowing interneuron in cat medulla. *Brain Research, 632,* 216–224.

Gestreau, C., Dutschmann, M., Obled, S., & Bianchi, A. L. (2005). Activation of XII motoneurons and premotor neurons during various oropharyngeal behaviors. *Respiratory Physiology Neurobiology, 147,* 159–176.

Guyton, A. C. (1981). *Textbook of medical physiology.* (6th ed., pp. 803-804), Philadelphia: W. B. Saunders.

Hamdy, S., Aziz, Q., Rothwell, J. C., Hobson, A., Barlow, J., & Thompson, D. G. (1997). Cranial nerve modulation of human cortical swallowing pathways. *American Journal of Physiology, 272,* G802–G808.

Hamdy, S., Mikulis, D. J., Crawley, A., Xue, S., Lau, H., Henry, S., et al. (1999). Cortical activation during human volitional swallowing: An event related fMRI study. *American Journal of Physiology:*

*Gastrointestinal Liver Physiology*, 277, G219–G225.

Hamdy, S., Rothwell, J. C., Brooks, D. J., Bailey, D., Aziz, Q., & Thompson, D.G. (1999). Identification of the cerebral loci processing human swallowing with H₂(15)O PET activation. *Journal of Neurophysiology*, 81, 1917–1926.

Hrycyshyn, A. W., & Basmajian, J. V. (1972). Electromyography of the oral sage of swallowing in man. *American Journal of Anatomy*, 133, 333–340.

Jean, A. (1990). Brainstem control of swallowing: localization and organization of the central pattern generator for swallowing. In A. Taylor (Ed.), *Neurophysiology of the jaws and teeth* (pp. 294–321), London: MacMillan.

Jean, A. (2001). Brain stem control of swallowing: Neuronal network and cellular mechanisms. *Physiological Reviews*, 81, 929–969.

Jean, A., Car, A., & Roman, C. (1975). Comparison of activity in pontine versus medullary neurons during swallowing. *Experimental Brain Research*, 22, 211–220.

Jean, A., Kessler, J. P., & Tell, F. (1994). Nucleus tractus solitarii and deglutition: Monoamines, excitatory amino acids, and cellular properties. In R. A. Baracco (Ed.), *Nucleus of the solitary tract* (pp. 362–375), Boca Raton, FL: CRC.

Kendall, K. (2002). Oropharyngeal swallowing variability. *Laryngoscope*, 112, 547–551.

Kendall, K., Leonard, R., & McKenzie, S. W. (2001). Accommodation to changes in bolus viscosity in normal deglutition: A videofluoroscopic study. *Annals of Otology, Rhinology and Laryngology*, 110, 1059–1065.

Kendall, K., Leonard, R., & McKenzie, S. (2003). Sequence variability during hypopharyngeal bolus transit. *Dysphagia*, 18, 1–7.

Kendall, K., McKenzie, S., Leonard, R., Gonçalves, M., & Walker, A. (2000). Timing of events in normal swallowing: A

videofluoroscopic study. *Dysphagia*, 15, 74–83.

Kessler, J. P., & Jean, A. (1985). Identification of the medullary swallowing regions in the rat. *Experimental Brain Research*, 57, 256–263.

Kidder, T. M. (1995). Esophago/pharyngo/laryngeal interrelationships: Airway protection mechanisms. *Dysphagia*, 10, 228–231.

Larson, C. R., Yajima, Y., & Ko, P. (1994). Modification in activity of medullary respiratory-related neurons for vocalization and swallowing. *Journal of Neurophysiology*, 71, 2294–2304.

Lawn, A. M. (1966).The localization in the nucleus ambiguus of the rabbit of the cells of origin of motor nerve fibres in the glossopharyngeal nerve and various branches of the vagus nerve by means of retrograde degeneration. *Journal of Comparative Neurology*, 127, 293–305.

Lawn, A. M. (1988). The nucleus ambiguus of the rabbit. *Journal of Comparative Neurology*, 127, 307–320, 1966.

McConnel, F. M. S. (1988a). Analysis of pressure generation and bolus transit during pharyngeal swallowing. *Laryngoscope*, 98, 71–78.

McConnel, F. M. S. (1988b). Timing of major events of pharyngeal swallowing. *Archives of Otolaryngology-Head and Neck Surgery*, 114, 1413–1418.

Miller, A. J. (1982). Deglutition. *Physiologic Reviews*, 62, 129–184.

Moore, K. L., & Dalley, A. F. (2002). The head, the neck, the cranial nerves. In: *Clinically oriented anatomy* (3rd ed., pp. 637–875), Baltimore: Williams & Wilkins.

Moore, K. L., & Dalley, A. F. (2006). *Clinicaly oriented anatomy* (5th ed.). Baltimore: Williams & Wilking.

Mosier, K., & Bereznaya, I. (2001). Parallel cortical networks for volitional control of swallowing in humans. *Experimental Brain Research*, 140, 280–289.

Ono, T., Ishiwata, Y., Kuroda, T., & Nakamura, Y. (1998). Swallowing-related perihypoglossal neurons projecting to hypoglossal motoneurons in the cat. *Journal of Dental Research, 77,* 351–360.

Ootani, Umezaki,T., Shin, T., & Murata, Y. (1995). Convergence of afferents from the SLN and GPN in cat medullary swallowing neurons. *Brain Research Bulletin, 37,* 397–404.

Roda, F., Gestreau, C., & Biachi, A. L. (2002). Discharge patterns of hypoglossal motoneurons during fictive breathing, coughing, and swallowing. *Journal of Neurophysiology, 87,* 1703–1711.

Tomomune, N., & Takata, M. (1988). Excitatory and inhibitory postsynaptic potentials in cat hypoglossal motoneurons during swallowing. *Experimental Brain Research, 71,* 262-272.

Zald, D. H., & Pardo, J. V. (1999). The functional neuroanatomy of voluntary swallowing. *Annals of Neurology, 46,* 281–286.

Zoungrana, O. R., Amri, M., Car, A., & Roman, C. (1997). Intracellular activity of motoneurons of the rostral nucleus ambigus during swallowing in sheep. *Journal of Neurophysiology, 77,* 909–922.

# APPENDIX 1A

## Muscles Involved in Swallowing (Head and Neck)

### Muscles of the velopharyngeal valve

| Muscle | Superior Attachment | Inferior Attachment | Innervation | Main Action |
|---|---|---|---|---|
| Tensor veli palatini | Scaphoid fossa of medial pterygoid plate, spine of sphenoid bone, and cartilage of pharyngotympanic tube | Palatine aponeurosis | Medial pterygoid nerve (a branch of mandibular nerve, CN V$_3$) via otic ganglion | Tenses soft palate and opens mouth of pharyngotympanic tube during swallowing and yawning |
| Levator veli palatini | Cartilage of pharyngotympanic tube and petrous part of temporal bone | | | Elevates soft palate during swallowing and yawning |
| Palatoglossus | Palatine aponeurosis | Side of tongue | Pharyngeal branch of vagus nerve (CN X) via pharyngeal plexus | Elevates posterior part of tongue and draws soft palate onto tongue |
| Palatopharyngeus | Hard palate and palatine aponeurosis | Lateral wall of pharynx | | Tenses soft palate and pulls walls of pharynx superiorly, anteriorly, and medially during swallowing. |
| Musculus uvulae | Posterior nasal spine and palatine aponeurosis | Mucosa of uvula | | Shortens uvula and pulls it superiorly |

*(continues)*

# Muscles of the pharynx

| Muscle | Origin | Insertion | Innervation | Main Action |
|---|---|---|---|---|
| **External layer** | | | | |
| Superior constrictor | Pterygoid hamulus, pterygomandibular raphe; posterior end of mylohyoid line of mandible and side of tongue | Pharyngeal tubercle on basilar part of occipital bone | Pharyngeal branch of vagus (CN X) and pharyngeal plexus | Constrict walls of pharynx during swallowing |
| Middle constrictor | Stylohyoid ligament and greater and lesser horns of hyoid | Pharyngeal raphe | Pharyngeal branch of vagus (CN X) and pharyngeal plexus, plus branches of external and recurrent laryngeal nerves of vagus | |
| Inferior constrictor (including cricopharyngeus m) | Oblique line of thyroid cartilage and side of cricoid cartilage | Pharyngeal raphe; cricopharyngeal part encircles pharyngo-esophageal junction without forming a raphe | | |
| **Internal Layer** | | | | |
| Palatopharyngeus | Hard palate and palatine aponeurosis | Posterior border of lamina of thyroid cartilage and side of pharynx and esophagus | Pharyngeal branch of vagus (CN X) and pharyngeal plexus | Elevate (shorten and widen) pharynx and larynx during swallowing and speaking |
| Salpingopharyngeus | Cartilaginous part of pharyngotympanic tube | Blends with palatopharyngeus | | |
| Stylopharyngeus | Styloid process of temporal bone | Posterior and superior borders of thyroid cartilage with palatopharyngeus | Glossopharyngeal nerve (CN IX) | |

**Muscles of mastication**

| Muscle(s) | Proximal Attachment | Distal Attachment | Innervation | Action on mandible |
|---|---|---|---|---|
| Temporal | Triangular muscle with broad attachment to floor of temporal fossa and deep surface of temporal fascia | Narrow attachment to tip and medial surface of coronoid process and anterior border of ramus of mandible | Anterior trunk of mandibular nerve (CN $V_3$) via deep temporal branches | Elevates mandible, closing jaws, posterior, more horizontal fibers are 1° retractors of mandible |
| Masseter | Quadrate muscle attaching to inferior border and medial surface of maxillary process of zygomatic bone and the zygomatic arch | Angle and lateral surface of ramus of mandible | Anterior trunk of mandibular nerve (CN $V_3$) via masseteric nerve | Elevates mandible, closing jaws, superficial fibers make limited contribution to protrusion of mandible |
| Lateral pterygoid | Triangular two-headed muscle from (1) infratemporal surface and crest of greater wing of sphenoid and (2) lateral surface of lateral pterygoid plate | Upper head attaches primarily to joint capsule and articular disc of TMJ; inferior head attaches primarily to pterygoid fovea on anteromedial aspect of neck of condyloid process of mandible | Anterior trunk of mandibular nerve (CN $V_3$) via lateral pterygoid nerves | Acting bilaterally, protracts mandible and depresses chin; acting unilaterally, swings jaw toward contralateral side; alternate unilateral contraction produces larger lateral chewing movements |
| Medial pterygoid | Quadrangular two headed muscle from (1) medial surface of lateral pterygoid plate and pyramidal process of palatine bone and (2) tuberosity of maxilla | Medial surface of ramus of mandible, inferior to mandibular foramen; in essence, a "mirror image" of the ipsilateral masseter, the two muscles flanking the ramus | Anterior trunk of mandibular nerve (CN $V_3$) via medial pterygoid nerve | Acts synergistically with masseter to elevate mandible; contributes to protrusion; alternate unilateral activity produces smaller grinding movements |

*(continues)*

Muscles of the neck and larynx

| Muscle | Origin | Insertion | Innervation | Action |
|---|---|---|---|---|
| **Suprahyoid muscles** | | | | |
| Digastric | *Anterior belly:* Digastric fossa of mandible *Posterior belly:* Mastoid notch of temporal bone | Intermediate tendon to body and greater horn of hyoid bone | *Anterior belly:* Nerve to mylohyoid, a branch of inferior alveolar nerve *Posterior belly:* Digastric branch of (preparotid) CN VII | Working with infrahyoid muscles, depresses mandible against resistance; elevates and steadies hyoid during swallowing and speaking |
| Stylohyoid | Styloid process of temporal bone | Body of hyoid bone | Stylohyoid branch of (preparotid) CN VII | Elevates amd retracts hyoid, thus elongating floor of mouth |
| Mylohyoid | Mylohyoid line of mandible | Myloid raphe and body of hyoid bone | Mandibular nerve of CN V | Elevates hyoid, floor of mouth and tongue during swallowing and speaking |
| Geniohyoid | Inferior mental spine of mandible | Body of hyoid bone | C1 via CN XII | Pulls hyoid anterosuperiorly; shortens floor of mouth; widens pharynx |
| **Infrahyoid muscles** | | | | |
| Omohyoid | Superior border of scapula near suprascapular notch | Inferior border of hyoid | C1–C3 by a branch of ansa cervicalis | Depresses, retracts, and steadies hyoid |
| Sternohyoid | Manubrium of sternum | Body of hyoid bone | C1–C3 by a branch of ansa cervicalis | Depresses hyoid after elevation during swallowing |
| Sternothyroid | Posterior surface of manubrium of sternum | Oblique line of thyroid cartilage | C2 and C3 by a branch of ansa cervicalis | Depresses hyoid and larynx |
| Thyrohyoid | Oblique line of thyroid cartilage | Inferior border of body and greater horn of hyoid | C1 via CN XII | Depresses hyoid and elevates larynx |

| Muscle | Origin | Insertion | Innervation | Main Action(s) |
|---|---|---|---|---|
| *Intrinsic laryngeal muscles* | | | | |
| Cricothyroid | Anterolateral part of cricoid cartilage | Inferior margin and inferior horn of thyroid cartilage | External laryngeal nerve (from CN X) | Stretches and tenses vocal ligament |
| Thyroarytenoid | Lower half of posterior aspect of angle of thyroid laminae and cricothyroid ligament | Anterolateral arytenoid surface | Inferior laryngeal nerve (terminal part of recurrent laryngeal nerve, from CN X) | Relaxes vocal ligament |
| Posterior cricoarytenoid | Posterior surface of lamina of cricoid cartilage | Muscular process of arytenoid cartilage | | Abducts vocal folds |
| Lateral cricoarytenoid | Arch of cricoid cartilage | Vocal process of arytenoid cartilage | | Adducts vocal folds (interligamentous portion) |
| Transverse and oblique arytenoids | One arytenoid cartilage | Contralateral arytenoid cartilage | | Adduct arytenoid cartilages (adducting intercartilaginous portion of vocal folds, closing posterior rima glottidis) |
| Vocalis | Lateral surface of vocal process of arytenoid cartilage | Ipsilateral vocal ligament | | Relaxes posterior vocal ligament while maintaining (or increasing) tension of anterior part |

*(continues)*

31

# Muscles of lower face (CN VII)

| Muscle | Origin | Insertion | Main Action(s) |
|---|---|---|---|
| Orbicularis oris (oral sphincter) | Medial maxilla and mandible; deep surface of perioral skin; angle of mouth (modiolus) | Mucous membrane of lips | Tonus closes rima oris; phasic contraction compresses and protrudes lips (kissing) or resists distension (when blowing) |
| Levator labii superioris | Infraorbital margin (maxilla) | Skin of upper lip | Part of dilators of mouth; retract (elevate) and/or evert upper lip; deepen nasolabial sulcus (showing sadness) |
| Zygomaticus minor | Anterior aspect, zygomatic bone | | |
| Buccinator (cheek muscle) | Mandible, alveolar processes of maxilla and mandible, pterygomandibular raphe | Angle of mouth (modiolus); orbicularis oris | Presses cheek against molar teeth; works with tongue to keep food between occlusal surfaces and out of oral vestibule; resists distension (when blowing) |
| Zygomaticus major | Lateral aspect of zygomatic bone | Angle of mouth (modiolus) | Part of dilators of mouth; elevate labial commissure bilaterally to smile (happiness); unilaterally to sneer (disdain) |
| Levator anguli oris | Infraorbital maxilla (canine fossa) | | |
| Risorius | Parotid fascia and buccal skin (highly variable) | | Part of dilators of mouth; widens rima oris, as when grinning or grimacing |
| Depressor anguli oris | Anterolateral base of mandible | | Part of dilators of mouth;depresses labial commissure bilaterally to frown (sadness) |
| Depressor labii inferioris | Platysma and anterolateral body of mandible | Skin of lower lip | Part of dilators of mouth;retracts (depresses) and/or everts lower lip (pouting, sadness) |
| Mentalis | Body of mandible (anterior to roots of inferior incisors) | Skin of chin (mentolabial sulcus) | Elevates and protrudes lower lip; elevates skin of chin (showing doubt) |
| Platysma | Subcutaneous tissue of infraclavicular and supraclavicular regions | Base of mandible; skin of cheek and lower lip; angle of mouth (modiolus); orbicularis oris | Depresses mandible (against resistance); tenses skin of inferior face and neck (conveying tension and stress) |

**Muscles of the Tongue (primarily CN XII)**

| Muscle | Shape and Position | Proximal Attachment | Distal Attachment | Main Action(s) |
|---|---|---|---|---|
| *Extrinsic muscles of the tongue* | | | | |
| Genioglossus | Fan-shaped muscle; constitutes bulk of tongue | Via a short tendon from superior part of mental spine of mandible | Entire dorsum of tongue; inferior most and posterior most fibers attach to body of hyoid bone | Bilateral activity depresses tongue, especially central part, creating a longitudinal furrow; posterior part pulls tongue anteriorly for protrusion, most anterior part retracts apex of protruded tongue; unilateral contraction deviates ("wags") tongue to contralateral side |
| Hyoglossus | Thin, quadrilateral muscle | Body and greater horn of hyoid bone | Inferior aspects of lateral part of tongue | Depresses tongue, especially pulling its sides inferiorly; helps shorten (retrude) tongue |
| Styloglossus | Small, short triangular muscle | Anterior boder of distal styloid process; stylohyoid ligament | Sides of tongue posteriorly, interdigitating with hyoglossus | Retrudes tongue and curls(elevates) its sides working with genioglossus to form a central trough during swallowing |
| Palatoglossus (CN X) | Narrow crescent-shaped palatine muscle; forms posterior column of isthmus of fauces | Palatine aponeurosis of soft palate | Enters posterolateral tongue transversely, blending with intrinsic transverse muscles | Capable of elevating posterior tongue or depressing soft palate; most commonly acts to constrict isthmus of fauces |

*(continues)*

**Muscles of the Tongue (primarily CN XII)** *(continued)*

| Muscle | Shape and Position | Proximal Attachment | Distal Attachment | Main Action(s) |
|---|---|---|---|---|
| *Intrinsic muscles of the tongue* | | | | |
| Superior longitudinal | Thin layer deep to mucous membrane of dorsum | Submucous fibrous layer and median fibrous septum | Margins of tongue and mucous membrane | Curls tongue longitudinally upward, elevating apex and sides of tongue; shortens (retrudes) tongue |
| Inferior longitudinal | Narrow band close to inferior surface | Root of tongue and body of hyoid bone | Apex of tongue | Curls tongue longitudinally downward, depressing apex; shortens (retrudes) tongue |
| Transverse | Deep to superior longitudinal muscle | Median fibrous septum | Fibrous tissue at lateral lingual margins | Narrows and elongates (protrudes) tongue |
| Vertical | Fibers intersect transverse muscle | Submucous fibrous layer of dorsum of tongue | Inferior surface of borders of tongue | Flattens and broadens tongue |

*Source: Adapted from Clinically Oriented Anatomy by K. L. Moore & A. F. Dailey, 2006. Williams and Wilkins, Baltimore.*

# 2

# *Head and Neck Physical Exam*

## Katherine Kendall

Dysphagia is the sensation that solids or liquids are not being swallowed correctly. Possible etiologies of dysphagia include neuromuscular disease involving the oral and pharyngeal musculature normally active during swallowing, altered anatomy such as occurs after surgical resections, radiation therapy, trauma, cervical osteophytes, pharyngeal diverticuli, cricopharyngeal spasm, foreign bodies, tumors, and mucosal irritation or injury.

## INDICATIONS

A thorough history and head and neck examination is indicated in all patients suffering from dysphagia but may not provide enough information to gain a complete understanding of the pathophysiologic process. Flexible fiberoptic endoscopy may be required to complete the examination. A dynamic videofluoroscopic swallow study complements the physical examination and is usually indicated.

## HISTORY

### Chief Complaint

Symptoms of dysphagia may include a history of coughing or choking while eating. These symptoms indicate the patient may be aspirating during deglutition. Patients may have required that a Heimlich maneuver be performed on them when the airway became blocked by a food bolus. Patients may have noticed an increased need to clear their throat, may complain of increased mucus or phlegm production or the sensation of something sitting on their vocal cords. They may note a change to a wet or gargling vocal quality as saliva or residual bolus drips onto the vocal folds. Patients may complain that foods get stuck at various locations in the pharynx. It is important to determine where this sensation occurs as it can focus the physical examination on the areas most likely to be involved or abnormal. It is also important to determine if difficulty is experienced with solids only, or with both liquids and solids. Dysphagia for solids only is often caused by an obstruction or narrowing of the alimentary passage and a history of dysphagia for both liquids and solids may indicate generalized neuromuscular incoordination, or a very advanced obstructive process. Dysphagia for liquids only is often seen with a vocal fold paralysis or paresis because liquids tend to drip into the airway where a solid bolus holds together better and usually causes little difficulty. A history of weight loss underscores the severity of the problem and a history of pneumonia indicates the occurrence of intolerable aspiration. Meal duration may be prolonged in these patients and they may avoid certain types of food they know to worsen their symptoms (Castell & Donner, 1987).

A sudden onset of dysphagia is more likely to occur with trauma or ingestion of a foreign body. Careful questioning of the patient may be required to elicit a history of chicken or fish in the recent diet.

## Past Medical History

A history of heartburn, indigestion, or known gastroesophageal reflux is significant in that chronic irritation of the pharyngeal mucosa can enhance a foreign-body sensation. A long exposure of the esophageal mucosa to stomach acid may lead to poor relaxation of the upper esophageal sphincter and subsequent solid-food dysphagia. Over time, failure of upper esophageal sphincter relaxation can lead to the development of pharyngeal diverticuli. Gastroesophageal reflux can also lead to aspiration of an extremely caustic nature that is not necessarily associated with swallowing (Leonard, & Kendall, 1999; Shaker, 1995).

A history of neuromuscular disease is important as this may be the primary etiology of the swallowing abnormality and give an indication of the prognosis for improvement. Past surgical procedures involving structures of the oral cavity and pharynx may be responsible for altered swallowing function. Head and neck radiation therapy can lead to fibrosis of structure whose mobility is required for adequate swallowing and will cause xerostomia (Kendall, McKenzie, Leonard, & Jones, 1998).

A detailed medication history may shed light on factors contributing to the patient's symptoms of dysphagia. Many medications cause decreased salivary production and contribute to poor bolus lubrication and clearing. These medications act primarily through their effects on the parasympathetic nervous system, responsible for the stimulation of salivation. Drugs may be "parasympathomimetic" meaning that they stimulate or simulate the parasympathetic nervous system. This results in increased salivation, occasionally to the point of drooling. Drugs that are "parasympatholytic" block or decrease parasympathetic stimulation causing a decrease in salivary output and a dry mouth. "Anticholinergic" drugs fall into this category. Antihistamines and antinausea medications commonly have anticholinergic side effects. The use of multiple drugs, a common finding in older patients, may result in drug interactions that potentiate the anticholinergic effects of those drugs. The side effect of a dry mouth can reduce the patient's ability to communicate, predispose to malnutrition, promote mucosal damage, denture misfit, or dental caries, and increase the risk of serious respiratory infection secondary to the loss of antimicrobial activity of saliva (Feinberg, 1993; Narhi et al., 1992).

Other drug categories also have dry mouth as a side effect. The following discussion provides a partial list of examples of these drug categories. The side effects of any drug can usually be investigated by referencing any of a number of drug handbooks or the Physicians Desk Reference (Arky, 1996).

Drugs that increase brain dopamine levels by stimulating the release of dopamine may cause a dry mouth. An example of this type of medication is Symmetrel, a drug that is used in the treatment of Parkinson's disease. Antipsychotic medications that act by blocking dopamine receptors also cause a dry mouth. Tricyclic antidepressants are basic in the treatment of depression. These drugs are thought to block serotonin and norepinephrine reuptake. They include Elavil, Senequan, and Tofranil. Some patients taking this type of medication experience dry mouth as these drugs produce a significant reduction in salivary flow. Newer antidepressants that block seratonin reuptake are also known to cause dry mouth. Examples of these medications include Prozac, Zoloft, Desyrel, and Paxil. Lithium carbonate used to treat manic-depressive disorders causes a dry mouth. Benzodiazepines are drugs used to treat symptoms of anxiety. The drugs act by potentiating the effect of GABA, a brain inhibitory neurotransmitter. Dry mouth is a side effect of many of these compounds (Hunter & Wilson, 1995; Vogel & Carter, 1995).

Diabetes mellitus is also associated with reduced salivary flow. In the case of diabetes, oral dryness is not associated with a malfunction of the parasympathetic nervous system but appears to be caused by disturbances in glycemic control (Sreebny, Yu, Green, & Valdini, 1992).

## EXAMINATION

The patient should be sitting upright for the examination. A bright light source is required to illuminate the oral cavity, pharynx, and hypopharynx. A head mirror or headlight is recommended. The patient should be seated at a level so that he or she is slightly higher than the examiner. The legs should be uncrossed and the patient should be sitting up straight, leaning slightly forward at the hip.

The face of the patient should be examined for any obvious asymmetries or outward signs of trauma. Facial musculature and sensation should be tested to rule out abnormalities of cranial nerves V and VII. The eyes and orbits should be evaluated for deficits of cranial nerves II, III, IV, or VI. Abnormalities of cranial nerve function and facial sensation may be clues to the diagnosis of central or neuromuscular disease. A nasal exam should rule out any masses that could impinge upon the soft palate and therefore preclude complete closure of the velum.

The lips should be first inspected and evaluated in terms of sensation and competency. Salivary leak should be noted. Two tongue blades aid in the examination of the oral cavity. The patient is asked to open the mouth and the tongue blades are employed to move structures allowing complete inspection of all the mucosal surfaces. Upon opening, the interincisal distance can be evaluated. Trismus can be a sign of temporomandibular joint disease or pterygoid muscle abnormalities. Tumors invading the pterygoid muscles are a cause of trismus. Trismus may interfere with mastication and proper bolus preparation. The dentition should be inspected. Carious, broken, and missing teeth may also lead to difficulty with bolus preparation. The mucosal surfaces should be inspected for irregularities, lesions, and moisture. Saliva quantity and quality should be noted.

Adequate tongue mobility is paramount to effective swallowing. The tongue should be inspected for any surface irregularities, fasciculations, or atrophy. The patient should be asked to protrude the tongue and to move it from side to side in order to judge mobility. The lingual sulci should be examined to rule out tethering of the tongue to the inner surface of the mandible. Palpation of the tongue allows detection of any masses that are not evident on visual inspection alone.

Examination of the oral pharynx also should begin with a visual inspection of the mucosal surfaces to rule out any obvious abnormalities. The soft palate should elevate symmetrically when the patient is asked to say "ah." The presence or absence of enlarged tonsillar tissue should be noted.

The hypopharyngeal exam requires indirect laryngoscopy. This method enables the visual inspection of the tongue base as well as the larynx and region of the upper esophageal inlet. The patient must be properly positioned to carry out the examination in such a manner as to provide the best visualization with the least discomfort to the patient. The patient should be asked to sit up straight. The head of the patient should be above the head of the examiner. The patient should be asked to extend the neck anteriorly so that the mandible is forward. This position moves the tongue base anteriorly and brings the larynx into view. The patient is then asked to protrude the tongue maximally. The examiner holds the tongue with a thin gauze sponge and stabilizes the position of the patient with the same hand. A warmed mirror is introduced into the oral pharynx with the other hand using care not to touch the tongue base. As we have previously mentioned, the tongue base is extremely sensitive and a region involved in the swallowing reflex initiation. It is also involved in airway protection and the initiation of the gag reflex. The soft palate, however, is not as sensitive and the mirror can be placed against it as it is positioned posteriorly in the oral pharynx for viewing of the hypopharynx.

The mirror can be pivoted back and forth to allow full examination of the hypopharyngeal structures. Starting with the base of the tongue, the vallecula, and the epiglottis, evaluation for any anatomical abnormalities is carried out. The presence or absence of saliva pooling in the vallecula, piriform fossae or glottic opening is then noted. Pooling of saliva suggests significant dysfunction of the swallowing mechanism and identifies patients at significant risk for aspiration. The piriform fossae are also evaluated in terms of asymmetries, mucosal lesions, or masses.

The larynx is then inspected and vocal fold mobility and closure are assessed. The patient is asked to say "ee," which closes the vocal folds and further elevates the larynx for inspection. A higher frequency "ee" will often elevate the larynx even further for viewing. Any vocal-fold lesions that inhibit full vocal-fold closure are noted. The patient may be asked to perform a rapid "ee-ee-ee" sequence to assess fine control of vocal-fold movement and closure. The vocal folds should be evaluated during inspiration, as well, to allow visualization of the vocal-fold medial surfaces that are obscured during phonation. The interarytenoid region should be evaluated for color and character of tissues, as erythema of this region may indicate irritation by chronic gastroesophageal reflux.

Once hypopharyngeal inspection has been carried out, a test of sensation in the oral pharynx can be performed. By touching the tongue base and posterior pharyngeal wall, a gag reflex should be elicited.

The final part of the physical examination involves palpation of the neck for anatomic abnormalities, especially masses.

The routine physical examination is limited in that the evaluation of the nasopharynx and hypopharyngeal sensation cannot be performed adequately. To complete these parts of the evaluation, a flexible nasopharyngoscope is used. One nostril can be spayed with topical neosynephrine (0.25%) and/or topical anesthetic such as lidocaine (4%). The scope is lubricated and dipped in an antifog solution. It is then passed along the nasal floor to allow inspection of the nasopharynx.

All mucosal surfaces should be inspected. Palatal mobility is evaluated along with velopharyngeal closure by asking the patient to perform a forceful "sss" sound. Once this portion of the examination is complete, the patient is asked to breathe through his nose and thus open the nasopharyngeal passage for further advancement of the flexible scope and evaluation of hypopharyngeal sensation. This technique can also be employed to visually inspect the hypopharynx in patients who are unable to cooperate with an indirect examination.

The tip of the flexible scope is used to touch the tongue, piriform fossae, lateral pharyngeal walls, aryepiglottic folds, laryngeal surface of the epiglottis, and the vocal folds themselves. The examination is carried out bilaterally and the two sides are compared. Patients with normal sensation will cough or swallow when touched with the scope. Abnormal sensation can contribute significantly to abnormalities of initiating a swallow and control of the bolus.

## REVIEW

The head and neck physical examination allows an assessment of alterations in anatomy, motor function, and sensory function that affect a patient's ability to swallow. The following is a list reviewing the information that may be gained during the physical examination.

- Obvious tumor, surgical changes, or other anatomic abnormalities.
- Abnormalities of tongue, palatal, and vocal fold mobility.
- Inadequate sphincteric functions such as oral incompetence, velopharyngeal incompetence, and poor laryngeal closure.
- Loss of sensation.
- Pooling of secretions.

## LIMITATIONS

In patients with subtle abnormalities of sensation, the gross nature of the physical examination will be inadequate to detect them. Yet, these sensory deficits may be responsible for delayed swallow-reflex triggering and poor bolus control. The same problems exist in the evaluation of subtle motor deficits that may not be detected on the physical examination. The complex coordination of swallowing may be abnormal in patients with central control deficits who present with normal anatomy, sensation, and apparent muscular function. Thus, the physical examination may not provide enough information to fully understand the nature of the patient's swallowing problems. A dynamic videofluoroscopic swallow study is often required to further elucidate subtle abnormalities of the swallowing mechanism.

## STUDY QUESTIONS

1. Discuss three symptoms consistent with severe dysphagia.
2. What important information is learned from the past medical history with respect to complaints of dysphagia? Name three specific examples.
3. How does gastroesophageal reflux disease cause dysphagia?
4. Describe the limitations of the physical examination and what testing can be done to complement the physical examination.

## REFERENCES

Arky, R. (1996). *Physician's desk reference*. Montvale, NJ: Medical Economics.

Castell, D. O., & Donner, M. W. (1987). Evaluation of dysphagia: A careful history is crucial. *Dysphagia, 2*, 65–71.

Feinberg, M. (1993). The problems of anticholinergic adverse effects in older patients. *Drugs and Aging, 3*, 335–348.

Hunter, K. D., & Wilson, W. S. (1995). The effects of antidepressant drugs on salivary flow and content of sodium and potassium ions in human parotid saliva. *Archives of Oral Biology, 40*, 983–989.

Kendall, K., McKenzie, S., Leonard, R., & Jones, C. (1998). Structural mobility in deglutition after single modality treatment of head and neck carcinomas with radiation therapy. *Head and Neck, 20*, 720–725.

Leonard, R., & Kendall, K. (1999). Dysphagia secondary to cricopharyngeal achalasia. *Phonoscope: Voice-Speech-Swallowing Clinics in Head and Neck Practice, 2*, 123–128.

Narhi, T. O., Meurman, J. H., Ainamo, A., Nevalainen, J. M., Schmidt-Kaunisaho, K. G., Siudosaari P., et al. (1992). Association between salivary flow rate and the use of systemic medication among 76-, 81-, and 86-year-old inhabitants in Helsinki, Finland. *Journal of Dental Research, 71*, 1875–1880.

Shaker, R. (1995). Airway protective mechanisms: Current concepts. *Dysphagia, 10*, 216–227.

Sreebny, L. M., Yu, A., Green A., & Valdini, A. (1992). Xerostomia in diabetes mellitus. *Diabetes Care, 15*, 900–904.

Vogel, D., & Carter, J. E. (1995). *The effects of drugs on communication disorders*. San Diego, CA: Singular Publishing Group.

# 3

# *Dysphagia in Head and Neck Surgery Patients*

## Katherine Kendall

Successful swallowing depends on the smooth and coordinated functioning of multiple structures in the head and neck region. Although the swallowing sequence can be influenced by input from higher cortical centers, it is primarily a semiautomatic mechanism. The swallowing mechanism relies on sensory input from the muscles and mucosal surfaces of the structures involved to help regulate and fine tune the sequence of muscular contractions that results in a swallow. It makes sense that disruption of the sensory, muscular, or structural integrity of the oral cavity, pharynx, and larynx may result in dysphagia. Any surgical procedure involving the head and neck region, therefore, has the potential to cause dysphagia. The discussion in this chapter focuses on the difficulty experienced by patients after surgery for head and neck cancer. These patients are the most common head and neck population to experience dysphagia,

and the concepts involved in understanding the etiology of dysphagia in this group can be generalized to other patient populations.

During the last several years, greater emphasis has been placed on improving functional outcomes for head and neck cancer patients. This trend has been highlighted by the development of several "quality of life" measurement tools (Hammerlid et al., 1997; Hassan & Weymuller, 1993; Terrell, 1999). Patients have indicated through the use of these tools that their lives are most impacted by poor swallowing function and the presence of a stoma (Terrell, 1999). The development of "organ sparing" protocols employing combined chemo- and radiation therapy as a primary treatment modality for head and neck cancer is a step toward providing treated patients with improved speech and swallowing and freedom from a stoma (Eisbruch et al., 1999; Urba et al., 2000; Wolf et al., 1999).

Yet, despite increasing use of organ-sparing protocols, surgical therapy followed by radiation remains a primary treatment modality for head and neck cancer and is used as a salvage modality for patients who fail organ-sparing treatments. In keeping with the goal of improved functional outcomes, surgeons need to continue to focus their efforts on improved reconstruction techniques that maximally restore function.

The development of improved reconstructive techniques depends on a clear understanding of what is required for normal functioning and how it is disrupted by surgical extirpation of a tumor. This is particularly true for deglutition, a complex function involving modulation through sensory input, development of adequate pulsive forces, and competency of multiple valves. The advent of several techniques for the objective evaluation of deglutition, such as videofluoroscopy, has allowed for the in-depth analysis of normal deglutition and can be applied to the study of patients after head and neck cancer resection (Baker, Fraser, & Baker, 1991; Kendall, McKenzie, & Leonard, 2000; McConnel & O'Connor, 1994; Stachler et al., 1994). These techniques afford the ability to identify crucial functional elements lacking in specific patients or groups of patients. In particular, videofluoroscopy can provide information about the timing of bolus transit and swallowing gestures and the extent of structural displacements. In addition, multiple published studies provide normative data for comparison purposes and interobserver reliability for measurements made with this technique is typically greater than 90% (Kendall, McKenzie, Leonard, Goncalves,

& Walker, 2000; Leonard, Kendall, McKenzie, Goncalves, & Walker, 2000). Many of the studies cited in this chapter involve the use of videofluoscopy for patient evaluation.

Despite the availability of quantitative assessment techniques, investigations of swallowing function in cancer patients that have focused on the objective evaluation of specific alterations in swallowing and/or causes of dysphagia, and not just the presence or absence of aspiration, are relatively few. Reasons for this include the difficulty in grouping patients because of variability in tumor size and location and the involvement of other structures. However, it may be possible to identify general trends in swallowing function measured with videofluoroscopy based on the anatomical structures removed at the time of surgery and to develop reconstructive principles accordingly while tailoring the reconstructive design to each individual patient.

## INTRODUCTION

In patients with head and neck cancer, interference with normal swallowing can result from the growth of the tumor that invades structures and impairs their functioning, or from the obstructive effects of the tumor, itself. Surgery to excise the tumor with a margin of normal tissue results in a defect and loss of structures, which typically also produces dysphagia. The chosen method of reconstruction of the defect will subsequently influence the character and the severity of the dysphagia. When radiation therapy is added to the regimen postoperatively, dysphagia may worsen secondary to xerostomia and fibrosis of soft tissues in the field of radiation exposure (Baker et al., 1991; Kendall, McKenzie, Leonard, & Jones, 1998).

All patients undergoing surgery for head and neck cancers involving the oral cavity, pharynx, and larynx should be considered to be at risk for dysphagia in the postoperative period. These patients must be evaluated accordingly before embarking on attempts at oral feeding. Patients' perceptions of the types of difficulty they experience may be erroneous, and they tend to understate their actual swallowing difficulties (Pauloski et al., 1993). For this reason, a bedside swallow evaluation should be followed by a dynamic videofluoroscopic swallow study to document actual swallowing function and to rule out silent aspiration.

In our center, a swallow study is done in every patient before attempting oral feeding. Initially, we made an effort to perform a swallow study before the patient's discharge from the hospital. Often patients studied this early have extreme difficulty with dysphagia. Many of the same patients will do much better a few weeks later. We have now modified our protocol so that patients are studied later in the postoperative course. This minimizes the number of studies performed on an individual patient and improves the chance that the patient will be well enough to participate in attempts to identify strategies for safe swallowing. Each patient must be considered on an individual basis in terms of deciding when the swallow study, and thus oral feeding, should be attempted. Healing from surgery, local edema, other medical conditions, the development of oro-

or pharyngocutaneous fistulae, and the psychological condition of the patient must be weighed into the decision.

Several studies have found little improvement of swallowing function when the immediate postoperative swallowing is compared to swallowing function as long as 1 year later (Pauloski et al., 1993; Pauloski et al.; 1994; Pauloski, Logemann, Fox, & Colangelo, 1995). However, Pauloski and colleagues were able to demonstrate some functional adaptation and the development of secondary coping strategies in patients after anterior tongue and floor-of-mouth resections (McConnel et al., 1994).

## ORAL SPHINCTER

When the lips are involved in a surgical cancer resection, the subsequent functioning of the oral sphincter is influenced by the size, sensation, and structural support of the reconstructed ostium. Up to one half of the lower lip can be excised and closed primarily without serious cosmetic and functional consequences. If more than one half of the lip requires removal, local flaps are usually required for reconstruction. When microstomia results from extensive resection of the lips, difficulty in bolus introduction is experienced by the patient. When the mental nerve on one or both sides is involved in the resection, the subsequent loss of sensation of the lower lip results in difficulty in maintaining oral competence even if the sphincter mechanism remains largely intact. Lip sensory deficits also cause difficulty in bolus manipulation and the patient may experience drooling or loss of the bolus during bolus preparation for swallowing.

## ANTERIOR FLOOR OF MOUTH

Floor-of-mouth structures important for deglutition include the muscles responsible for hyoid elevation and tongue stabilization. An inability to open the pharyngoesophageal sphincter occurs when the hyoid no longer elevates and is a prominent characteristic of the dysphagia experienced by this group of patients. The pliability of the floor of the mouth region and the attachments of the tongue musculature to the anterior mandible allow for tongue mobility in the anterior and posterior directions. When tissue is lost from this area, difficulty in bolus preparation and propulsion from the oral cavity into the pharynx results from a loss of tongue maneuverability (McConnel et al., 1994). If the lingual nerve and the hypoglossal nerve are involved in the resection, problems with tongue sensation, taste, and tongue mobility will result.

Reconstruction of floor-of-mouth defects can have a significant impact on patients' functional outcomes. Any closure that results in tethering of the tongue or further loss of tongue bulk, such as the use of local tongue flaps, will amplify the disability. Care must be taken not to limit posterior tongue mobility, in particular its ability to contact the posterior pharyngeal wall, by closing the defect in such a way that the tongue is pulled anteriorly. Similarly, if large or bulky regional flaps are inset into the defect, they may displace the tongue too far posteriorly and prevent normal oral manipulation of the bolus. Skin grafting, local nasolabial flaps, and free tissue transfer such as the radial forearm or jejunal flaps are alternatives for closure of floor-of-mouth defects. Surgeons performing this type of surgery may consider the addition of a hyoid suspension procedure to facilitate opening of the pharyngoesophageal sphincter.

## TONGUE

Loss of tongue bulk after tongue-cancer resection can significantly impact oral and pharyngeal movement of the bolus. The degree of impairment is influenced by the location and the extent of the resection (Doberneck & Antoine, 1974). Anterior defects are likely to lead to problems with oral bolus manipulation and difficulty in propelling the bolus into the pharynx, especially if the tongue cannot contact the palate. Loss of posterior tongue tissue affects the pharyngeal phase of the swallow and results in difficulty in generating the forces required to propel the bolus into the upper esophagus. Poor pharyngeal constriction is seen in these cases on the dynamic videofluoroscopic swallow study (see videoclips of patient studies in the materials folder for Chapter 17). Previous studies of swallowing function after oropharyngeal cancer resection have demonstrated that the percentage of oral tongue or base of tongue removed correlates with postoperative swallowing ability (Pruszewicz & Kruk-Zagajewska, 1984). This finding was confirmed in studies that considered patients in whom the primary tumor location was either the tonsillar fossa or the anterior floor of mouth (Doberneck & Antoine, 1974). Additional studies found that mobility of residual tongue is the most important consideration in the restoration of swallowing function (Doberneck & Antoine, 1974; Logemann &

Bytell, 1979; McConnel & Mendelsohn, 1987; Pruszewicz & Kruk-Zagajewska, 1984).

Clearly, when considering the best technique for reconstruction after a tongue-cancer resection, restoration of tongue mobility and bulk must be a primary consideration. Several options exist, including closure by secondary intention or granulation, skin grafts, regional flaps, or free tissue transfer. McConnel reported that, after excision of oral tongue tumors greater than 2 cm in size without involvement of other oral-cavity structures, the best swallowing results were achieved in patients who had skin-graft reconstructions (McConnel & O'Connor, 1994; McConnel, 1996). For base-of-tongue defects, McConnel found that primary closure resulted in better swallowing function than pectoralis myocutaneous flaps or radial forearm free flaps (Freeman, Marks, & Ogura, 1979). Irrespective of the reconstructive method, some alteration of tongue function is likely after partial glossectomy.

Research from our own laboratory has attempted to compare swallowing in normal controls to swallowing in patients with resections for oral cavity or oropharyngeal cancer, and across subgroups of patients with oropharyngeal resection involving the tongue (Leonard & Gonçalves, unpublished data). The resection categories are designated unilateral limited, unilateral extensive, anterior, posterior, and subtotal, according to the site and extent of glossal resection. Timing and displacement characteristics of events and structures involved in swallow have been obtained from videofluoroscopic studies performed as uniformly as possible across patient and control subjects.

In a comparison of control to postoperative subjects, all measured swallowing parameters differed between the two groups except the duration of upper esophageal sphincter opening. Across categories of glossectomy patients, those with unilateral limited resections generally fared better on parameters investigated, while those in the posterior and subtotal categories performed most poorly.

A second study from our laboratory analyzed structural displacements measured by videofluoroscopy in a group of 28 patients after tongue-base resection who complained of dysphagia (Kendall & Leonard, unpublished data). The study analyzed the distance of hyoid movement, the size of the upper esophageal sphincter at maximal opening, and the extent of pharyngeal constriction. The measure of pharyngeal constriction is of particular interest because adequate pharyngeal contractile strength and tongue mobility are required for complete constriction of the pharynx behind the tail of the bolus. The action of the tongue against the contracting pharyngeal musculature drives the bolus inferiorly into the hypopharynx and esophagus. A lack of complete pharyngeal obliteration may be seen in the lateral projection of a videofluoroscopic study of swallowing. Normally, pharyngeal area measured from this view constricts down to approximately 0.02 cm$^2$ (Leonard et al., 2000). Failure of pharyngeal constriction may be caused by a lack of tongue bulk, such as after base-of-tongue resections. (Other instances where poor pharyngeal constriction may be observed include anterior tethering of the tongue after primary closure of anterior floor-of-mouth resections and in cases of pharyngeal muscular weakness after resection of the pharyngeal wall and reconstruction with an adynamic flap.) Weak or incomplete pharyngeal constriction usually results in difficulty transferring the bolus into the esophagus and in pharyngeal residue that may be inhaled after the swallow. The results of our study demonstrated no difference in the extent of hyoid bone elevation between the tumor patients and normal controls. The hyoid bone normally moves farther to accommodate a larger bolus size and this characteristic of normal swallowing was maintained in the patient group. The opening size of the upper esophageal sphincter tended to be larger in patients than in normal controls for the 1-cc bolus category. Perhaps this finding represents a strategy developed by patients in an attempt to accommodate other changes in their swallowing function. Pharyngeal area at maximum constriction, however, was significantly larger in tumor patients than in the normal controls ($p = .04$). Further analysis of the tongue-base cancer patients revealed that swallowing function measurements were not affected by the time since surgery or the method of reconstruction. The results of this study indicate that poor pharyngeal constriction may contribute to dysphagia in head and neck cancer patients irrespective of tumor location.

## MANDIBLE

Cancer that involves the anterior floor of the mouth, the tongue, or the lateral pharyngeal wall often invades the adjacent mandible, as well. Occasionally, a portion of the mandible is removed to provide an adequate margin for the tumor resection. The alveolar and the mental nerves run through the mandible and may be sacrificed along with a segment of the mandible, resulting in the loss of sensation to the remaining ipsilateral mandibular teeth and lower lip. When the angle of the mandible is removed, the contralateral masseter and medial pterygoid muscles are unopposed, resulting in jaw swing and malocclusion. If the anterior portion of the jaw is removed, an "Andy Gump" deformity results with oral incompetence and the loss of the chin contour. The hyoid elevators will have lost their attachment and consequent failure of the hyoid to elevate may produce poor pharyngoesophageal sphincter opening. The advent of mandibular plates for reconstruction of the mandible and the use of osseous free flaps has improved the outcomes in these patients in terms of the cosmetic defect. Unfortunately, the functional difficulties often remain.

## PALATE

Defects of the hard palate result in oronasal fistulae. A fistula effectively enlarges the oral cavity by the area of the nasal cavity and results in an open chamber instead of a closed structure. Bolus material can readily pass into the nasal cavity during preparation for swallowing. Manipulation of the bolus is more difficult as the tongue may be unable to retrieve material from the nasal cavity. The hard palate also serves as a surface against which the tongue pushes to propel the bolus into the pharynx in preparation for swallowing. Defects in the palate cause difficulty with pressure generation and inefficient bolus transfer. In general, obturation of a hard palate defect with a prosthesis is very successful in improving the dysphagia.

Soft-palate defects inhibit the dual sphincter function of the soft palate. During the oral phase of swallowing, the soft palate acts to divide the oral and pharyngeal cavities as it is fully relaxed and resting on the tongue base. The soft palate then elevates and divides the nasopharynx from the oropharynx during the pharyngeal phase of swallowing. Any loss of palate mobility will impact these functions of the soft palate. Any loss of palatal tissue will prevent full closure of these sphincters and allow pressure and bolus material to escape inappropriately through the defect. Soft-palate defects are difficult to reconstruct. Most techniques available cannot recreate the unique muscle configuration of the palate and mobility is diminished. Usually, palatal bulk can be restored with local flaps. Prosthetic obturators can help position the poorly mobile palate into a position that is more favorable for the pharyngeal phase of swallowing.

## PHARYNX

Removal of portions of the pharyngeal walls, such as occurs in resections of tonsillar-fossa cancer, results in the potential for weakness of the wall at the resection site. It must be kept in mind that in swallowing the pharynx acts as a chamber that provides resistance to the posterior movement of the tongue base, thereby generating the pressures needed to propel the bolus through the pharyngoesophageal sphincter. The subsequent sequential contraction of the pharyngeal musculature aids in clearing the bolus from the pharyngeal cavity. Dehiscence of the pharyngeal musculature may result in diverticuli and the potential for residue in the pharynx after the swallow. Surgery that affects the posterior pharyngeal wall may also produce tethering of the pharynx to the prevertebral fascia. Although elevation of the pharyngeal cavity is not thought to be a significant requirement for deglutition, patients who experience posterior pharyngeal-wall tethering complain of severe dysphagia and have poor pharyngeal constriction on the dynamic videofluoroscopic swallow study.

Reconstruction of pharyngeal-wall defects is best accomplished with primary closure if the size of the defect permits. When bulky, adynamic flaps are required, dysphagia may be worsened by lack of muscular tone in the flap area or by obstruction to bolus flow by flap bulk. An analysis, performed in our laboratory, of 43 patients who complained of dysphagia after lateral pharyngeal-wall resection for cancer revealed poor pharyngeal constriction ($p = .04$), but no difference in the extent of hyoid-bone elevation or the size of the upper esophageal sphincter opening, when compared to normal controls (Kendall & Leonard, unpublished data, 2003).

## LARYNX

The supraglottic laryngectomy was designed for removal of cancers involving supraglottic structures such as the epiglottis and false vocal folds. The surgical procedure usually involves the removal of the hyoid bone and includes resection of the structures superior to the petiole of the epiglottis and the laryngeal ventricles. The remaining laryngeal structures are sutured to the residual tongue base. Airway protection during swallowing is severely compromised by the removal of most of the structures responsible for directing the bolus away from the glottis. Prevention of aspiration is accomplished by the well timed closure of the vocal folds alone. Supraglottic laryngectomy patients must be trained in swallow techniques that insure timely vocal-fold closure and even so are at significant risk for the development of aspiration pneumonia (Calcaterra, 1971). Some surgeons have recommended that the remaining larynx be suspended anteriorly to the mandible during the reconstruction to improve airway protection provided by the bulk of the tongue base (Kronenberger & Meyers, 1994).

Partial laryngectomy surgery has been designed to remove cancers involving the structures of the larynx with the reconstruction of a voicing source using the residual tissues. Usually the aperture is too small to serve as an adequate airway and a permanent tracheostomy is required. The ability of the reconstructed vibratory source to prevent bolus penetration during deglutition is often incomplete. Again, these patients may require therapy to develop strategies for safe, effective swallowing.

After total laryngectomy, the mechanism usually responsible for the opening of the pharyngoesophageal sphincter, laryngeal elevation, no longer functions. Laryngectomy patients must rely on the forces generated by the base of the tongue against the pharyngeal walls to drive the bolus inferiorly. A "pumping" action of the tongue is often observed in these patients to help generate the increased pressures required to compensate for lack of pharyngoesophageal sphincter opening. If significant tongue-tissue resection is required for adequate cancer removal, patients can be expected to experience significant dysphagia. Laryngectomy reconstruction, however, results in complete separation of the airway from the digestive tract and obviates any concerns for aspiration.

## BASE OF SKULL

When head and neck cancers invade the base of the skull, the impact on swallowing is often primarily caused by the loss of cranial nerve function. Because of the anatomic proximity of the cranial nerves at the skull base, multiple nerve deficits are usually present (Jennings, Sirocky, & Jackson, 1992; Johnson, McKenzie, Rosenquist, Lieberman, & Sievers, 1992). Tumors in the region of the infratemporal fossa, near the foramen ovale, can be expected to impact the trigeminal nerve. The muscles of mastication and sensation to the tongue and soft palate will be impaired, thus affecting oral bolus preparation and manipulation. Tumors near the jugular fossa may involve the glossopharyngeal nerve (IX) and the vagus (X). As the glossopharyngeal nerve provides sensation to the posterior one third of the tongue, swallow initiation may be delayed. Both the glossopharyngeal and the vagus nerves provide innervation to the muscles of the pharynx. Once the pharyngeal swallowing sequence is initiated, weakness of the pharynx caused by tumor involvement of the tumor and glossopharyngeal nerves results in poor pharyngeal contraction with poor pharyngeal clearing and, in extreme cases, the inability to propel the bolus into the pharyngoesophageal sphincter. An ipsilateral vocal-fold paralysis is usually present in these already severely compromised patients. As tumors near the jugular foramen enlarge, the hypoglossal nerve (XII) will become involved. The resultant tongue weakness has obvious impact on both the oral and pharyngeal phases of swallowing.

When a patient is diagnosed with a vocal-fold (VF) paralysis, it is often assumed that vocal-fold medialization will prevent aspiration, even in the face of multiple cranial nerve deficits. Little objective data exist to support the belief that medialization of a paralyzed vocal fold decreases the risk of aspiration, however. There is an association, on the other hand, between prolonged bolus pharyngeal transit time and increased risk of aspiration pneumonia (Yip, Kendall, & Leonard, 2005). A study was done in our laboratory to assess the impact of medialization on the duration of pharyngeal transit and incidence of aspiration. Two groups of patients (1996–2000) with unilateral VF paralysis were identified. One group ($n = 12$) had isolated VF paralysis caused by recurrent laryngeal nerve injury. A second group ($n = 7$) had multiple cranial neuropathies secondary to skull base surgery or strokes. All patients underwent VF medialization with pre- and postmedialization videofluoroscopic swallow studies. Before medialization, the incidence of aspiration in the isolated vocal-cord paralysis group was 44% (8/18) and 100% in the multiple

cranial neuropathy group for an overall incidence of 58%. Both patient groups demonstrated prolonged pharyngeal transit times (overall mean = 1.3 seconds ± 0.32) compared to normal controls (mean = 0.84 seconds ± 0.15) ($p < .0001$). Postmedialization, the incidence of aspiration in the isolated vocal-cord paralysis group decreased to 27% (5/18) and to 67% (4/6) in the multiple cranial neuropathy group for an overall incidence of 37%. Bolus pharyngeal transit times were significantly improved after medialization ($p = .0098$) but remained significantly prolonged compared to normal controls (1.04 seconds ± 0.44) ($p = .0015$) (Yip et al., 2005).

Aspiration occurs in patients with isolated unilateral VF paralysis and in patients with multiple cranial neuropathies, although the incidence is higher in patients with multiple cranial nerve deficits. VF medialization reduces the overall incidence of aspiration in both groups by 50% but does not eliminate it. Prolonged pharyngeal transit following medialization suggests that the risk of aspiration pneumonia is not eliminated even when aspiration is not identified.

## RADIATION THERAPY

The addition of postoperative radiation therapy to the treatment regimen will likely worsen dysphagia. During the treatment period, patients experience significant mucositis resulting in pain, swelling, mucus production, and xerostomia. Oral feeding may be extremely difficult during the treatment period. Acute effects of radiation therapy usually last for approximately 8 to

12 weeks after the final treatments. Swallowing therapy may be limited during this period by the patient's inability to participate. Generally, the use of exercises during this period has not yet been shown to be effective in limiting the resulting dysphagia (see discussion in Chapter 18). However, further study of the effects of swallowing therapy in this patient population is sorely needed (Pauloski et al., 1995).

The long-term effects of radiation therapy involve the fibrosis of residual soft tissues and xerostomia. Tissue fibrosis of the muscles involved in deglutition limits the normal range of muscle motion resulting in decreased tongue mobility and lack of larynx and hyoid elevation. A study of 20 patients treated for head and neck cancer with radiation therapy alone revealed that the most common abnormality identified 1 year after the completion of therapy on the dynamic videofluoroscopic swallow study was poor pharyngeal constriction, likely secondary to a decrease of tongue range of motion (Kendall, McKenzie, & Leonard, 1998). Xerostomia will predispose to dental caries as well as diminished lubrication of the bolus.

## CONCLUSION

Surgical resections in the head and neck region for cancer often require the resection of more than one anatomic subunit. The defects described in this chapter are often combined or only partial. The variability inherent in this disease results in significant difficulty in the categorization of patients into groups for comparison in outcome studies involving deglutition. Each

patient must be considered individually. Other factors, including the overall medical condition, social situation, and support system, will likely impact the patient's ability to achieve adequate safe oral intake to maintain nutritional requirements.

## STUDY QUESTIONS

1. How does tongue tethering impact swallowing function? For example, if the tongue is tethered to the anterior oral cavity (as in primary closure of an anterior floor-of-mouth defect), how does that affect the movement of the bolus through the pharynx?
2. What are the consequences (for swallowing) of a palatal defect?
3. What reconstructive options are available to repair a tongue defect and what is the potential impact of each option on swallowing function?
4. How does poor hyoid bone elevation impact swallowing function?

## REFERENCES

Baker, B. M., Fraser, A. M., & Baker, C. D. (1991). Long-term postoperative dysphagia in oral/pharyngeal surgery patients: subjects' perceptions vs. videofluoroscopic observations. *Dysphagia*, 6, 11–16.

Calcaterra, T. (1971). Laryngeal suspension after supraglottic laryngectomy. *Archives of Otolaryngology*, 94, 306–309.

Doberneck, R., & Antoine, J. (1974). Deglutition after resection of oral, laryngeal and pharyngeal cancers. *Surgery*, 1, 87–90.

Eisbruch, A., Dawson, L. A., Kim, H. M., Bradford, C. R., Terrell, J. E., Chepeha, D. B., et al. (1999). Conformal and intensity modulated irradiation of head and neck cancer: The potential for improved target irradiation, salivary gland function, and quality of life. *Acta Otorhinolaryngologica Belgica, 53,* 271–275.

Freeman, R. B., Marks, J. E., & Ogura, J. H. (1979). Voice preservation in treatment of carcinoma of the pyriform sinus. *Laryngoscope, 89,* 1855–1863.

Hammerlid, E., Bjordal, K., Ahlner-Elmqvist, M., Jannert, M. Kaasa, S., Sullivan, M., et al. (1997). Prospective, longitudinal quality-of -life study of patients with had and neck cancer: A feasibility study including the EORTC QLQ-C30. *Otolarygology-Head and Neck Surgery, 116,* 666–673.

Hassan, S. J., & Weymuller, E. A. (1993). Assessment of quality of life in head and neck cancer patients. *Head and Neck, 15,* 485–496.

Jennings, K. S, Sirocky, D., & Jackson, C. G. (1992). Swallowing problems after excision of tumors of the skull base: Diagnosis and management in 12 patients. *Dysphagia, 7,* 40–44.

Johnson, E. R., McKenzie, S. W., Rosenquist, C. J., Lieberman, J. S., & Sievers, A. (1992). Dysphagia following stroke: Quantitative evaluation of pharyngeal transit times. *Archives of Physical Medicine and Rehabilitation, 73,* 419–423.

Kendall, K., McKenzie, S., Leonard, R. , & Jones, C. (1998). Structural mobility in deglutition after single modality treatment of head and neck carcinomas with radiation therapy. *Head and Neck, 20,* 720–725.

Kendall, K. A., McKenzie, S., & Leonard, R. (2000). Timing of swallowing events after single modality treatment of head and neck carcinomas with radiation therapy. *Annals of Otology, Rhinology and Laryngology, 109,* 767–775.

Kendall, K. A., McKenzie, S., Leonard, R., Goncalves, M., & Walker, A. (2000). Timing of events in normal swallowing: A videofluoroscopic study. *Dysphagia, 15,* 146–152.

Kronenberger, M. B., & Meyers, A. D. (1994). Dysphagia following head and neck cancer surgery. *Dysphagia, 9,* 236–244.

Leonard, R., Kendall, K. A., McKenzie, S., Goncalves, M., & Walker, A. (2000). Stuctural mobility in normal swallowing: A videofluoroscopic study. *Dysphagia, 15,* 146–152.

Logemann, J. A., & Bytell, D. E. (1979). Swallowing disorders in three types of head and neck surgical patients. *Cancer, 44,* 1095–1105.

McConnel, F. M. S. (1996). *Evaluation of the reconstruction of the oropharynx with modified barium swallow and manofluorography,* Presentation at the First International Neurolaryngology Symposium; Bethesda, MD.

McConnel, F. M. S., Logemann, J. A., Rademaker, A. W., Pauloski, B. R., Lewin, J. Shedd, D., et al. (1994). Surgical variables affecting postoperative swallowing efficiency in oral cancer patients: A pilot study. *Laryngoscope, 104,* 87–90.

McConnel, F. M. S., & Mendelsohn, M. (1987). The effects of surgery on pharyngeal deglutition. *Dysphagia, 1,* 145–151.

McConnel, F. M. S., & O'Connor, A. (1994). Dysphagia secondary to head and neck cancer surgery. *Acta Otorhinolaryngologica Belgica, 48,* 165–170.

Pauloski, B. R., Logemann, J. A., Fox, J. C., & Colangelo, J. A. (1995). Biomechanical analysis of the pharyngeal swallow in postsurgical patients with anterior tongue and floor of mouth resection and distal flap reconstruction. *Journal of Speech and Hearing Research, 38,* 110–123.

Pauloski, B. R., Logemann, J. A., Rademaker, A. W., McConnel, F. M., Beery, Q., Johnson, J., et al. (1994). Speech and swallowing function after oral and oropharyngeal resections: One-year follow-up. *Head and Neck, 16,* 313–322.

Pauloski, B. R., Logemann, J. A., Rademaker, A. W., McConnel, F. M. S., Heiser, M. A., Cardinale, S., et al. (1993). Speech and swallowing function after anterior tongue and floor of mouth resection with distal flap reconstruction. *Journal of Speech and Hearing Research, 36,* 267–276.

Pruszewicz, A., & Kruk-Zagajewska, A. (1984). Phoniatric disturbances in patients after partial tongue resection for malignant neoplasms. *Folia Phoniatrica et Logopaedica, 36,* 84–92.

Stachler, R. J., Hamlet, S. L., Mathog, R. H., Jones, L., Heilbrun, L. K., Manov, J. M., et al. (1994). Swallowing of bolus types by postsurgical head and neck cancer patients. *Head and Neck, 16,* 413–419.

Terrell, J. E. (1999). Quality of life assessment in head and neck cancer patients. *Hematology/Oncology Clinics of North America, 13,* 849–856.

Terrell J. E, Fisher, S. G., & Wolf, G. T. (1998). Long-term quality of life after treatment of laryngeal cancer: The Veterans Affairs Laryngeal Cancer Study Group. *Archives of Otolaryngology-Head and Neck Surgery, 124,* 964–971.

Urba, S. G., Wolf, G. T., Bradford, C. R., Thornton, A. F., Eisbruch, A., Terrell, J. E., et al. (2000). Neoadjuvant therapy for organ preservation in head and neck cancer. *Laryngoscope, 110,* 2074–2080.

Wolf, G. T., Forastiere, A., Ang, K., Brockstein, B. Conley, B., Goepfert, H. D., et al. (1999).Workshop report: Organ preservation strategies in advanced head and neck cancer—current status and future directions. *Head and Neck, 21,* 689–693.

Yip, H., Kendall, K. A., & Leonard, R. J. (2006). Impact of vocal fold medialization on pharyngeal transit time and incidence of aspiration, *Journal of Otolaryngology.* Manuscript submitted for publication.

# 4

# *Dysphagia in Neurogenic Disorders*

## E. Ralph Johnson

Swallowing problems occur in a wide variety of neurological and neuromuscular disorders. The intent of this chapter is to review specific swallowing problems associated with the major categories of neurogenic disorders and to discuss concerns related to diagnostic strategies, and the timing of these strategies, in patients experiencing central nervous system or neuromuscular diseases.

Particular attention is given to diagnostic strategies that provide both qualitative and quantitative information regarding dysphagia in neurogenic patient populations. Bedside and clinical evaluations and dynamic radiographic studies of swallow function represent major components of this diagnostic protocol. Information obtained from bedside and clinical evaluations is particularly useful for identifying and monitoring patients experiencing swallowing disorders, and in determining the timing of more comprehensive diag-

nostic studies. The "gold standard" of these studies is the dynamic videofluoroscopic evaluation, also called a dynamic swallow study. The dynamic swallow study (Chapters 15–18) provides objective and quantitative data that can elaborate the nature and severity of a swallowing problem, provide insights into prognosis in individual patients, and be used to develop remedial treatment programs. However, the radiographic study requires exposure to ionizing x-irradiation (approximately that of two cervical spine x-rays). Consequently, the use and timing of the dynamic swallow study must be considered with respect to minimizing both diagnostic costs and x-ray exposure. A battery of diagnostic strategies that permits the most efficacious use of radiographic studies is of particular concern in patient populations that experience frequent and significant change, sometimes rapid and for the better, sometimes prolonged and for the worse. Of necessity, these issues must be considered in any discussion of swallowing problems in neurogenic patients, and are a major focus of this chapter.

## CENTRAL NERVOUS SYSTEM DISORDERS

### Stroke

Dysphagia is seen in unilateral cortical lesions on either the right or left side, subcortical lesions, and brainstem lesions. Tongue motor function is rarely affected in cortical strokes because the nucleus of cranial nerve XII is in the median medulla and is not often impaired by vascular lesions. Problems are generally apparent in the pharyngeal component of swallow. The oropharyngeal (or mesopharyngeal) component (described as beginning at the juncture between the hard and soft palates and extending to the valleculae) is primarily involved, although the hypopharyngeal component (from the valleculae to the upper esophageal sphincter) may also be compromised (Donner, Bosma, & Robertson, 1985). Problems may relate to poor sensation, poor pharyngeal peristalsis, or discoordination or delay in the timing of bolus propulsion through the pharynx. Predicting those acute stroke patients likely to develop dysphagia from clinical signs alone is difficult (Mann & Hankey, 2001). In one report, more than half of patients with medullary strokes presented with clinical indications of dysphagia. Aspiration pneumonia appeared as an early complication in these patients, and dietary modifications did not prevent aspiration pneumonia. (Teasdale, Foley, Fisher, & Finestone, 2002).

Swallowing problems in stroke have been the subject of numerous dysphagia studies. However, until the past few years, the information available for dysphagia after stroke has been primarily qualitative. More recently, quantitative studies have provided additional useful information (Johnson, Mckenzie, Rosenquist, Sievers, & Lieberman, 1992). With clinical or bedside evaluation alone, aspiration is missed in approximately one half of patients with neurological or neuromuscular disease (Splaingard, Hutchins, Sulton, & Chaudhuri, 1988). Thus, the need for more definitive assessment, including videofluoroscopy, is clear.

Significant differences exist between the swallow-respiration patterns of patients with poststroke dysphagia and healthy volunteers. However, there is no evidence linking poststroke swallow-respiration characteristics with aspiration on simultaneous videofluoroscopy (Leslie, Drinnen, Ford, & Wilson, 2002). Because recovery from stroke is a time-related process, the timing of specific evaluation procedures is also important. In general, there is a need for early speech pathology assessment within the first week in order to evaluate the patient's ability to handle oral intake and to provide a baseline for consistent follow-up assessment. Speech pathology and nursing personnel are then prepared to watch for evidence of aspiration, assess the need for more definitive diagnostic studies, and provide for a rational progression of dietary intake. Clinical factors that suggest the need for evaluation with a dynamic swallow study include: (a) aspiration pneumonia, (b) cough and "wet lung" following swallowing, and (c) inability to maintain oral hydration and nutrition.

The dynamic swallow study is of value in identifying the presence of aspiration and the effects of various remedial strategies, even with no quantitative assessment. Our experience, however, suggests that the extra time and expense associated with obtaining objective measures can contribute significantly to patient care. As an example, our research has demonstrated that a kinematic pharyngeal transit time of more than 5 seconds (normal $1.00 \pm .15$ sec) is highly associated with aspiration pneumonia risk in stroke patients, whereas a time of less than 2 seconds has a low association (Johnson & McKenzie, 1993a).

There is only a rare indication for a dynamic swallow study in stroke before 2 weeks after onset. During this time, the patient stabilizes and time is allowed for recovery. This waiting period is particularly important in individuals with cerebral hemorrhage because excessive diagnostic study before 1 week may increase the risk for additional bleeding. Careful monitoring of patients during this time period will help determine the patient's need and readiness for comprehensive evaluation. Well-timed and appropriate dynamic swallow studies will then prove to be valuable tools for management of dysphagia in stroke.

## Brain Injury

Problems with swallowing and nutrition are significant difficulties in the management of individuals with traumatic brain injuries, in postoperative individuals after resection of brain tumors, and in patients with brain injury from hypoxia, encephalitis, or meningitis (Field & Weiss, 1989; Lazarus & Logemann, 1987). The evaluation techniques are the same as for individuals with stroke. Clinical factors such as aspiration pneumonia, cough or "wet lung" following feeding, or inability to maintain oral hydration and nutrition should trigger consideration for a dynamic swallow study. As with stroke, no individual with brain injury should have a dynamic swallow study if the sensorium is not clear enough to permit following instructions for the study or if trunk balance does not permit sitting upright in a chair. The time of day the study is done should include consideration of any diurnal variation in cognitive alertness. Irradiation exposure is, of course, significantly and directly related to the length of the procedure, which can be prolonged in these patients. Total exposure time of less than 5 minutes is preferred with a mean exposure time goal for all patients of 3 minutes.

In head injury, the most common problems identified with a dynamic swallow study are prolonged oral transit and delayed swallowing initiation. Aspiration is common. Pharyngeal peristalsis is reduced. Vallecular and piriform residue are prominent features of the dynamic swallow study (Leslie et al., 2002).

## Cerebral Palsy

Cerebral palsy produces significant nutrition and swallowing problems for patients and their families (Field &

Weiss, 1989; Rogers, Arvedson, Buck, Smart, & Msall, 1994). Individuals with cerebral palsy are now living longer and attaining adulthood, often because of dedicated families who over the years feed the children with love and care. Adults with cerebral palsy are frequently housed in skilled nursing and long-term care facilities. These facilities are concerned about the risks of feeding orally and often do not have the personnel to provide the same amount of time for feeding as previously provided by the family. These caregivers' most common concerns relate to airway protection during oral feedings. More than 50% of individuals with cerebral palsy may experience coughing, choking, and troubled breathing during meals. Silent aspiration has also been reported as common, with aspiration of specific textures significantly more common than aspiration of all food textures (Taniguchi & Moyer, 1994). Dynamic swallow studies can provide extensive information for determining appropriate consistencies and techniques to prevent or minimize aspiration. Such studies are indicated in individuals who develop aspiration pneumonia, fail to maintain hydration or nutrition, or require more time for feeding than caregivers have available. The study requires a subject who can sit upright with bolsters. Spastic or athetoid movements may produce a suboptimal study; however, even suboptimal studies may give valuable information regarding remedial techniques, including best head position for feeding and most manageable food textures. As in head injury, care should be taken regarding the timing of the study to optimize volitional assistance from the patient.

## Parkinson's Disease

Swallowing is frequently influenced by the bradykinesia and rigidity of Parkinsonism (Lieberman, Horowitz, & Redmond, 1980; Logemann, Blonsky, & Boshes, 1975; Stroudley & Walsh, 1991). Parkinsonism is associated with neuronal degeneration and subsequent depletion of dopamine and its metabolites within the basal ganglia. Dysphagia may be present in as many as 50% of Parkinson patients, but rarely is severe enough to require a feeding gastrostomy. Logemann and her colleagues reviewed the neuromuscular control of swallowing in more than 100 Parkinson patients (Rogers et al., 1994). Approximately 20% complained of swallowing problems; however, when examined videofluoroscopically, 95% showed specific quantifiable disturbances in neuromuscular control. Specific problems were found in all three stages of the swallow and included slowed oral transit, slowed pharyngeal transit times, and vallecular pooling. Tracheal aspiration was present on fluoroscopy in 46% of 24 patients (Taniguchi & Moyer, 1994).

Although oral agents that pass the blood/brain barrier to increase dopamine stores in the basal ganglia have greatly improved function in Parkinson's disease, a significant percentage of patients will need dysphagia evaluation, including a dynamic swallow study. These studies should be scheduled after an optimal medical treatment regimen has been attained; that is, when maximal benefit from medication is seen in the hypokinesia of skeletal muscle function. If at that time significant problems with dysphagia persist, a dynamic swallow study will give useful clinical information for remedial techniques.

## Multiple Sclerosis

Multiple sclerosis is a disease that usually begins in early adulthood and is characterized by numerous sequential areas of central nervous system demyelination and sclerosis. Multiple sclerosis produces a protean set of symptoms that "wax and wane" but produce slowly progressive spastic neurologic deficits. The time course for progression of symptoms is as long as 20 years. Swallowing evaluations should be primarily clinical in the first years of the illness as the pathological lesion often "heals" (but with a plaque scar remaining). In one study of 29 multiple sclerosis patients, 16 experienced swallowing difficulties (Daly, Dode, & Andersen, 1962). Choking was a frequent complaint. Difficulty in initiating the pharyngeal phase of swallowing was also described. There was no nasal regurgitation. Hypernasality of speech was noted in only one patient although spastic or ataxic dysarthria was present in 15. Poor relaxation of the lower esophageal sphincter and disturbances of esophageal motility were present in 42% of patients assessed. Dynamic swallow studies should be delayed until clinical evaluation is no longer sufficient to adequately assess and treat the swallowing problem, and more specific individual remedial techniques are required.

On videofluoroscopy in multiple sclerosis, laryngopharyngeal dysmotility includes shorter than normal intervals from onset of laryngeal excursion to return to rest, and longer than normal time intervals between airway closure at the arytenoids to epiglottic base and upper pharyngeal sphincter opening (Abraham & Inn, 2002).

## NEUROMUSCULAR DISEASE

Swallowing difficulties in varying degrees are present in a wide range of neuromuscular diseases (Willig, Paulus, Lacau Saint Guilly, Beon, & Navarro, 1994). The following are representative of those diseases.

## Polymyositis/Dermatomyositis

Polymyositis is an acquired myopathy in which muscle undergoes degeneration with inflammation resulting in proximal skeletal muscle weakness. In approximately one third of individuals with polymyositis, there are associated skin changes, in which case the disease is called dermatomyositis. Polymyositis and dermatomyositis have long been recognized as diseases with dysphagia as a major problem. The swallowing difficulties in polymyositis/dermatomyositis occur early and are severe (Johnson & McKenzie, 1993b; Metheny, 1988). Dysphagia may be the only presenting complaint (Metheny et al., 1988). Nutrition is impaired by the swallowing difficulty. Aspiration is frequent. Aspiration pneumonia is a significant early risk. In polymyositis, transit times of the bolus are slowed through both the mesopharynx and the hypopharynx. In many other neurological and neuromuscular diseases the slowing is primarily through the hypopharynx.

The swallowing disorder in polymyositis may be marked early in the disease and require assessment and treatment within 6 months of onset of the disease (Metheny, 1988). As in Parkinson syndrome, dynamic swallow study should await the maximum effect of pharmacologic treatment. Corticosteroids may improve swallowing to the point where the study can be delayed. The development of pneumonia or inability to maintain hydration or nutrition are indications for more immediate radiologic study.

## Myasthenia Gravis

As with polymyositis, dysphagia may be a presenting complaint in myasthenia gravis. Myasthenia gravis produces symptoms of weakness and fatigue. The pathophysiologic problem is a muscle receptor antibody that blocks the muscle acetylcholine receptor. Acetylcholine stimulates the muscle receptor and initiates muscle contraction after crossing the neuromuscular junction. In myasthenia gravis, muscle weakness is produced by the decreased number of unblocked muscle receptors available for muscle fiber stimulation. Pharyngeal and pharyngoesophageal impairments are a problem (Joshita, Yoshida, & Kimura, 1990). Dysphagia can be pronounced. Dysphagia frequently improves with treatment with anticholinesterase inhibitors such as pyridostigmine. It may also improve with corticosteroids or thymectomy. Radiological swallow studies should be delayed if thymectomy has been scheduled.

## Muscular Dystrophies

The muscular dystrophies are a series of muscle diseases produced by different specific genetic abnormalities. The neuropathology varies but generally involves muscle breakdown and atrophy, producing weakness and dysfunction. The dysfunction may involve skeletal, cardiac, or smooth muscle. Many of the muscular dystrophies have associated swallowing problems (Willig et al., 1994). Limb girdle dystrophy, Duchenne muscular dystrophy, myotonic muscular dystrophy, and limb girdle syndromes show delay of transit time primarily through the hypopharynx. Dysphagia in facioscapulohumeral syndrome is uncommon.

### Myotonic Muscular Dystrophy

There are multiple reports of abnormalities in the swallowing mechanism in myotonic muscular dystrophy (MMD), (Pruzanski, 1962; Salomonson, Kawamoto, & Wilson, 1988). The return time for hyoid movement is prolonged (Bosma & Brodie, 1969). Vallecular/piriform pooling and prolongation of pharyngeal transit times may also be present, as well as small intestinal hypomotility and velopharyngeal incompetence. Leonard, Kendall, Johnson, and McKenzie (2001) reported prolonged bolus transit times and delays in the onset of a number swallow gestures (Jaffe, McDonald, Ingram, & Haas, 1990). Pharyngeal constriction was markedly reduced. The authors concluded that weakness associated with the disease, and not myotonia, was the most significant contributor to impairment. Swallowing abnormalities in MMD occur after several years disease duration and are slowly progressive.

Dynamic swallow studies are indicated when there is prolongation of eating time, unexplained weight loss, coughing with swallowing, or episodes of pneumonia. Many myotonic dystrophy patients have a cardiac conduction defect through the bundle of His and develop first-degree heart block. In the majority of cases, this produces no cardiac symptom. However, a small percentage may develop more advanced heart block. Cardiac resuscitation drugs and equipment should be immediately available during the dynamic swallow study. If a myotonic patient develops syncope during the swallow study, blood pressure and pulse should be taken. If the pulse drops below 60 per minute, an electrocardiogram is indicated to check for atrioventricular block.

### Limb Girdle Syndrome

Swallowing abnormalities are present in limb girdle syndrome (Johnson & McKenzie, 1993b; Willig et al., 1994). If a cricopharyngeal bar is present there may be improvement following a surgical cricopharyngeal myotomy (Johnson & McKenzie, 1993b). As with the other muscular dystrophies, hypopharyngeal transit times are impaired while mesopharyngeal transit times are not significantly different from normal controls. Limb girdle syndromes are slowly progressive muscular dystrophies. The need for dynamic swallow studies is usually not present before 10 years' duration. The general clinical indications for the study are the same as for the previous disease categories. Cardiac dysrhythmias are not as prominent as with myotonic dystrophy.

### Duchenne Muscular Dystrophy

Swallowing difficulties are present in individuals with Duchenne muscular dystrophy (Hillel & Miller, 1989; Willig et al., 1994). Individuals with Duchenne muscular dystrophy lack dystrophin, a muscle protein that is thought to be significant in muscle repair. There is decreased biting force and esophageal motility is also impaired. Pharyngeal transit times are normal to mildly prolonged, and mild vallecular and piriform pooling are typical. Hyoid displacement, maximal pharyngeal constriction, and pharyngoesophageal segment opening are typically normal. The incidence of pneumonia in individuals with Duchenne muscular dystrophy (which has previously been ascribed to respiratory muscle failure) may have a component of aspiration secondary to the myopathic swallowing problem. The optimal timing for dynamic swallow studies in Duchenne muscular dystrophy is not clear. Weight loss and inability to maintain hydration are not prominent clinical findings. Acute cardiorespiratory failure is a significant clinical problem and is often the cause of death before the age of 20 years. That failure has previously been ascribed to the ventricular cardiac hypokinesia; however, the importance of aspiration in the early deaths in Duchenne muscular dystrophy is unclear.

## MOTOR NEURON DISEASE

### Amyotrophic Lateral Sclerosis

Amyotrophic lateral sclerosis and primary lateral sclerosis are degenerative neurological diseases that cause atrophy of anterior horn cells in the spinal cord and bulbar motor neurons in the brain stem. The bulbar motor neuron lesions produce profound and difficult swallowing problems early in the disease process. Dysphagia may be the presenting symptom, occurring before the onset of muscle weakness and fasciculations so characteristic of the illness. In the early stages of amyotrophic lateral sclerosis, dysphagia severity tends to be significantly influenced by posterior tongue dysfunction secondary to degeneration atrophy. Although amyotrophic lateral sclerosis usually produces death within 3 years after onset, management of nutrition and aspiration may be helped with dynamic swallow evaluation. The progression of the swallowing deficit may require evaluation within 1 year of onset to assist in determining nutrition management strategies.

There are marked abnormalities in swallowing mechanisms in amyotrophic lateral sclerosis, including pharyngeal weakness, pharyngeal and esophageal hypomotility, increased transit times, and aspiration (Buchholz & Jones, 1991; Leighton, Burton, Lund, & Cochrane, 1994). Dysphagia, aspiration pneumonia, and severe nutritional deficits are a part of the rapid progression of this disease. The patient's difficulty in managing saliva can present a serious problem. Aggressive surgical procedures, including laryngeal diversion, have been used with varying success in prevention of aspiration.

## Congenital Spinal Muscular Atrophy

Congenital spinal muscular atrophy is a progressive disorder involving degeneration of motor neurons in the spinal cord and brainstem. Muscle weakness and atrophy are a result. Dysphagia is secondary to the loss of bulbar neurons. In many cases, the course of the illness is of several years' duration and requires ongoing attention to the swallowing disorder. The clinical indications for dynamic swallow study in those cases are the same as described for amyotrophic lateral sclerosis.

## Postpolio Syndrome

Anterior poliomyelitis is a degeneration of spinal cord anterior horn cells and bulbar motor neurons produced by an acute viral infection of those cells. Although anterior poliomyelitis has become a rare disease in the United States, it is still present in the world. Furthermore, many adults born in the United States before the development of polio vaccines have had poliomyelitis and may develop postpolio syndrome with increased swallowing problems (Leonard et al., 2001). Postpolio syndrome is the development of additional muscle weakness occurring several years after the acute viral infection has been cleared. The exact etiology of postpolio syndrome has not been established, but it may result from additional loss of motor neurons associated with the aging process. Particular attention should be given to a clinical swallow evaluation in individuals who have had polio and who develop progressive late onset skeletal muscle weakness. Subsequent dynamic swallow studies may identify useful compensatory strategies for those patients.

## SUMMARY

Dysphagia is a significant clinical problem requiring evaluation and treatment in many individuals with neuromuscular and neurologic degenerative diseases. A thorough clinical examination and appropriate diagnostic imaging studies are necessary to develop an appropriate treatment regimen. Thoughtful timing of these studies is required to limit irradiation exposure.

## STUDY QUESTIONS

1. What types of stroke produce dysphagia?
2. Which is more likely to be affected by stroke, mesopharynx (or oropharynx) or hypopharynx function for swallowing?
3. What is the most optimal time for DSS in an acute stroke patient?
4. What are typical features of dysphagia in head injured patients?
5. If a DSS is recommended for a patient with Parkinson disease, what might the clinician want to consider in scheduling it?
6. Have significant features of swallowing difficulty been identified for patients with muscular dystrophy? Multiple sclerosis? Polymyositis or dermatomyositis?
7. Are there differences in the onset time of swallowing disorders in patients with polymyositis/dermatomyositis as compared to patients with limb girdle syndrome?
8. Are the effects of postpolio syndrome thought to be solely related to aging that renders compensatory mechanisms previously developed by a patient less effective?

## REFERENCES

Abraham, S., & Inn, P. (2002). Laryngopharyngeal dysmotility in multiple sclerosis. *Dysphagia, 16,* 69–74.

Bosma, J., & Brodie, D. (1969). Cineradiographic demonstration of pharyngeal area myotonia in myotonic dystrophy patients. *Radiology, 92,* 104–109.

Buchholz, D., & Jones, B. (1991). Dysphagia occurring after polio. *Dysphagia, 6,* 165–169.

Daly, D., Dode, C., & Andersen, H. (1962). Disturbance of swallowing and esophageal motility in patients with multiple sclerosis. *Neurology, 12,* 250–256.

Donner, M., Bosma, J., & Robertson, D. (1985). Anatomy and physiology of the pharynx. *Gastrointestinal Radiology, 10,* 196–212.

Field, L., & Weiss, C. (1989). Dysphagia with head injury. *Brain Injury, 3,* 19–26.

Hillel, A. & Miller, R. (1989). Bulbar amyotrophic lateral sclerosis: Patterns of progression and clinical management. *Head and Neck, 11,* 51–59.

Jaffe, K., McDonald, C., Ingram, E., & Haas, J. (1990). Symptoms of upper gastrointestinal dysfunction in Duchenne muscular dystrophy: Case control study. *Archives of Physical Medicine and Rehabilitation, 71,* 742–744.

Johnson, E., & McKenzie, S. (1993a). Aspiration pneumonia in stroke. *Archives of Physical Medicine and Rehabilitation, 74,* 973–976.

Johnson, E., & McKenzie, S. (1993b). Kinematic pharyngeal transit times in myopathy. *Dysphagia, 8,* 35–40.

Johnson, E., McKenzie, S., Rosenquist, C., Sievers, A., & Lieberman, J. (1992). Dysphagia following stroke: Quantitative evaluation of pharyngeal transit times. *Archives of Physical Medicine and Rehabilitation, 73,* 419–423.

Joshita, Y., Yoshida, M., & Kimura, K. (1990). Manometric study of the pharynx and pharyngoesophageal sphincter in myasthenia gravis [in Japanese]. *Rinsho Shineigaku, Clinical Neurology, 30,* 944–951.

Lazarus, C., & Logemann, J. (1987). Swallowing disorders in closed head trauma patients. *Archives of Physical Medicine and Rehabilitation, 68,* 79–84.

Leighton, S., Burton, M., Lund, W., & Cochrane, G. (1994). Swallowing in motor neurone disease. *Journal of the Royal Society of Medicine, 87,* 801–805.

Leonard R, J., Kendall K. A., Johnson R., & McKenzie, S. (2001). Swallowing in myotonic muscular dystrophy: A videofluoroscopic study. *Archives of Physical Medicine and Rehabilitation, 82,* 979–85.

Leslie, P., Drinnen, M., Ford, G., & Wilson, J. (2002). Swallow respiration patterns in dysphagic patients following acute stroke. *Dysphagia, 17,* 202–207.

Lieberman, A., Horowitz, L., & Redmond P. (1980). Dysphagia in Parkinson's disease. *American Journal of Gastroenterology, 74,* 157–160.

Logemann, J., Blonsky, E., & Boshes, B. (1975). Dysphagia in parkinsonism. *Dysphagia, 231,* 69–70.

Mann, G., & Hankey, G. (2001). Initial clinical and demographic predictors of swallowing impairment following acute stroke. *Dysphagia, 16,* 208–215.

Metheny, J. (1988). Dermatomyositis. A vocal and swallowing entity. *Laryngoscope, 98,* 414–417.

Pruzanski, W. (1962). Respiratory tract infections and silent aspiration in myotonic dystrophy. *Diseases of the Chest, 42,* 608–610.

Rogers, B., Arvedson, J., Buck, G., Smart, P., & Msall, M. (1994). Characteristics of dysphagia in children with cerebral palsy. *Dysphagia, 9,* 69–73.

Salomonson, J., Kawamoto, H., & Wilson, L. (1988). Velopharyngeal incompetence as the presenting symptom of myotonic dystrophy. *Cleft Palate Journal, 25,* 296–300.

Splaingard, M., Hutchins, B., Sulton, L., & Chaudhuri, G. (1988). Aspiration in rehabilitation patients: Videofluoroscopy vs. bedside clinical assessment. *Archives of Physical Medicine and Rehabilitation, 69,* 637–640.

Stroudley, J., & Walsh, M. (1991). Radiological assessment of dysphagia in Parkinson's disease. *British Journal of Radiology, 64,* 890–893.

Taniguchi, M. & Moyer, R. (1994). Assessment of risk factors for pneumonia in dysphagic children: Significance of videofluoroscopic swallowing evaluation. *Developmental Medicine and Child Neurology, 36,* 495–502.

Teasdale, R., Foley, N., Fisher, J. & Finestone, H. (2002). The incidence, management, and complications of dysphagia in patients. *Dysphagia, 17,* 115–120.

Willig, T., Paulus, J., Lacau Saint Guilly, J., Beon, C. & Navarro, J. (1994). Swallowing problems in neuromuscular disorders. *Archives of Physical Medicine and Rehabilitation, 75,* 1175–1181.

# 5

# *Esophageal Phase Dysphagia*

## Peter C. Belafsky
## Catherine J. Rees

The esophageal phase of deglutition begins with passage of the food bolus through the most distal aspect of the pharyngoesophageal segment. Gravity and esophageal peristalsis are responsible for moving the bolus 25 cm along the esophageal body, through the lower esophageal sphincter, and into the proximal stomach. An esophageal etiology of dysphagia can be found in 60% of individuals presenting to a tertiary Swallowing Center. Up to 30% of individuals with an oropharyngeal swallowing disorder may have comorbid esophageal pathology. Patients are not always successful at localizing the site of their swallowing problem (Roeder, Murray, & Dierkhising, 2004). An individual pointing to the suprasternal notch may, in fact, have distal esophageal pathology responsible for their swallowing problem. A thorough knowledge of all causes of esophageal phase dysphagia is necessary to adequately care for individuals with swallowing complaints.

## ESOPHAGITIS

The most common cause of esophageal phase dysphagia is gastroesophageal reflux disease (GERD). Reflux has been estimated to affect over 59 million Americans. Up to 50% of individuals with GERD suffer from dysphagia. Dysphagia in persons with GERD appears to be more prevalent as the severity of esophagitis increases (Vakil, Traxler, & Levine, 2004) (Figure 5–1). The cause of dysphagia is probably secondary to edema and diminished esophageal body motility caused by the chronic inflammation. The swallowing difficulty will resolve in over 80% of individuals after 4 weeks of antireflux therapy with proton pump inhibitors. Persistent dysphagia indicates failed healing of the esophagitis (Wetscher et al., 1997). Dysphagia in persons with GERD may also be caused by the presence of a peptic stricture or a hiatal hernia (HH). An HH has been shown to cause dysphagia because of

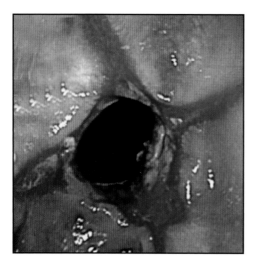

**Figure 5-1.** High-grade erosive esophagitis (Grade D) in a person presenting with solid-food dysphagia.

**Figure 5-2.** Hiatal hernia sac in a person with solid-food dysphagia. The dysphagia resolved after surgical reduction of the hernia.

impingement of the hernia sac by the diaphragm (Figure 5–2). Surgical repair of the HH can relieve dysphagia in over 90% of individuals (Kaul et al., 1990).

Gastroesophageal reflux is not the only cause of esophageal inflammation. Infection, pills and other foreign bodies, allergy, chemotherapy and radiation therapy, and caustic injury can all result in esophagitis, as well as dysphagia and stricture. Infection with *Candida albicans* is the most common cause of infectious esophagitis. Patients may present solely with the complaint of dysphagia or odynophagia and some may report symptoms such as throat clearing, globus, or excessive throat mucus. Fiberoptic laryngoscopy may display pharyngeal candidiasis but is often normal. A fluoroscopic swallow evaluation is usually unremarkable. Esophagoscopy with biopsy is necessary to confirm the diagnosis (Figure 5–3). Risk factors for esophageal candidiasis

**Figure 5-3.** Florid esophageal candidiasis in a person presenting with solid food dysphagia and globus.

include diabetes mellitus, corticosteroid use (inhaled, oral, and systemic), immunodeficiency, and a history of chemotherapy or radiation therapy. Other less common causes of infectious esophagitis include histoplasmosis, actinomycetes, cytomegalovirus, and herpes simplex virus.

Pills can produce esophageal phase dysphagia through their systemic effects or by directly causing caustic injury. Medications may systemically cause dysphagia by inducing reflux, by impairing esophageal motility and clearance, and by compromising the immune system and predisposing the individual to esophageal infection. Table 5–1 displays a list of medications that relax the lower esophageal sphincter (LES) and promote reflux. With prolonged esophageal mucosal contact, many pills can cause caustic esophageal injury and dysphagia. In a study of 98 consecutive upper gastrointestinal radiologic examinations, over 50% of barium tablets taken by individuals while supine remained in the esophagus for more than 5 minutes (Evans & Roberts, 1976). This is ample time for many medications to produce esophageal injury. Medications most likely to cause pill-induced esophagitis include slow-release potassium, the tetracyclines, nonsteroidal anti-inflammatory drugs (NSAIDS), and alendronate (Fosamax). To prevent pill-induced esophagitis, patients should be instructed to take pills with a relatively large quantity of water (120 cc), take pills upright, avoid a double swallow if possible, and avoid lying down for 30 minutes after consumption.

Eosinophilic esophagitis (EE) is an emerging cause of esophageal phase dysphagia in children and adults. Although the exact etiology of EE is unknown, the disorder is believed to be atopic in nature. Persons typically present with dysphagia and/or odynophagia that is unresponsive to antireflux medication. Forty percent may suffer from food impactions. Most individuals have a prior history of allergic rhinitis, eczema, or asthma. Endoscopy may reveal a corrugated, ringed, or "trachealized" esophagus. Esophageal strictures are common. The diagnosis is made by demonstrating more than 20 eosinophils per high-powered field on esophageal biopsy. The mucosa can often look normal so it is important to emphasize the need to biopsy an ordinary appearing esophagus in an individual with dysphagia and no other apparent cause. Treatment with topical and systemic corticosteroids, montelukast, proton pump inhibitors, histamine antagonists, and cromolyn sodium have all shown varying degrees of success. Esophageal dilation may occasionally be necessary but should be performed with caution, as the mucosa is often extremely friable with an increased risk of perforation and laceration.

**Table 5–1.** Medications that Relax the Lower Esophageal Sphincter and Promote Reflux

- Oral contraceptives
- Ethanol
- Tobacco
- Theophylline
- Alpha-antagonists
- Anticholinergic agents
- Dopamine
- Nitrates
- Meperidine
- Morphine
- Calcium channel blockers
- Diazepam

## ESOPHAGEAL WEBS AND RINGS

Esophageal webs and rings are another frequent cause of esophageal phase dysphagia. An esophageal B-ring or Schatzki's ring is the most common cause of solid-food dysphagia in adults (Figure 5–4). Schatzki's rings can be found in up to 14% of patients on fluoroscopic swallow evaluations (DeVault, 1996). They occur at the gastroesophageal junction and have squamous esophageal mucosa on the proximal margin and columnar gastric mucosa on the distal margin of the ring. They usually occur in the presence of a hiatal hernia and frequently become symptomatic when the diameter of the lumen is less than 13 mm. Esophageal dilation is the treatment of choice. In comparison to the B-ring, which is membranous and occurs at the gastroesophageal junction (GEJ), the esophageal A-ring is a thick muscular ring that is present 2 cm above the GEJ. It marks the upper border of the lower esophageal sphincter. Esophageal A-rings are an infrequent cause of dysphagia. Treatment with dilation is usually unsuccessful, and the treatment of choice is injection of botulinum toxin into the muscular ring.

Esophageal webs are mucosal constrictions that occur above the gastroesophageal junction. Unlike a Schatzki's ring, they have squamous mucosa on both sides. An esophageal web usually occurs in the proximal esophagus. A web in the postcricoid region may be associated with Plummer-Vinson syndrome. Dilation is curative. Other less frequent causes of esophageal dysphagia include vascular rings, diverticula, and large esophageal varices.

## ESOPHAGEAL MOTILITY DISORDERS

Occasionally esophageal endoscopy and fluoroscopy fail to reveal an etiology of the solid food dysphagia. In these cases esophageal body and LES manometry is essential in identifying the causative disorder. Manometric causes of dysphagia include ineffective esophageal motility (IEM), a hypertensive LES, diffuse esophageal spasm (DES), nutcracker esophagus, and achalasia.

Ineffective esophageal motility is defined as low amplitude (<30 mm Hg) but peristaltic esophageal contractions in more than 30% of swallows tested on manometry. IEM is the most common esophageal motor abnormality in persons with GERD. Although many clinicians suspect that reflux causes IEM,

**Figure 5–4.** Schatzki's B-ring (*black arrows*) in an individual with solid food dysphagia. Also present are low-grade esophagitis and a small hiatal hernia. Treatment with proton pump inhibitors resolved the dysphagia and healed the esophagitis. Dilation and surgical correction of the hernia was not necessary.

the precise cause and effect relationship has not been defined. A diagnosis of IEM does not guarantee ineffective passage of barium on fluoroscopic swallow study. Forty-five percent of persons with manometric IEM will have normal transit of barium through the esophagus (Shakespear, Blom, Huprick, & Peters, 2004).

A hypertensive LES (HTLES) is defined as a LES resting pressure of more than 45 mm Hg. Symptoms associated with a HTLES include dysphagia, regurgitation, heartburn, and chest pain (Gockel, Lord, Bremner, Crookes, & Hamrah, et al., 2003). Unlike achalasia, which is associated with absent esophageal body motility and incomplete LES relaxation, a HTLES is associated with ineffective or normal esophageal body peristalsis and complete LES relaxation. Manometric parameters suggest the hypertensive sphincter is causing outlet obstruction. An association with GERD has been reported. Treatment options include sildenafil (which has been shown to relax the LES), botulinum toxin, dilation, and surgical myotomy.

Nutcracker esophagus is defined as high amplitude (>180 mm Hg) peristaltic esophageal contractions. Presenting symptoms include dysphagia and atypical chest pain (Csendes, Carcamo, & Henriquez, 2004). An association with GERD has been reported although causality remains uncertain. Antireflux medication is utilized to treat comorbid GERD, although it has not been shown to have a significant effect on pain relief (Borjesson, Rolny, Mannheimer, & Pilhall, 2003). Sildenafil has been shown to decrease the amplitude of peristaltic contractions in persons with nutcracker esophagus and may be con-

sidered a treatment option (Lee, Park, Kim, Lee, & Conklin, 2003).

In comparison to nutcracker esophagus, which displays high amplitude peristaltic contractions, distal esophageal spasm (DES) is characterized by high amplitude nonperistaltic or simultaneous contractions. Presenting symptoms include dysphagia and atypical chest pain. The pain is often worse with the consumption of food at extremes of temperature. The pain may be indistinguishable from that of a heart attack. The simultaneous hyperkinetic esophageal contractions can give the appearance of a "corkscrew esophagus" on barium esophagram (Figure 5–5). The diagnosis is made by a combination of manometry and radiography. Treatment options include botulinum toxin, smooth muscle relaxants such as sildenafil, nitrates, and calcium channel blockers, and surgical myotomy. Variable success with pain control has been reported with tricyclic antidepressants, selective serotonin reuptake inhibitors,

**Figure 5–5.** Barium esophagram displaying a corkscrew esophagus in an individual with distal esophageal spasm.

and trazodone. Comorbid GERD is treated with antireflux medication. DES may progress to achalasia in some individuals.

Achalasia is a disorder of unknown etiology characterized by the absence of esophageal peristalsis and by failure of lower esophageal sphincter relaxation. Patients present with a history of slowly progressive dysphagia. Regurgitation and weight loss are also frequent. Diagnosis is made by barium esophagram and esophageal manometry. The esophagram shows a dilated tortuous esophagus with a "bird's beak" appearance at the LES (Figure 5–6). Manometry shows an absence of esophageal peristalsis and failure of LES relaxation. Endoscopy is performed to exclude cancer that can produce a similar appearance on fluoroscopy (pseudoachalasia). Treatment options include endoscopic injection of botulinum toxin to relax the LES, dilation, and surgical myotomy.

**Figure 5–6.** Barium esophagram displaying a dilated, tortuous esophagus with a "bird's beak" appearance at the lower esophageal sphincter (*at arrow*) in an individual with achalasia.

## Systemic Causes of Esophageal Phase Dysphagia

There are various connective tissue diseases that can affect the esophagus. Systemic sclerosis (scleroderma), polymyositis, dermatomyositis, and systemic lupus erythematosus can all affect esophageal motility to varying degrees. Scleroderma affects the smooth muscle portion of the esophagus while sparing the proximal skeletal portion. The LES is often affected and may become hypotensive and incompetent. Severe GERD is frequent. In contrast to scleroderma, the inflammatory myopathies affect the proximal skeletal muscle portion of the esophagus. The cricopharyngeus and pharyngeal musculature may be involved. The distal esophagus and LES are spared. For this reason, associated GERD is less common than with scleroderma.

Patients with Sjögren's syndrome often complain of dysphagia. Although esophageal peristalsis may be affected, patients often develop severe swallowing problems as a result of xerostomia. Breads and other dry foods can be extremely difficult to consume. Salivary bicarbonate is very important in neutralizing even physiologic amounts of reflux. All persons with Sjögren's syndrome lack this important buffering capacity and are prone to develop severe GERD.

Other systemic diseases affecting the esophagus include diabetes mellitus, Parkinson's disease, and hypothyroidism. The autonomic dysfunction associated with diabetes can result in esophageal dysmotility with delayed esophageal emptying and in gastroparesis with delayed gastric emptying. Parkinson's disease can result in oropharyngeal and esophageal phase swallowing problems. Hypothyroidism can produce esophageal dysmotility and LES dysfunction that should normalize with appropriate thyroid replacement therapy (Eastwood, Braverman, White, & Vander, 1982).

## ESOPHAGEAL NEOPLASMS

The majority of esophageal tumors are malignant. Squamous cell carcinoma used to be the most common esophageal cancer. Adenocarcinoma, however, has now overrun squamous cell cancer as the most frequent esophageal malignancy. In fact, adenocarcinoma of the esophagus is the most rapidly expanding cancer in the United States. Early diagnosis by endoscopy and biopsy is critical. Benign esophageal tumors include leiomyomas, papillomas, cysts, fibrovascular polyps, lipomas, hemangiomas, and granular cell tumors. The most common presenting symptom for all esophageal tumors is dysphagia. Patient localization for the site of dysphagia is often inaccurate. We advocate esophagoscopy for all persons with solid food dysphagia to rule out esophageal neoplasia and its premalignant precursors.

## CONCLUSION

The causes of esophageal phase dysphagia are diverse, and a detailed understanding of esophageal pathology is necessary to properly evaluate and manage patients presenting with dysphagia. Even patients complaining of suprasternal dysphagia symptoms may have esophageal pathology. Esopha-geal manometry and fluoroscopic studies can be useful in detecting anatomic and motility abnormalities. A low threshold for esophageal endoscopy should be maintained so that neoplasms or potentially treatable infectious causes are not missed. Endoscopy is mandatory in any patient with solid food dysphagia to rule out esophageal carcinoma.

## STUDY QUESTIONS

1. What is the most common cause of esophagitis?
2. Match each of the following esophageal motility disorders with the description that best fits:

   1. Achalasia    a. high amplitude, nonperistaltic esophageal contractions

   2. IEM    b. lower esophageal sphincter (LES) hypertension, absence of esophageal peristalsis

   3. DES    c. high-amplitude esophageal contractions, peristaltic

   4. Nutcracker    d. low-amplitude esophageal contractions, peristaltic

3. Does scleroderma affect the proximal esophagus?
4. What is one medication that is a common cause of pill-induced esophagitis?

## REFERENCES

Borjesson, M., Rolney, P., Mannheimer, C., & Pilhall, M. (2003). Nutcracker esophagus: A double-blind, placebo-controlled, cross-over study of the effects of lansoprazole. *Alimentary Pharmacology Therapy, 18*, 1129–1135.

Csendes A., Carcamo, C., & Henriquez, A. (2004). Nutcracker esophagus: Analysis of 80 patients. *Revista Medica de Chile, 132*, 160–164.

DeVault K. R. (1996). Lower esophageal (Schatzki's) ring: Pathogenesis, diagnosis and therapy. *Digestive Diseases, 14*, 323–329.

Eastwood, G. L., Braverman, L. E., White, E. M., & Vander Salm, T. J. (1982). Reversal of lower esophageal sphincter hypotension and esophageal aperistalsis after treatment for hypothyroidism. *Journal of Clinical Gastroenterology, 4*, 307–310.

Evans, K. T., & Roberts, G. M. (1976). Where do all the tablets go? *Lancet, 2*, 1237.

Gockel, I., Lord, R. V., Bremner, C. G., Crookes, P. F., Hamrah, P., & DeMeester, T. R. (2003). The hypertensive lower esophageal sphincter: A motility disorder with manometric features of outflow obstruction. *Journal of Gastrointestinal Surgery, 7*, 692–700.

Kaul, B. K., DeMeester, T. R., Oka, M., Ball, C. S., Stein, H. J., Kim, C. B., et al. (1990). The cause of dysphagia in uncomplicated sliding hiatal hernia and its relief by hiatal herniorrhaphy, A roentgenographic, manometric, and clinical study. *Annals of Surgery, 211*, 406–410.

Lee, J. I., Park, H., Kim, J. H., Lee, S. I., & Conklin, J. L. (2003). The effect of sildenafil on oesophageal motor function in healthy subjects and patients with nutcracker oesophagus. *Neurogastroenterology and Motility, 15*, 617–623.

Roeder, B. E., Murray, J. A., & Dierkhising, R. A. (2004). Patient localization of esophageal dysphagia, *Digestive Diseases and Sciences, 49*, 697–701.

Shakespear, J. S., Blom, D., Huprich, J. E., & Peters, J. H. (2004). Correlation of radiographic and manometric findings in patients with ineffective esophageal motility. *Surgical Endoscopy, 18*, 459–462.

Vakil, N. B., Traxler, B., & Levine, D. (2004). Dysphagia in patients with erosive esophagitis: Prevalence, severity, and response to proton pump inhibitor treatment. *Clinical Gastroenterology and Hepatology, 2*, 665–668.

Wetscher, G. J., Glaser, K., Wieschemeyer, T., Gadenstaetter, M., Prommegger, R., & Profanter, C. (1997). Tailored antireflux surgery for gastroesophageal reflux disease: Effectiveness and risk of postoperative dysphagia. *World Journal of Surgery, 21*, 605–610.

# 6

# *Laryngopharyngeal Reflux*

## Catherine J. Rees
## Peter C. Belafsky

## DEFINITION AND NOMENCLATURE OF LARYNGOPHARYNGEAL REFLUX (LPR)

*Laryngopharyngeal reflux (LPR)* is the backflow of stomach contents into the laryngopharynx (Koufman, Aviv, Casiano, & Shaw, 2002). LPR has been implicated in the pathophysiology of numerous disorders of the upper aerodigestive tract, including dysphonia, laryngeal granulomas, and subglottic stenosis. Although laryngopharyngeal reflux is currently the term endorsed by the American Academy of Otolaryngology Head and Neck Surgery, multiple synonyms are used, including reflux laryngitis, posterior laryngitis, laryngeal reflux, gastroesophagopharyngeal reflux, esophagopharyngeal reflux, pharyngoesophageal reflux, gastroesophageal-laryngeal reflux, atypical reflux, silent reflux, and supraesophageal reflux. Perhaps the most common synonym for LPR is *extra-esophageal reflux* (Belafsky, 2003; Koufman, Belafsky, Bach, Daniel, & Postma, 2002).

The idea that acidic gastric contents can affect structures above the upper esophageal sphincter was put forth in 1968 (Cherry & Marguilies, 1968; Delahunty & Cherry, 1968; Koufman, 2002a). At this time, LPR was postulated to relate to contact ulcers and granulomas, and the mechanism was felt to be vagally mediated from acidic contents contacting the lower esophagus. Although this theory has not entirely lost favor, actual drops in the pH of the pharynx in patients with LPR symptoms were demonstrated in 1987 and 1989 (Wiener, Koufman, & Wu, 1987; Wiener, Koufman, Wu, Cooper, & Richter, et al., 1989). These findings suggested that the physical presence of gastric contents in the laryngopharynx was to blame in the disease process. It is likely that both theories of causality play a role in LPR disease.

## EPIDEMIOLOGY OF REFLUX

The incidence of laryngopharyngeal reflux is not clearly understood, but it has been estimated that up to 4% to 10% of patients with otolaryngologic complaints have underlying LPR (Toohill, Mushtag, & Lehman, 1990). In a community cohort of 100 patients without any history of voice or laryngeal complaints, 35% had symptoms of LPR and 64% demonstrated one or more physical finding of LPR on laryngoscopic examination (Reulbach, Belafsky, Blalock, Koufman, & Postma, 2001). This study suggested that physical findings and symptoms of LPR frequently are found in the general population and that some degree of LPR may be normal. In a prospective cohort of 113 new patients with laryngeal and voice disorders, 50% were found to have abnormal results on 24-hour dual pH probe testing (Koufman, Amin, & Panetti, 2000, 2001). LPR was highest in patients presenting with laryngeal neoplasia (88%) and muscle tension dysphonia (70%).

Reflux to a certain degree is ubiquitous in adults, and clinical disease only occurs in the presence of excessive reflux and/or a breakdown of mucosal defenses. In the lower esophagus, up to 50 reflux episodes at or below pH 4 in a 24-hour period is considered normal (Demeester, Johnson, Joseph, Toscano, & Hall, et al., 1976). In the pharynx, the normal or physiologic limit of reflux is not as clear. Generally, up to two episodes of reflux with pH less than 4 may be seen in healthy controls without LPR disease (Merati, Lim, Ulualp, & Toohill, 2005; Vincent, Garrett, Radionoff, Reussner, & Stasney, 2000; Ylitalo, Lindestad, & Ramel, 2001; Ylitalo & Ramel, 2002a, 2002b). However, animal studies have suggested that as few as three pharyngeal reflux episodes per week are sufficient to produce laryngeal damage in the face of a pre-existing mucosal injury (Koufman, 1991).

## DIFFERENCE BETWEEN LPR AND GERD

Laryngopharyngeal reflux must be distinguished from classic gastroesophageal reflux disease (GERD). The primary characteristics of GERD include heartburn and esophagitis. The majority of patients with LPR deny heartburn (70%), (Koufman, Aviv, et al., 2002) and the incidence of esophagitis only is about 25% in the LPR population (Koufman, 1991; Koufman et al., 2002; Koufman, Sataloff, & Toohill, 1996; Koufman, Belafsky, et al., 2002; Wiener et al., 1989). GERD patients tend to have primarily nighttime supine reflux, whereas LPR patients tend to have daytime upright reflux. Episodes of pathologic esophageal reflux may be prolonged, but LPR episodes are typically brief. Patients with GERD are more frequently obese, whereas body mass index is not related to LPR prevalence (Halum, Postma, Johnston, Belafsky, & Koufman, 2005). GERD is thought to be a result of lower esophageal sphincter dysfunction and/or esophageal dysmotility, but this does not appear to be true for LPR. Esophageal acid clearance is better in LPR patients than in classic GERD patients, (Postma, Tomek, Belafsky, & Koufman, 2001a) and LPR may be related to dysfunction of the upper esophageal sphincter (Celik, Alkan, & Ercan, 2005; Gerhardt, Shuck, Bordeaux, & Winship, 1978; Helm, Dodds, Riedel, Teeter, Hogan, & Arndorfer, 1983; Koufman, Belafsky, et al., 2002; Koufman, 2002a; Orsmeth & Wong, 1999; Ulualp, Toohill, Kern, & Shaker, 1998).

In the healthy adult, the esophagus is well-equipped to handle intermittent exposure to acidic gastric contents (Koufman, 1991). Lower esophageal sphincter competence is physically supported by: the muscular diaphragm; the acute angle of entry of the esophagus into the stomach (i.e., the cardiac angle); and the high abdominal pressure imposed on the intra-abdominal segment of the esophagus. LES pressure is also regulated by hormonal mechanisms and in response to alkalinization of gastric contents.

Primary peristalsis clears the majority of a distal esophageal bolus, and secondary peristalsis as a result of repeat swallows every 30 to 60 seconds allows for improved clearance as well as buffering by saliva. Salivary bicarbonate bathing the esophagus helps to neutralize refluxate within the esophageal lumen. Increased acid in the distal esophagus stimulates an increase in salivary production in the normal individual (Koufman, 1991).

The esophageal lining displays innate tissue resistance to physiologic reflux events. Mucus lining the esophageal lumen prevents the penetration of large molecules such as pepsin. The "unstirred water layer" below is rich in bicarbonate and buffers the environment adjacent to the esophageal mucosal cells. Furthermore, the esophageal epithelium itself is capable of blocking both acid and pepsin with cell membranes and intracellular bridges. Local blood flow is increased in the

event of esophageal injury to facilitate recovery (Orlando, 1986).

In stark contrast, the larynx is poorly protected from injury by gastric refluxate, specifically acid and pepsin (Axford, Sharp, Ross, Pearson, & Dettmar, 2001; Johnston et al., 2003; Koufman, 1991). The upper airways are exquisitely sensitive to acid and especially to activated pepsin. Pepsin has been shown to be active above pH 4, suggesting that a smaller drop in pH is required to cause laryngeal injury than esophageal injury (Johnston, Knight, Dettmar, Lively, & Koufman, 2004). As noted above, very few episodes of pharyngeal reflux (three per week) can damage the larynx in the setting of a mucosal injury (Koufman, 1991; Little, Koufman, Kohut, & Marshall, 1985). The larynx is not protected by salivary bicarbonate, endogenous tissue buffering, or peristalsis. The larynx has poor intrinsic tissue defenses as well. Carbonic anhydrase isoenzyme III (CA III) is an enzyme with buffering capacity that is increased in the esophagus in response to acid. However, CA III is actually reduced in laryngeal tissue damaged by acid and pepsin, further decreasing laryngeal protection (Axford et al., 2001; Johnston et al., 2003, 2004).

## DIAGNOSIS OF LPR

### Patient Symptoms

The diagnosis of LPR is primarily based on a constellation of clinical signs and physical findings. In a 2002 survey sent to 415 members of the American Broncho-Esophagological Association, the responders were in agreement about certain symptoms of LPR (Book, Rhee, Toohill, & Smith,

2002). These include throat clearing (98%), chronic cough (97%), globus (95%), dysphonia (95%), and postnasal drip (57%). The Reflux Symptom Index (RSI) has been shown to be a reliable and valid patient-administered questionnaire for identifying patient symptoms (Table 6–1) (Belafsky, Postma, & Koufman, 2002b). One group, however, has reported sensitivity and specificity for the RSI of 80.7% and 37.5%, respectively, in patients with hypopharyngeal reflux documented by pH studies (Park, Choi, Kwon, Yoon, & Kim, 2006).

The most common complaint of LPR patients appears to be dysphonia, followed by chronic throat clearing, cough, globus sensation, and dysphagia (Koufman, 1991; Woo, Noordzij, & Ross, 1996). Most LPR patients do not complain of heartburn. LPR has been implicated in the etiology of a multitude of otolaryngologic disorders, including subglottic stenosis, chronic sinusitis, chronic otitis media, laryngeal granulomas, paroxysmal laryngospasm, Reinke's edema, Zenker's diverticulum, and laryngeal carcinoma (Maronian, Azadeh, Waugh, & Hillel, 2001; Cohen, Bach, Postma, & Koufman, 2002; DelGaudio, 2005; Koufman, 1991; Lewin et al., 2003; Sasaki, Ross, & Hundal, 2003;).

## Physical Findings

Laryngeal examination with a flexible or rigid laryngoscope is essential to the diagnosis of LPR. Findings associ-

**Table 6-1.** Reflux Symptom Index (maximum score 45)

| Within the past month, how did the following problems affect you? | 0 = No problem 5 = Severe problem | | | | | |
|---|---|---|---|---|---|---|
| Hoarseness or a problem with your voice | 0 | 1 | 2 | 3 | 4 | 5 |
| Clearing your throat | 0 | 1 | 2 | 3 | 4 | 5 |
| Excess throat mucus or postnasal drip | 0 | 1 | 2 | 3 | 4 | 5 |
| Difficulty swallowing food, liquids, or pills | 0 | 1 | 2 | 3 | 4 | 5 |
| Coughing after you ate or after lying down | 0 | 1 | 2 | 3 | 4 | 5 |
| Breathing difficulties or choking episodes | 0 | 1 | 2 | 3 | 4 | 5 |
| Troublesome or annoying cough | 0 | 1 | 2 | 3 | 4 | 5 |
| Sensations of something sticking in your throat or a lump in your throat | 0 | 1 | 2 | 3 | 4 | 5 |
| Heartburn, chest pain, indigestion, or stomach acid coming up | 0 | 1 | 2 | 3 | 4 | 5 |
| | Total | | | | | |

*Source:* From Belafsky, P. C., Postma, G. N., & Koufman, J. A. (2002). Validity and reliability of the reflux symptom index (RSI). *Journal of Voice, 16,* 274–277. Reproduced with permission.

ated with LPR include erythema, laryngeal and vocal fold edema, subglottic edema/pseudosulcus vocalis, ventricular obliteration, posterior commissure hypertrophy, laryngeal granulomas, lymphoid hypertrophy, and excessive pharyngeal mucus. Endoscopic findings can be succinctly described with the Reflux Findings Score (RFS) (Table 6–2),

which is an indicator of overall laryngeal inflammation.

It is important to recognize that the diagnosis is based on a constellation of findings rather than any one finding. For example isolated posterior commissure hypertrophy does not correlate well with LPR, but it is felt to be an important sign of LPR when associated

**Table 6-2.** Reflux Findings Score (maximum score 26)

| | |
|---|---|
| Pseudosulcus (infraglottic edema) | 0 = Absent<br>2 = Present |
| Ventricular obliteration | 0 = None<br>2 = Partial<br>4 = Complete |
| Erythema/hyperemia | 0 = None<br>2 = Arytenoids only<br>4 = Diffuse |
| Vocal fold edema | 0 = None<br>1 = Mild<br>2 = Moderate<br>3 = Severe<br>4 = Polypoid |
| Diffuse laryngeal edema | 0 = None<br>1 = Mild<br>2 = Moderate<br>3 = Severe<br>4 = Obstructing |
| Posterior commissure hypertrophy | 0 = None<br>1 = Mild<br>2 = Moderate<br>3 = Severe<br>4 = Obstructing |
| Granuloma/granulation | 0 = Absent<br>2 = Present |
| Thick endolaryngeal mucus | 0 = Absent<br>2 = Present |
| | **Total** |

*Source:* From Belafsky, P. C., Postma, G. N., & Koufman, J. A. (2001). Validity and reliability of the reflux findings score (RFS). *Laryngoscope, 111,* 1313–1317. Reproduced with permission.

with other laryngeal findings listed in the RFS. Laryngeal erythema has been described in LPR (Hanson, Jiang, & Chi, 1998), but this may be highly variable depending on the examiner's video equipment. Diffuse laryngeal erythema is thought to be a stronger indicator of LPR than erythema localized to the arytenoids (Belafsky, 2003).

Endoscopic findings isolated to the true vocal folds can range from mild edema to Reinke's edema, also known as polypoid degeneration or polypoid corditis (Figure 6–1) (Belafsky, 2003). Obliteration of the laryngeal ventricle is the result of edema of the true and false vocal folds (Figure 6–2). This may be one of the first signs to improve after the initiation of antireflux therapy. Posterior commissure hypertrophy, or posterior laryngeal edema, is graded from mild, producing a mustachelike appearance of the posterior larynx, to severe, producing an actual obstruction of the posterior airway by the edematous mucosa (Figure 6–3). Patients with LPR and posterior laryngeal edema appear to have a higher incidence of laryngeal sensory deficits on functional endoscopic evaluation of swallowing with sensory testing (FEEST), which improves with LPR treatment (Aviv, Liu, Parides, Kaplan, & Close, 2000). Pseudosulcus vocalis is also known as infraglottic edema (Figure 6–4) (Koufman, 1995). This finding represents edema of the ventral surface of the vocal folds and extends along the entire length of the true vocal fold. This detail differentiates pseudosulcus vocalis from sulcus vergeture, which stops at the vocal process rather than extending to the posterior larynx. The presence of pseudosulcus is at least 70% sensitive and 77% specific for LPR (Belafsky, Postma, & Koufman, 2002a; Hickson, Simpson, & Falcon, 2001).

**Figure 6-1.** Reinke's edema.

**Figure 6-2.** Ventricular obliteration and Reinke's edema.

**Figure 6-3.** Posterior commissure hypertrophy.

**Figure 6–4.** Pseudosulcus vocalis.

**Figure 6–5.** Vocal fold granuloma.

Vocal fold granulomas are typically seen on the vocal process and have a high recurrence rate (Figure 6–5). LPR has recently been identified as an etiologic factor in the development of granulomas. Lymphoid hyperplasia, especially seen as hypertrophy of the lingual tonsils (Mamede, De Mello-Filho, Vigario, & Dantas, 2000) and cobblestoning of the posterior pharyngeal wall, can also be related to LPR, although these findings are nonspecific. Finally LPR may be associated with the sensation of increased mucus in the throat, which can often be confused with postnasal drip (Belafsky, 2003).

## pH Monitoring

Twenty-four hour dual-probe pH testing is currently the gold standard for diagnosis of LPR. The upper pH probe should be in the hypopharynx above the upper esophageal sphincter, not in the proximal esophagus. The lower probe is ideally 5 cm above the lower esophageal sphincter, which is the standard position used by gastroenterologists. The hypopharyngeal probe should be no more than 2 cm above the upper esophageal sphincter (UES) to prevent drying of the probe and false-positive readings. Esophageal manometry is very helpful in determining proper probe placement, and a variety of pH catheter lengths should be available. Placement of the upper probe under endoscopic visualization does not allow confirmation of the lower probe position (Harrell et al., 2005; Postma, Belafsky, Aviv, & Koufman, 2002).

Although up to 50 episodes of reflux in the distal esophagus are normal, when these reflux events reach the pharynx, the diagnosis of LPR may be made. In a recent meta-analysis of 24-hour dual-probe pH monitoring, the technique was found to be consistent between multiple studies. Up to 20% of normal subjects had brief reflux events at the upper probe when the probe was in the hypopharynx, and this number increased when the probe was at the UES (Merati et al., 2005).

The exact cutoff for number of reflux events in the pharynx is controversial (Richardson, Heywood, Sims, Stoner, & Leopold, 2004). It is clear that in the setting mucosal airway injury, even one episode of LPR is enough to exacerbate the injury (Little et al., 1985). However, in an asymptomatic individual without voice or airway concerns, one or two episodes of LPR may be physiologic rather than clinically significant. The results of 24-hour pH monitoring should be reviewed on an individual patient basis. Intake of meals and beverages will give false readings and must be considered in interpretation of pH studies. Finally, both number of LPR events and acid exposure time should be considered. Although pH 4 or less is the accepted cutoff for reflux events in the esophagus, it has been suggested that pH 5 or less may be clinically important in the laryngopharynx, given the persistent activation of pepsin at this pH (Postma, 2000).

## Other Diagnostic Studies

Cinefluoroscopy is used as an adjunct by some clinicians to diagnose LPR. Esophageal reflux can often be seen with this study, but LPR may be missed. Impedance testing is a relatively new tool in the diagnosis of LPR, and its utility is not yet clear. Impedance testing is performed with an intraluminal catheter much like pH testing. However, the impedance monitor measures all refluxate, regardless of acidity. The importance of nonacid reflux in LPR is an area of current research. As the role of pepsin in LPR is further elucidated, demonstration of pepsin in laryngeal tissues may prove to be a reli-able way to diagnose LPR in the future (Johnston et al., 2004).

Many clinicians also believe that an evaluation of the esophagus, either by the otolaryngologist or the gastroenterologist, is critical in any patient diagnosed with LPR. This recommendation is based on findings of esophageal pathology, in particular Barrett's esophagus, in a significant proportion of patients with LPR (Postma et al., 2005). LPR symptoms may be more predictive of esophageal adenocarcinoma than typical GERD symptoms (Reavis, Morris, Gopal, Hunter, & Jobe, 2004). Esophageal adenocarcinoma is a devastating disease with an often-delayed diagnosis, and evaluation of the esophagus when LPR is present may result in earlier diagnosis in some patients.

## TREATMENT OF LPR

Patients with suspected LPR should be counseled about the standard lifestyle changes recommended for GERD patients (Table 6–3). Perhaps the most important of these recommendations are smoking cessation and alcohol avoidance. Chewing gum has been shown to increase both pharyngeal and esophageal pH because of an increase in salivary bicarbonate, salivary flow, and swallowing frequency. Bicarbonate gum is an even more effective adjunctive antireflux therapy (Smoak & Koufman, 2001). Over-the-counter antacids and liquid alginate certainly have a role in mild GERD, but their effectiveness in treating LPR is not clear. Liquid alginate, especially thoe formulation available in Europe, forms a physical barrier to help prevent reflux (Mandel, Daggy, Brodie, & Jacoby, 2000).

**Table 6–3.** Recommended Lifestyle Modifications in LPR.

| |
|---|
| Elevate head of bed 6 inches |
| Smoking cessation |
| Low-fat diet |
| Weight loss |
| Avoid lying down within 3 hours of eating |
| Eat small frequent meals |
| Avoid refluxogenic foods: |
|   Alcohol |
|   Chocolate |
|   Peppermint |
|   High-fat foods |
|   Tomato-based products |
|   Spicy foods |
|   Citrus |

Most patients with symptomatic LPR require pharmacologic treatment with H2-receptor antagonists and/or proton-pump inhibitors. According to the position statement on LPR by the American Academy of Otolaryngology-Head and Neck Surgery, LPR treatment should be more aggressive and of longer duration than GERD treatment. Mild symptoms may be appropriately treated with lifestyle modifications and H2-receptor antagonists.

Most LPR patients require twice-daily proton-pump inhibitor (PPI) therapy, although this therapy has not been well supported in placebo-controlled trials (Koufman, Aviv, et al., 2002; Noordzij et al., 2001; Park et al., 2005; Postma & Johnson, 2002; Steward et al., 2004;). Twice-daily dosing is important because none of the PPIs suppress gastric acid for more than 16 hours (Pegh-ini, Katz, Bracy, & Castell, 1998). Some investigators suggest using high dose H2-receptor antagonists at night in addition to twice daily PPI therapy, but the efficacy of this approach is controversial (Pan, Wang, & Guo, 2004; Tutuian & Castel, 2004). More than 2 months therapy may be necessary for LPR symptom improvement, and more than 6 months therapy may be required to see resolution of laryngeal findings (Belafsky, Postma, & Koufman, 2001a). Patients should be carefully counseled about the need for prolonged therapy and the proper timing of medication doses. PPIs should be taken 30 to 45 minutes before a meal for maximum efficacy. Resistance to PPI therapy should be considered in patients without improvement after 6 months therapy, and this can be documented by repeat pH testing while on medication (Amin, Postma, Johnson, Digges, & Koufman, 2001).

In refractory LPR, especially in life-threatening cases such as subglottic stenosis, surgical therapy may be considered as an alternative to PPIs. There are limited data supporting endoscopic antireflux procedures in LPR at this point. LPR symptoms often improve after Nissen fundoplication or hiatal hernia repair (Lindstrom, Wallace, Loehrl, Merati, & Toohill, et al., 2002; Westcott, Hopkins, Bach, Postman, & Belafsky, et al., 2004; Wright & Rhodes, 2003).

## CONCLUSION

Laryngopharyngeal reflux should be considered as a contributing factor in most disorders of the upper aerodigestive tract. LPR is different from classic gastroesophageal reflux disease in that most patients do not experience heart-burn or have findings or esophagitis. A constellation of patient symptoms and physical findings are important in diagnosing LPR. Twenty-four-hour dual-probe pH monitoring with the upper probe in the hypopharynx is the gold standard for LPR diagnosis. Twice-daily proton pump inhibitor therapy for at least 6 months is the mainstay of LPR therapy.

## STUDY QUESTIONS

1. Which is most damaging to tissues: pepsin, acid, or both combined?
2. Describe the mechanism of reflux.
3. What is the most typical sign of laryngopharyngeal reflux (LPR)?
4. What is more important in the diagnosis of reflux, a single sign, or a constellation of signs? What would constitute a constellation of signs?
5. Is any reflux in the esophagus considered normal?
6. In the treatment of reflux, which typically improve first, signs or symptoms?

## REFERENCES

Amin, M. R., Postma, G. N., Johnson, P., Digges, N., & Koufman, J. A. (2001). Proton pump inhibitor resistance in the treatment of laryngopharyngeal reflux, *Otolaryngology Head and Neck Surgery*, *125*, 374–378.

Aviv, J. E., Liu, H., Parides, M., Kaplan S. T., & Close, J. G., (2000). Laryngopharyngeal sensory deficits in patients with laryngopharyngeal reflux and dysphagia. *Annals of Otology, Rhinology and Laryngology, 1099*, 1000–1006.

Axford, S. E., Sharp, N., Ross, P. E., Pearson, J. P., Dettmar, P. W., Panetti, M., et al. (2001a). Cell biology of laryngeal epithelial defenses in health and disease: Preliminary studies. *Annals of Otology Rhinology and Laryngology, 110*, 1099–1108.

Belafsky, P. C. (2003). Abnormal endoscopic pharyngeal and laryngeal findings attributable to reflux. *American Journal of Medicine, 115*, 90S–96S.

Belafsky, P. C., Postma, G. N., & Koufman, J. A. (2001a). Laryngopharyngeal reflux symptoms improve before changes in physical findings. *Laryngoscope, 111*, 979–981.

Belafsky, P. C., Postma, G. N., & Koufman, J. A. (2001b). Validity and reliability of the reflux findings score (RFS). *Laryngoscope, 111*, 1313–1317.

Belafsky, P. C., Postma, G. N., & Koufman, J. A. (2002a). The association between laryngeal pseudosulcus and laryngopharyngeal reflux, *Otolaryngology Head and Neck Surgery, 126*, 649–652.

Belafsky, P. C., Postma, G. N., & Koufman, J. A. (2002b). Validity and reliability of the reflux symptom index (RSI). *Journal of Voice, 16*, 274–277.

Book, D. T., Rhee, J. S., Toohill, R. J., & Smith T. L. (2002). Perspectives in laryngopharyngeal reflux: An international survey. *Laryngoscope, 112*, 1399–1406.

Celik, M., Alkan, Z. S., & Ercan, I. (2005). Cricopharyngeal muscle electromyography in laryngopharyngeal reflux, *Laryngoscope, 115*, 138–142.

Cherry, J., & Margulies, S. I. (1968). Contact ulcer of the larynx. *Laryngoscope, 78*, 1937–1940.

Cohen, J. T., Bach, K. K., Postma, G. N., & Koufman, J. A.(2002). Clinical manifestations of laryngopharyngeal reflux, *Ear Nose and Throat Journal, 81*(Suppl. 2), 19–23.

Delahunty, J. E., & Cherry, J. (1968). Experimentally produced vocal cord granulomas. *Laryngoscope, 78*, 1941–1947.

DelGaudio, J. M., (2005). Direct nasopharyngeal reflux of gastric acid is a contributing factor in refractory chronic sinusitis. *Laryngoscope, 115*, 946–956.

Demeester, T. R., Johnson, L. F., Joseph, G. J., Toscano, M. S., Hall, A. W., & Skinner, D. B. (1976). Patterns of gastroesophageal reflux in health and disease. *Annals of Surgery, 184*, 459–470.

Gerhardt, D. C., Shuck, T. J., Bordeaux, R. A., & Winship, D. H. (1978). Human upper esophageal sphincter. Response to volume, osmotic, and acid stimuli. *Gastroenterlogy, 75*, 268–274.

Halum, S. L., Postma, G. N., Johnston, C., Belafsky, P. C., & Koufman, J. A. (2005). Patients with isolated laryngopharyngeal reflux are not obese. *Laryngoscope, 115*, 1042–1045.

Hanson, D. G., Jiang, J., & Chi, W. (1998). Quantitative color analysis of laryngeal erythema in chronic posterior laryngitis. *Journal of Voice, 12*, 78–83.

Harrell, S., Evans, B., Goudy, S., Winstead, W., Lentsch, E., Koopman, J., et al. (2005). Design and implementation of an ambulatory pH monitoring protocol in patients with suspected laryngopharyngeal reflux. *Laryngoscope, 115*, 89–92.

Helm, J. F., Dodds, W. J., Riedel, D. R., Teeter, B. C., Hogan, W. J., & Arndorfer, R. C. (1983). Determinants of esophageal acid clearance in normal subjects. *Gastroenterology, 85*, 607–612.

Hickson, C., Simpson, C. B., & Falcon, R. (2001). Laryngeal pseudosulcus as a predictor of laryngopharyngeal reflux. *Laryngoscope, 111*, 1742–1745.

Hill, R. K., Simpson, C. B., Velazquez, R., & Larson, M. (2004). Pachydermia is not diagnostic of active laryngopharyngeal reflux disease. *Laryngoscope, 114*, 1557–1561.

Johnston, N., Bulmer, D., Gill, G., Panetti, M., Ross, P. E., Pearson, J. P., et al. (2003). Cell biology of laryngeal epithelial defenses in health and disease: Further studies. *Annals of Otology, Rhinology, and Laryngology, 112*, 481–491.

Johnston, N., Knight, J., Dettmar, P. W., Lively, M. O., & Koufman, J. A. (2004).

Pepsin and carbonic anhydrase isoenzyme III as diagnostic markers for laryngopharyngeal reflux disease. *Laryngoscope, 114*, 2129–2134.

Koufman, J. A. (1991).The otolaryngologic manifestations of gastroesophageal reflux disease (GERD): A clinical investigation of 225 patients using ambulatory 24-hour pH monitoring and an experimental investigation of the role of acid and pepsin in the development of laryngeal injury. *Laryngoscope, 101*(Suppl. 53), 1–78.

Koufman, J. A. (1995). Gastroesophageal reflux and voice disorders. In: J. S. Rubin, R. T. Sataloff, & G. Korovin (Eds.), *Diagnosis and Treatment of Voice Disorders* (pp. 161–175), New York: Igaku-Shoin.

Koufman, J. A. (2002a). Laryngopharyngeal reflux is different from classic gastroesophageal reflux disease. *Ear Nose Throat Journal, 81*(Suppl. 2), 7–9.

Koufman, J. A. (2002b).Laryngopharyngeal reflux 2002: A new paradigm of airway disease. *Ear Nose and Throat Journal, 81*(Suppl. 2), 2–6.

Koufman, J. A., Amin, M. R., & Panetti, M. (2000, 2001) Prevalence of reflux in 113 consecutive patients with laryngeal and voice disorders. *Otolaryngology Head and Neck Surgery, 123*, 385–388. Erratum in: *Otolaryngology Head and Neck Surgery, 124*, 104.

Koufman, J. A., Aviv, J. E., Casiano, R. R., & Shaw, G. Y. (2002). Laryngopharyngeal reflux: Position statement of the Committee on Speech, Voice, and Swallowing Disorders of the American Academy of Otolaryngology-Head and Neck Surgery. *Otolaryngology-Head and Neck Surgery, 127*, 32–35.

Koufman, J. A., Belafsky, P. C., Bach, K. K., Daniel, E., & Postma, G. N. (2002). Prevalence of esophagitis in patients with pH-documented laryngopharyngeal reflux. *Laryngoscope, 112*, 1606–1609.

Koufman, J. A., Sataloff, R. T., & Toohill, R. (1996). Laryngopharyngeal reflux: Consensus report. *Journal of Voice, 10*, 215–216.

Koufman, J. A., Weiner, G. J., & Wu, W. C. et al. (1988). Reflux laryngitis and its sequelae: The diagnostic role of ambulatory 24-hour pH monitoring. *Journal of Voice, 2,* 78–89.

Lewin, J. S., Gillenwater, A. M., Garrett, J. D., Bishop-Leone, J. K., Nguyen, D. D., Callender, D. L., et al. (2003). Characterization of laryngopharyngeal reflux in patients with premalignant and early carcinomas of the larynx. *Cancer, 97,* 1010–1014.

Lindstrom, D. R., Wallace, J., Loehrl, T. A., Merati, A. L, & Toohill, R. J. (2002). Nissen fundoplication surgery for extraesophageal manifestation of gastroesophageal reflux (EER). *Laryngoscope, 112,* 1762–1765.

Little, F. B., Koufman, J. A., Kohut, R. I., & Marshall, R. B. (1985). Effect of gastric acid on the pathogenesis of subglottic stenosis. *Annals of Otology, Rhinology and Laryngology, 94,* 516–519.

Mamede, R. C., De Mello-Filho, F. V., Vigario, L. C., & Dantas, R. O. (2000). Effect of gastroesophageal reflux on hypertrophy of the base of tongue. *Otolaryngology-Head and Neck Surgery, 122,* 607–610.

Mandel, K. G., Daggy, B. P., Brodie, D. A., & Jacoby, H. I. (2000). Review article: alginate-raft formulations in the treatment of heartburn and acid reflux. *Alimentary Pharmacology Therapy, 14,* 669–690.

Maronian, N. C., Azadeh, H., Waugh, P., & Hillel, A., (2001). Association of laryngopharyngeal reflux disease and subglottic stenosis. *Annals of Otology, Rhinology and Laryngology, 110,* 606–612.

Merati, A. L., Lim, H. J., Ulualp, S. O., & Toohill, R. J. (2005). Meta-analysis of upper probe measurements in normal subjects and patients with laryngopharyngeal reflux. *Annals of Otology, Rhinology, and Laryngology, 114,* 177–182.

Noordzij, J. P., Khidr, A., Evans, B., Desper, E., Mittal, R. K., Reibel, J. F., et al. (2001). Evaluation of omeprazole in the treatment of reflux laryngitis: A prospective, placebo-controlled, randomized, double-blind study. *Laryngoscope, 111,* 2147–2151.

Orlando, R. C. (1986). Esophageal epithelial resistance. *Journal of Clinical Gastroenterology, 8*(Suppl. 1), 12–16.

Orsmeth, E. J. & Wong, R. K. H. (1999). Reflux laryngitis: Pathophysiology, diagnosis, and management. *American Journal of Gastroenterology, 94,* 2812–2817.

Pan, T., Wang, Y., & Guo, Z. (2004). Additional bedtime H2-receptor antagonist for the control of nighttime gastric acid breakthrough. *Cochrane Database System Review, 4,* CD004275.

Park, K. H., Choi, S. M., Kwon, S. U., Yoon, S. W., & Kim, S. U. (2006). Diagnosis of laryngopharyngeal reflux among globus patients. *Otolaryngology-Head and Neck Surgery, 134,* 81–85.

Park, W., Hicks, D. M., Khandwala, F., Richter, J. E., Abelson, T. I., Milstein C., et al. (2005). Laryngopharyngeal reflux: Prospective cohort study evaluating optimal dose of proton-pump inhibitor therapy and pretherapy predictors of response. *Laryngoscope, 115,* 1230–1238.

Peghini, P. L., Katz, P. O., Bracy, N. A., & Castell, D. O. (1998). Nocturnal recovery of gastric acid secretion with twice-daily dosing of proton pump inhibitors. *American Journal of Gastroenterology, 93,* 763–767.

Postma, G. N. (2000). Ambulatory pH monitoring methodology. *Annals of Otology, Rhinology and Laryngology, 109,* 10–14.

Postma, G. N., Belafsky, P. C., Aviv, J. E., & Koufman, J. A. (2002).Laryngopharyngeal reflux testing. *Ear Nose and Throat Journal, 81*(Suppl. 2), 14–18.

Postma, G. N., Cohen, J. T., Belafsky, P. C., Halum, S. L., Gupta, S. K., Bach, K. K., et al. (2005).Transnasal esophagoscopy: Revisited (over 700 consecutive cases). *Laryngoscope, 115,* 321–323.

Postma, G. N., & Johnson, L. F. (2002).Treament of laryngopharyngeal reflux. *Ear Nose and Throat Journal, 81*(Suppl. 2), 24–26.

Postma, G. N., Tomek, M. S., Belafsky, P. C., & Koufman, J. A. (2001). Esophageal motor function in laryngopharyngeal reflux is superior to that in classic gastroesophageal reflux disease. *Annals of Otology, Rhinology and Laryngology, 110,* 114–116.

Reavis, K. M., Morris, C. D., Gopal, D. V., Hunter, J. G., & Jobe, B. A. (2004). Laryngopharyngeal reflux symptoms better predict the presence of esophageal adenocarcinoma than typical gastroesophageal reflux symptoms. *Annals of Surgery, 239,* 849–858.

Reulbach, T. R., Belafsky, P. C., Blalock, P. D., Koufman, J. A., & Postma, G. N. (2001). Occult laryngeal pathology in a community-based cohort. *Otolaryngology-Head and Neck Surgery, 124,* 448–450.

Richardson, B. E., Heywood, B. M., Sims, H. S., Stoner, J., & Leopold, D. A. (2004). Laryngopharyngeal reflux: Trends in diagnostic interpretation criteria. *Dysphagia, 19,* 248–255.

Sasaki, C. T., Ross, D. A., & Hundal, J. (2003). Association between Zenker diverticulum and gastroesophageal reflux disease: Development of a working hypothesis. *American Journal of Medicine, 18* (Suppl. 3A), 169S–171S.

Smoak, B. R., & Koufman, J. A. (2001). Effects of gum chewing on pharyngeal and esophageal pH. *Annals of Otology, Rhinology and Laryngology, 110,* 1117–1119.

Steward, D. L., Wilson, K. M., Kelly, D. H., Patil, M. S., Schwartzbauer, H. R., Long, J. D., et al. (2004). Proton pump inhibitor therapy for chronic laryngo-pharyngitis: randomized placebo-control trial. *Otolaryngology-Head and Neck Surgery, 131,* 342–350.

Toohill, R. J., Mushtag, E., & Lehman, R. H. (1990). Otolaryngologic manifestations of gastroesophageal reflux. In T. Sacristan, J. J. Alvarez-Vincent, & J. Bartual (Eds.), *Proceedings of XIV World Congress of Otolaryngology-Head and Neck Surgery* (pp. 3005–3009). Amsterdam, The Netherlands: Kugler & Ghedini.

Tutuian, R., & Castell, D. O. (2004). Nocturnal acid breakthrough—approach to management. *Medscape General Medicine, 6,* 11.

Ulualp, S. O., & Toohill, R. J. (2000). Laryngopharyngeal reflux: state of the art diagnosis and treatment. *Otolaryngology Clinics of North America, 33,* 785–802.

Ulualp, S. O., Toohill, R. J., Kern, M., & Shaker, R. (1998). Pharygo-UES contractile reflux in patients with posterior laryngitis. *Laryngoscope, 108,* 1354–1357.

Vincent, D. A., Jr., Garrett, J. D., Radionoff, S. L., Reussner, L. A., & Stasney, C. R. (2000). The proximal probe in esophageal pH monitoring: development of a normative database. *Journal of Voice, 14,* 247–254.

Wiener, G. J., Koufman, J. A., & Wu, W. C. (1987). The pharyngo-esophageal dual ambulatory pH probe for evaluation of atypical manifestations of gastroesophageal reflux (GER). *Gastroenterology, 92,* 1694.

Wiener, G. J., Koufman, J. A., Wu, W. C., Cooper, J. B., Richter, J. E., & Castel, D. O. (1989). Chronic hoarseness secondary to gastroesophageal reflux disease: Documentation with 24-h ambulatory pH monitoring. *American Journal of Gastroenterology, 84,* 1503–1508.

Westcott, C. J., Hopkins, M. B, Bach, K., Postma, G. N., Belafsky, P. C., & Koufman, J. A. (2004). Fundoplication for laryngopharyngeal reflux disease. *Journal of the American College of Surgery, 199,* 23–30.

Woo, P., Noordzij, P., & Ross, J. (1996). Association of esophageal reflux and globus symptom: Comparison of laryngoscopy and 24-hour pH manometry. *Otolaryngology-Head and Neck Surgery, 115,* 502–507.

Wright, R. C., & Rhodes, K. P. (2003). Improvement of laryngopharyngeal reflux symptoms after laparoscopic Hill repair. *American Journal of Surgery, 185,* 455–461.

Ylitalo, R., Lindestad, P. A., & Ramel, S. (2001). Symptoms, laryngeal findings, and 24-hour pH monitoring in patients with suspected gastroesophago-pharyngeal reflux. *Laryngoscope. 111,* 1735–1741.

Ylitalo, R. & Ramel, S. (2002a & 2002b). Gastroesophagopharyngeal reflux in patients with contact granuloma: A prospective controlled study. *Annals of Otology, Rhinology and Laryngology, 111,* 178–183; Corrected and republished in: *Annals of Otology, Rhinology and Laryngology, 111*(5 Pt. 1), 441–446.

# 7

# Nursing Evaluation and Care of the Patient with Dysphagia

## Ann E. F. Sievers

Early identification of patients with dysphagia is important to maintain nutritional requirements, to protect the airway during swallow, and to prevent complications. In a hospitalized patient, a nurse may be the first person to recognize signs and symptoms of dysphagia. The nurse also plays a major role in implementing strategies for treatment, particularly as these relate to alternative feeding methods or monitoring of dietary restrictions. Communication of pertinent information to the physician managing the patient's care, other professionals, the patient, and his or her family members or significant others in the patient's life is an integral part of the nurse's responsibility. It is therefore incumbent on the dysphagia team nurse and the staff nurse, to be knowledgeable about the person with dysphagia, including symptoms, risk factors, complications, and possible treatments. This chapter will address, first, the role of the nurse in observing and evaluating patients with, or at risk for, dysphagia and, second, the role of the nurse in the ongoing care and monitoring of patients with dysphagia, particularly as it relates to hospitalized patients.

## INDICATIONS

### Patients at Risk for Dysphagia: Discussion

Patients at risk for dysphagia may have an underlying medical condition that obviously predisposes them to difficulty in swallowing, such as head trauma, neuromuscular disease, brain tumor, head and neck cancer, or stroke (Table 7–1). More difficult to identify are patients with dysphagia with conditions that may not clearly signal dysphagia.

**Table 7-1.** Risk Factors for Aspiration

- Decreased level of consciousness.
- Supine position.
- Presence of a nasogastric tube.
- Tracheal intubation and mechanical ventilation.
- Bolus or intermittent feeding delivery methods.
- Malpositioned feeding tube.
- Vomiting.
- High-risk disease and injury conditions.
- Neurologic disorders.
- Major abdominal and thoracic trauma/surgery.
- Diabetes mellitus.
- Poor oral health.
- Inadequate R.N. staffing levels.
- Advanced age.

*Source:* Reprinted with permission from Metheny (2002). Risk factors for aspiration. *Journal of Parenteral and Enteral Nutrition, 26*(Suppl. 6), S26–S33.

Patients recovering from stroke, patients with dementia or other mental debilitation, elderly patients, and malnourished patients may fall into this category. All critically ill patients are at risk for dysphagia because of the general deconditioning and weakness of musculature involved in bolus propulsion and airway protection during deglutition. Poor oral care and the influences of intubation, changes in oral flora and bacterial overgrowth, and poor dentition lead to ventilator associated pneumonias (Munroe, 2004; Trieger, 2004). Deconditioned patients generally lack breath support and have a poor cough in response to airway penetration by food or liquid, making them less able to respond effectively to even mild aspiration. Evidence of repeated fevers or pneumonia in a patient should also stimulate concern if there is a possibility these symptoms could be related to aspiration.

## Pulmonary Risk Factors

Patients with pre-existing pulmonary disease who become dysphagic have a diminished ability to tolerate even mild aspiration. Aspiration insults are very poorly tolerated by an already compromised pulmonary system. Pulmonary diseases include all the smoking-related lung diseases, for example, emphysema, chronic bronchitis, or lung cancer. Patients with cardiopulmonary pathologies such as cardiomyopathies, pulmonary hypertension, and cardiovascular diseases are also at heightened risk for pulmonary complications from dysphagia.

## Aspiration Pneumonia

True aspiration pneumonia has a typical radiographic pattern. Aspirated materials are most often located in the right lower lobe, next most often in the right upper lobe, and less frequently in the left lower lobe. Rarely are all three lobes involved at once. This distribution is a consequence of the angle of the tracheobronchial tree into the parenchyma of the lung. The right lower lobe represents a straight line of descent from the trachea and right main stem bronchus. In a patient who is supine, or lying on the right side, the right upper lobe takeoff from the right main stem bronchus represents a dependent position. The left lobe is in a dependent position in the left side lying position. The site of aspirated materials is thus influenced largely by gravity and human anatomy.

Symptoms of aspiration pneumonia in a patient must be thoroughly explored, both clinically and radiographically. To ensure appropriate treatment, pneumonia related to dysphagia, or to difficulty eating and drinking, must be differentiated from a pneumonia related to aspiration related to other etiologies. Aspiration pneumonia may be a result of material entering the lungs during a period of unconsciousness, such as can occur in trauma, diabetic coma, or acute myocardial infarction with loss of consciousness. Aspiration can also occur when patients who have been instructed to remain NPO (*non per os*, nothing by mouth) before surgery do not comply with the instructions. Under general anesthesia, or even conscious sedation, the patient is unable to protect the airway. Reflux occurs as the lower esophageal sphincter is relaxed and the patient aspirates. Similarly, individuals who have eaten a meal and then experience a traumatic event leading to unconsciousness are at very high risk for aspiration. This aspiration is preceded by vomiting or reflux, and may have devastating consequences for the pulmonary system (Metheny, 2002).

Repeated aspiration occurs when the airway is unable to maintain its normal hygiene. Long-term endotracheal intubation heightens a patient's risk for repeated aspiration by the presence of an artificial tube that interferes with the normal cough, impairs the ciliary action of the lining of the trachea, and precludes the normal filtration and humidification of the nose and mouth. Even with cuffed endotracheal tubes and tracheostomy tubes, microaspiration into the tracheobronchial tree does occur. This is a consequence of the constant expansion and contraction of the trachea during normal respiration, and subsequent movement of the cuff in the airway.

Repeated aspiration may also be related to a patient's inability to protect the airway during eating and drinking. For example, a larynx that is incompetent as a consequence of paralysis or radiation effects may not be able to close quickly or completely enough to prevent swallowed materials from aspiration. An insensate larynx, caused by stroke, cranial nerve injury, or other factors, may precipitate aspiration of foods, liquids, or the patient's own secretions. "Silent" aspiration can be particularly difficult to diagnose (Horner & Massey, 1988). In one study, only 42% (18/43) of a group of inpatients with documented aspiration on videofluoroscopy were identified as aspirating on bedside swallow evaluations (Splaingard, Hutchins, Sulton, & Chaudhuri, 1988). Patients who chronically aspirate may become undernourished and unable to maintain their weight. Immunological risk is heightened because of the lack of adequate protein, albumin, and fat stores to maintain normal function. Clinical findings include fever, shortness of breath, weakness, and coughing. Sputum may be thick, colored, and difficult to expel by coughing. Chest auscultation may reveal rhonchi in the large airways, and the person with true pneumonia may have characteristic egophony, or "E" to "A" changes on auscultation (i.e., when patient produces the vowel "ee," sound heard through stethoscope sounds like the vowel in "bait," because of abnormally increased lung density.) Breath sounds are decreased over the consolidated lung (solidification of the lung secondary to pneumonia) and may even sound hollow (Bickley & Scizlaqyi, 2007). As noted, both an episode of severe, acute aspiration and chronic, repeated aspiration can cause pneumonia. Pneumonia is treated with appropriate antibiotic therapy. If not treated promptly, or with the correct antibiotic regimen, the patient can become dangerously ill. Today, some pneumonia may not be so easily treated because of resistant microorganisms. In a patient whose immune system has been threatened as a consequence of chemotherapy, significant deconditioning, or AIDS, pneumonia of any origin may be lethal.

If aspiration pneumonia is diagnosed, the dysphagia team must be able to differentiate its etiologies. A distinction should be made between aspiration caused by an inability to protect the airway during eating and swallowing because of motor and/or sensory factors, and aspiration from other causes. Whatever the etiology, early correct detection is tantamount to correct treatment and, ultimately, to recovery.

## DESCRIPTION OF NURSING EVALUATION

One goal of the nursing evaluation is to determine if a patient is able to attain normal oral nutrition, or if it has been impaired or altered. The evaluation also attempts to determine if aspiration is likely, possibly necessitating nonoral feeding as a precautionary measure until further diagnostic studies, such as comprehensive bedside swallow study or videofluoroscopy, can be completed. Components of the nursing assessment include the following.

## History/Medical Record Review

Comprehensive review of the patient's medical history should provide information about risk factors for dysphagia (Table 7–2). Significant flags for possi-

**Table 7-2.** Patient History

- Identification of the individual
- Chief Complaint
- History of Present Illness (HPI)
  - Onset, symptoms, chronology
- Past Medical History (PMH)
  - Illnesses, child, adult,
  - Hospital admits
  - PHM Medical
  - PHM Surgical
  - Immunizations
  - Health Maintenance
- Allergies
  - Medications, Food, Other
- Medications
  - Type and diagnosis
- Social History
  - Smoking
  - Alcohol
  - Lifestyle
  - Occupation
  - Education
  - Marital Status
  - Diet
  - Exercise
- Family History
- OB-GYN History

ble dysphagia include cranial nerve deficits, structural anomalies, or medical or surgical conditions that may contribute to a swallowing abnormality. All *medical diagnoses* are noted, specifically those pertaining to a recent change in the health status of the patient (Bates, 1979). *Surgical procedures* are also noted, for example, carotid endarderectomy or open heart surgery may cause damage to the vagus nerve, cranial nerve X, as it courses through the neck and chest. Chart review should also consider documentation of the patient's *dietary status* and, if possible, calorie counts that may have been performed. (See Chapter 10 for further details regarding appropriate calorie counts.) The inability to attain caloric and protein goals may portend a significant problem. Also noted are the patient's *height, weight, usual weight, and the amount of weight loss or gain and over what period of time.* Standard laboratory assessment of hematocrit, hemoglobin, electrolytes, trace elements, albumin and protein also aids in the evaluation. Dietetics professionals play an indispensable role in the evaluation and treatment of individuals diagnosed with head and neck cancer as well as individuals who are at further risk such as the elderly, those with cachexia, or multiple trauma (Dixon 2005; van Borkhost-de van der Schueren, Quak, von Blomberg-van der Flier, Kuik, Langendoen, & Snow et al., 2001; White, 2006).

It may be helpful to organize medical history-taking or chart documentation according to a review of systems, in particular, cardiovascular, gastrointestinal, genitourinary, neurologic, skeletal, and endocrine. Consideration of this comprehensive overview makes it less likely that details that may have

implications for swallowing function will be overlooked. Pertinent information regarding systems should be available in the patient's chart or medical records, and can be reviewed with the physician managing the patient's care.

## Physical Exam

A hospitalized patient's clinical status is continually monitored by the physician and medical team managing his or her care. In some instances, for example, when the patient's condition is subject to significant and/or frequent change, nursing evaluation includes a physical exam directed to food management, swallowing issues, and airway protection. A particular focus of this assessment is on correlating the patient's current level of alertness with swallowing function and determining how changes in physical status, that is, pulmonary, neurologic, and gastrointestinal, may impact additional diagnostic tests, such as bedside swallow or videofluoroscopy, and the patient's ability to cooperate with the objectives of these tests.

Smell and taste have a huge impact on a person's ability to identify foods and support nutrition. Both are subjective for the patient and significant changes occur with medications, chemotherapy, or surgery (Bartoshuk, 1993). The inaccurate old tongue map has been discarded for the scientific study of the interactions among taste and the relevant cranial nerves, glossopharyngeal and chorda tympani (Bartoshuk, 1993). The sense of smell is innervated by cranial nerve I (olfactory ), and this function should not be excluded during the physical exam.

## Patient Interview

It is important to have the patient, if possible, describe his or her own complaints and experiences with swallowing and food management (Table 7–3). Patient complaints may be related to a single pathological process, or may suggest multiple problems. An important distinction is whether the patient

**Table 7–3.** Review of Symptoms.

| | |
|---|---|
| • General | • Musculoskeletal |
|    Height, Weight, Usual weight |    Posture |
|    Pain related to specific area |    Muscle aches |
| • HEENT, Head, Eyes, Ears, Nose, Throat |    Back/Neck/Hip pain |
|    Head |    Bone pain |
|    Eyes and Vision | • Neurological |
|    Nose, Sinuses |    Headache |
|    Mouth, dentition |    LOC (loss of consciousness) |
|    Throat |    Dizziness vertigo |
|    Larynx |    Seizures |
| • Cardiovascular |    Behavior |
|    Chest pain |    Memory |
|    SOB (shortness of breath) |    Thought content |
| • Respiratory |    Speech |
|    Cough |    Balance-gait |
|    SOB |    Sensation |
|    Sputum | • Psychiatric |
| • Endocrine |    Personality |
|    Weight, obesity, cachexia |    Affect |
|    Weight increase or decrease |    Depression |
|    from normal |    Anxiety |
| • Gastrointestinal | • Skin |
|    Mouth odynophagia, dysphagia |    Color-Turgor |
|    Swallowing |    Lesions |
|    Reflux, heartburn |    Masses |
|    Stomach complaints |    Rashes |
|    Bowel habits | • Pain |
| • Genitourinary |    Character |
|    Urine frequency, complaints |    Location |
|    Male genitalia |    Cause |
|    OB-GYN |    Onset/duration |
|    Breast |    Intensity (1–10 scale) |
| • Hematology-Oncology |    Treatment |
|    Pallor, red, bruising, bleeding |    Medications, other Rx |

experiences difficulty swallowing or pain on swallowing, or rather describes symptoms suggesting penetration or aspiration of materials into the airway. Examples of patient complaints, which may be significant, include:

- *Food sticking*—Reflecting possible inability to propel bolus material properly, failure of the upper esophageal sphincter to relax, changes in mucosal integrity, esophageal conditions, or other etiological factors.
- *Changes in taste*—Suggesting altered sensation related to neurogenic factors, changes in oral or pharyngeal mucosa, medications, and/or treatment programs, such as chemotherapy or radiation therapy (Bartoshuk, 1993).
- *Cough with food or liquid before, during or after the swallow*—Most likely caused by aspiration, but may be caused by pulmonary disease.
- *Cough at rest or between feedings*—Indicating possible aspiration of residual food or saliva. A cough at rest may be also be indicative of COPD (chronic obstructive pulmonary disease), chronic bronchitis, or other pre-existing pulmonary problems.
- *Excessive oral secretions*—Related to poor sensation, or to copious or thick secretions.
- *Impaired ability to manage foods of specific sensations or textures*—May provide clues useful to diagnosis.
- *Weight loss, acute or chronic*—Indicates inadequate nutrition, or metabolic needs in excess of nutritional intake, for example, undiagnosed cancer.
- *Social or behavioral changes related to meals*—May provide clues to patient's mental, emotional state, or to degree of debilitation, or to environmental or social factors that may be influencing patient's health, such as lack of care or nutrition (Kagan, 2004).
- *Family observation of any of above changes*

For the latter, an interview with a patient's family, friends, and other caregivers, if available, may be helpful. Family and friends may provide information related to observed changes in the patient's eating habits and changes in weight that the patient is not aware of or is unable or unwilling to communicate.

## Observations During Meals

The primary care nurse often identifies dysphagia and performs the initial bedside screening. A comprehensive bedside swallow evaluation may be performed by the dysphagia team nurse or by a swallowing or dysphagia therapist, most often a speech-language pathologist. Ideally, both specialists can see the patient together. This type of evaluation is discussed in depth in Chapter 8. The assessment reviewed here will focus primarily on the preliminary findings that suggest a patient is dysphagic and requires further diagnostic workup with bedside, videofluoroscopy, or other studies. For this purpose, the nurse observes the patient during one or more mealtimes. A representative sample of the patient's capabilities may require watching at different times of the day, before or after activities or medications. Any changes over time related to fatigue, medication administration, or other factors should be noted. Family interviews, or discussions with other caregivers, may be of help in obtaining significant information. The value of information obtained notwithstanding, it is important to remember limitations of the exam. For example, bedside evaluation alone has been reported to underestimate the frequency of aspiration in patients with neurologic dysfunction (Splaingard, Hutchins, Sultan, & Chauhuri, 1988).

Observations made of the patient during swallow can be of significance and should include the following:

- Change in vocal quality while eating (suggesting presence of material on vocal folds).
- Cough during or after swallow (suggesting aspiration).
- Wet or gurgling sound associated with respiration (suggesting food or liquids in airway, inability to clear pharynx or larynx).
- Change in ability to take routine medications, that is, pills more difficult, capsules and liquids easier.
- Apparent attempts to compensate for swallowing or food management difficulty, as by multiple swallows of one bolus, manipulating size or consistency of bolus, or by avoidance or preference of particular kinds of foods, or by assuming particular postures, that is, chin-tuck, head turning.

- Fatigue during meal; time needed to complete meal (amount of food or time).
- Alteration of normal laminar airflow during auscultation of the larynx.

## Chest and Cervical Auscultation

Auscultation of the chest and cervical airway is important in the clinical evaluation of any person suspected of dysphagia and aspiration. Airflow associated with normal respiration has a characteristic sound that can be detected by placing a stethoscope over various parts of the airway. Large airway sounds differ from small airway sounds because of the density of tissue the air is traveling through to reach the stethoscope (Bates, 1979), and each area of the chest has a unique sound dependent on its distance from the large airways.

Laryngeal auscultation may be especially useful in evaluating dysphagic, or possibly dysphagic, patients (Hamlet, Nelson, & Patterson, 1990; Penny, & Formolo, 1994; Selley, Ellis, Flack, Bayliss, & Pearce, 1994; Takahashi, Groher, & Michi, 1994a; Takahashi, Groher, & Michi, 1994b; Zenner, Losinski, & Mills, 1995). Placing the stethoscope gently on the lateral aspect of the larynx, and listening to airflow in normal breathing, during swallowing, or speech, will provide the listener with experience in identifying this sound and differentiating it from other sounds (Figure 7–1).

In a dysphagic patient who aspirates during swallow, the quality of sound

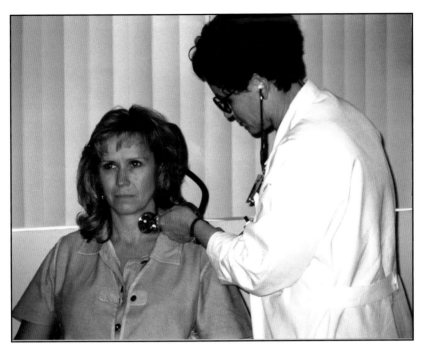

**Figure 7–1.** Laryngeal auscultation. Proper placement of bell of stethoscope while patient completes swallowing and speech maneuvers.

generated may be altered, as would be expected if fluids and air are mixed. In addition to airflow, some mechanical events associated with swallow have characteristic sounds. Such events may include elevation of the larynx and bolus flow through the pharyngoesophageal segment, although exact correspondences between sounds and events remain to be identified. A listener experienced with the characteristics of these mechanical "event" sounds may be able to differentiate normal and altered sound generation, however. Chest auscultation is of particular help in defining daily changes related to aspiration and aspiration pneumonia. Chest radiographs are indicated if pneumonia is suspected on auscultation.

## NURSING CARE IN PATIENTS WITH DYSPHAGIA

### Aspiration Precautions

Aspiration precautions may pertain to acute care hospitalized patients, patients in nursing home settings, and home health patients. However, precautions *must* be modified for each individual patient to match his or her type of dysphagia, nutritional needs, and treatment plan. Again, continual diligence is required because many patients with dysphagia aspirate without giving any external sign of food or liquid entering the airway (Logemann, 1986) (see Table 7–1).

*Inpatient aspiration precautions* are as follows:

Oral Feeding:

- Do not allow patient to eat unattended or unobserved.
- If patient is taking an oral diet, follow strict diet restrictions generated by dysphagia assessment.
    - (See physician's orders for consistency, amount, and frequency.)
- Position patient in optimally safe upper body position as recommended, or 90° in a chair with head or neck flexion, if possible.
- Observe for coughing, choking, throat clearing, or struggle during eating.
- Minimize distractions (maintain quiet environment, no television).
- Continually assess pulmonary function for fevers, rales, rhonchi, and clinical signs of aspiration.

Enteral Feeding:

- Ensure placement of tube is correct and monitor for evidence of change.
- Observe reflux precautions (limit nocturnal feeds, head of bed elevated).
- Check residuals before feeding.

*Outpatient aspiration precautions* include:
Oral Feeding:

- Avoid eating or drinking when alone.
- Minimize distractions (quiet environment, no television).
- Observe consistency, amount, and frequency restrictions imposed by team.

- Observe optimally safe upper body position as recommended, or use 90° upper body position with chin tuck.
- Ensure that family/caregivers are familiar with Heimlich maneuver, CPR, and signs of aspiration (cough, throat clear, "wet" voice, struggle associated with eating or drinking.
- Frequently assess for changes in pulmonary status reflective of aspiration (rales, fevers, rhonchi).

Enteral Feeding:

- Monitor tube position for evidence that it has changed.
- Observe reflux positions.
- Check residuals before feeding.

## Observation of Patients with Enteral Nutrition

Patients whose primary mode of feeding is by feeding tube are still susceptible to aspiration from gastroesophageal reflux and improper placement of the enteral tube. As early as 1986, Metheny, Eisenberg, and Spies stated that aspiration pneumonia is unquestionably the most potentially lethal complication of tube feeding. Reflux may occur with both continuous or bolus feeding and can also occur with gastric secretions, alone. Reflux and aspiration in patients with gastrostomy tubes can be caused by lower esophageal sphincter (LES) relaxation secondary to gastric distention of the stomach (Takahashi, Groher, & Michi, 1994b). These patients require rigorous monitoring because this type of aspiration may be silent and its symptoms elusive to cursory examination. The nurse must be alert to the position of the patient during feeding and the administering of medications via the tube. Antireflux precautions should also be maintained.

Coughing after feeding (especially bolus feeding), when the stomach is full, is a strong indication of reflux and aspiration. When feeding is administered lower in the gastrointestinal tract, via jejunostomy, reflux of gastric acid after feeding may still occur (Coben, Weintraub, DiMarino, & Cohen, 1994; Sands, 1991). The acidity of the gastric secretions is extremely damaging to the larynx and lungs (even more so than the content of tube feeds) and medications designed to decrease stomach acidity, such as antacids and H2-blockers, should be used. Elpern, Jacobs, and Bone (1987) found that 77% of patients with tubes in place aspirated material at some time during the study period.

Position of the tube is critical to the proper administration of enteral feeds. All tube placements should be confirmed by radiograph if there are any concerns regarding placement (Metheny, 2002). Ongoing routine checking for placement should be taught to family members if the patient is going home with an enteral tube. If a nasogastric tube is used, for example, the nasolabial tip should be protected with a skin barrier, and tape placement must be appropriate to avoid nasal tip necrosis (Figure 7–2). Similarly, gastrostomy and jejunostomy tubes necessitate protection of the anterior abdominal wall, and require skin barriers around the tube insertion site. Auscultation, measurement, instillation of air, and gastric contents checks are used to assess correct placement of enteral tubes. Radio-

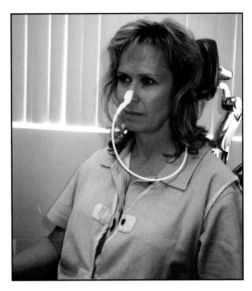

**Figure 7–2.** The correct method of securing a nasogastric tube to prevent dislodgement and nasal tip or alae necrosis.

graphic documentation is also required if there is any concern regarding clinical interpretation of the tube placement. Blue vegetable dye is never placed in the feeding tube formula of patients with a tracheostomy as a test for reflux and subsequent aspiration (Maloney, 2000). Glucose monitoring of pulmonary secretions is also not used as an indicator of formulas that have been refluxed into the airway, because of test discrepancies (Maloney, 2000; Metheny, Aud, & Wunderlich, 1999).

When drugs are mixed with enteral products, it is important to assess the mixture for physical compatibility. In some instances, there is a potential for the drugs and/or enteral products to undergo degradation and inactivation when combined (Cutie, Altman, & Lenkel, 1983). Another precaution with enteral tubes, concerns airway suctioning. Suctioning through a tracheostomy tube will cause a patient to cough. The increased intrathoracic pressure generated during a cough may cause reflux in some patients. Consequently, suctioning should be gentle, particularly if aspiration is suspected during a reflux episode. Following suctioning, a patient should be asked to cough voluntarily, without suction, to further determine if there is refluxed material in the airway. Timing of feedings and pulmonary therapies, such as chest physical therapy, and/or Trendelenburg positioning must also be considered.

In addition to monitoring patients for evidence of aspiration, the nurse charged with care of the enteral patient will need to work closely with the physician and dietitian to ensure the patient's tolerance and progression to feeding. Monitoring of fluctuations in weight, protein and albumin levels, and blood chemistry are important to this process. Similarly, it is critical to watch for alterations in the patient's level of consciousness as these may affect airway protection. Attention to the patient's physical well-being must, of course, also be accompanied by attention to maintaining the best quality of life possible in the face of what may represent a radical alteration in life style.

## Observation of Patients with Artificial Airways

In patients with an artificial airway in place, the disease process as well as the presence of the appliance may influence the patient's ability to swallow. The presence of food (or enteral feeding in the case of a tube-fed patient) in a tracheostomy, or endotracheal secre-

tions, are clear indicators of aspiration or reflux and should stimulate immediate concern. At the same time, patients with artificial airways can be suctioned readily in the event of a witnessed aspiration.

An artificial airway often intimidates the novice clinician, but is a safeguard to the protection of the patient. Clinicians involved in the care of the person with dysphagia must have an intimate knowledge of the kinds, uses, and complications of artificial airways used in their patient population (Lindholm, 1985). The following is an overview of the types of tracheostomy tubes used in acute care settings.

*Cuffed tubes* (Figure 7–3) are used to seal the airway for positive pressure ventilation and to attempt to prevent aspiration of secretions into the lungs (Lindholm, 1985). Cuff pressures are established at no more than 20 to 30 mm Hg in order not to exceed end capillary pressures (McGinnis, Shively, Patterson, & Magovern, 1971). These tubes are typically used in critical care

**Figure 7–3.** Cuffed tracheostomy tube. (Photo courtesy of Tyco Healthcare.)

settings and with patients on ventilators. Infrequently, patients are sent home with cuffed tubes because of the need for positive pressure ventilation, such as those with amyotrophic lateral sclerosis (ALS) or Guillain-Barré syndrome. When a patient does not require positive pressure ventilation, and is breathing independently, the cuff is deflated to avoid pressure and scarring of the tracheal walls (tracheal stenosis).

*Uncuffed/cuffless tubes* (Figure 7–4) are used to provide an airway when the patient is able to breathe on his or her own but still requires assistance with secretion removal and airway maintenance. These tubes are typically used for long-term tracheostomy patients. Aspiration may occur with these tubes, even in the presence of a normal aerodigestive tract. In addition, the tube itself may tether the larynx and interfere with its normal elevation during swallow (Johnson, Reilly, & Mallory, 1985).

*Fenestrated tubes* (Figure 7–5) are tubes that are occasionally used for weaning and decannulation, and are generally smaller in size than tubes used for airway maintenance. Their secondary benefit may be improved speech for selected individuals. When the inner cannula is removed and the tube is capped, the patient is breathing via the fenestra, as well as around the tube (Lindholm, 1985). Fenestrated (Latin for "window") tubes are not left in place for long periods of times, no more than 3 to 5 days, because of the possibility of invagination of fragile tracheal mucosa into the fenestra, therefore blocking the patient's airway (Figure 7–6). Before decannulation, the patient should have the tube capped for 18 to 24 hours to test tolerance, and then be decannulated early in the morning. This allows for the most hours of intense observation of the patient's accommodation and airway competence following decannulation.

**Figure 7-4.** Cuffless tracheostomy tube: Outer cannula; inner cannula; insertion obturator; decannulation plug (*red*). (Photo courtesy of Tyco Healthcare.)

**Figure 7-5.** Fenestrated tracheostomy tube: Outer cannula; decannulation plug (*red*); inner cannula unfenestrated; insertion obturator; inner cannula fenestrated. (Photo courtesy of Tyco Healthcare.)

**Figure 7-6.** Illustration of tube in place; site of narrowing (*at arrow*) caused by granulation tissue may require revision. (Photo courtesy of Tyco Healthcare.)

### Speech and Swallowing with a Tracheostomy

As soon as possible, the patient with a noncuffed tracheostomy should be taught to cover the tube opening and talk. (This should never be attempted with a cuffed tracheostomy tube, even with the cuff fully deflated.) The use of finger control speech, or the use of a one-way-valve speaking system is predicated upon the ability of the patient to use the technique. The patient and family should be instructed in the proper method of speech and breathing, that is, inhale through the tracheostomy tube, cover the tube at peak inhalation, and speak on exhalation. It is important to remind the patient to then release the cover and again breathe in through the tube. Once the technique is mastered, patients usually quickly become adept at speaking. The use of the vocal folds for speech is believed to facilitate function of the larynx for swallow. In addition, the patient's ability to communicate orally may be of great help in identifying problems, discussing needs, and maintaining interactions with significant others in the environment.

## Observation of Patients from Tube to Oral Feeding

Nursing intervention during transition from tube feeding to oral feeding includes assurance of adequate nutrition, monitoring of progress, and *slow, careful* advancement of the treatment plan. Patients who are in the process of transition from enteral feeding to oral feeding must be carefully followed for possible complications of aspiration. Aspiration and reflux precautions need to be carefully maintained throughout this period. Any alteration or acute changes of pulmonary function that may indicate aspiration should be quickly communicated to the physician managing the patient's care. Patients may initially view a return to oral eating as a huge success, and indeed it is. But, in their enthusiasm, they may also fail to observe necessary precautions. Patients must be monitored to ensure that they, and their families, understand and observe the precautions prescribed.

## Observation of Patients on Modified Oral Nutrition

When a treatment plan permits the patient to eat orally, but with modifications or restrictions, the nurse and dysphagia therapist can work together to ensure that the protocol is communicated to and understood by, the patient (to the extent possible), family members, other professionals and caregivers. This attention to implementation of dietary modifications, compensatory strategies, or other recommendations that comprise the treatment plan continues while the patient is in the hospital, and may also need to be extended to other environments (e.g., when the patient is transferred to another floor, discharged to another facility, or sent home.) Use of adaptive devices for feeding must be carefully monitored for safety (Sievers, Leonard, & McKenzie, 1992). Feedback regarding the effectiveness of the plan also needs to

be communicated regularly to other members of the dysphagia team, so that changes can be made as needed.

## PSYCHOSOCIAL FACTORS

Nurses are extremely influential in teaching patients how to cope with life's illnesses. This is true of the nurse in the acute care hospital, the skilled facility, the rehabilitation hospital, and the home. As part of a dysphagia team, the nurse should address a patient's psychosocial issues with concern, and with accurate information.

Quality of life issues are of great import for people who have a diagnosis of swallowing disorder, particularly after head and neck cancer resections (Dropkin, 1997; Dropkin et al., 2006). Patients with dysphagia, with or without aspiration, may experience a change in normally established eating habits. Issues related to safe nutrition, eating with friends and family, eating in public, alteration of normal routines, and the need for increased time for feeding may become pressing. The relationship between food and eating to quality of life, perhaps universally, is significant. Television has many advertisements emphasizing food; eating is a major part of holiday or just social activities. But for the dysphagic patient, and others in his or her environment, eating may be a stressful chore, not a pleasure. Coping skills can be sorely challenged during this time. Strategies for coping with the changes and the stressors they induce are a part of the patient education process, and the responsibility of all dysphagia team members who have contact with the patient. Nursing care, in particular, should include attention to these details, and to the resolution of issues that can separate rather than unite a family during a time of illness.

## TEAM COLLABORATION

As has been emphasized frequently in this manual, the best approach to the dysphagic patient is a team approach. The integration of many disciplines is needed for complete diagnosis and treatment, and the interaction of these professionals on a regular basis (i.e., daily or weekly) ensures that necessary feedback regarding the patient's progress is available to appropriately revise and update the plan as needed. The team approach represents the best care for patients, and allows members of the team to advance their own knowledge through shared experiences, skills, and information.

## STUDY QUESTIONS

1. The nurse's role in the treatment of dysphagia includes
   a. Critical observation
   b. Airway protection
   c. Adequate nutrition
   d. Intervention to prevent malnutrition
2. What is the optimum bed position recommended in the literature to prevent aspiration in critical patients?
   a. Head of bed elevated 30 degrees.
3. How does laryngeal auscultation help you in the evaluation of a patients swallow and airway?
   a. defines laminar versus turbulent airflow
   b. Information on the swallow response.
   c. Information on airway sounds, quiet vs. stridor or struggle.
4. How does a complete history help in the evaluation of a patient with a swallowing complaint?
   a. Better defines the patients issues
   b. Gives the clinician accurate and complete information with which to make informed therapy and intervention decisions.
5. What should be the first response if a patient is observed with significant swallowing difficulties?
   a. Stop oral nutrition
   b. Make the patient NPO
   c. Support the airway, by oxygen, positioning, and coughing to clear the airway, suctioning if necessary
   d. Consult the physician, dysphagia speech therapist.
6. Describe the correct method of securing a nasogastric tube in place.
   a. Clean the nose with acetone
   b. Swab the nose with benzoin
   c. Place a skin protector on the dry surface of the nose
   d. Secure the tube with tape in a figure-of-eight fashion.

## REFERENCES

August, D. (Chair), & Teitelbaum, D. (Co-Chair). (2002). Guidelines for the use of Parenteral and Enteral Nutrition in Adult and Pediatric Patients, ASPEN

Board of Directors and The Clinical Guidelines Task Force (pubs). *Journal of Parenteral and Enteral Nutrition, 26*(Suppl.), S1–S96.

Bartoshuk, L. M. (1993). Genetic and pathological taste variation: What can we learn from animal models and human disease? *CIBA Foundation Symposium, 179,* 251–262.

Bates, B. (1979). Interviewing the health history. In B. Bates, L. Bickley, & R. Hoekelman (Eds.), *A guide to physical examination and history taking* (4th ed., Chap. 1). Philadelphia: Lippincott Williams & Wilkins.

Bickley, L.& Scizlaqyi, P. (2007) *Bates pocket guide to physical examination and history taking.* Philadelphia: Lippincott Williams & Wilkins.

Coben, R., Weintraub A., DiMarino A., & Cohen, S. (1994). Gastroesophageal reflux during gastrostomy feeding. *Gastroenterology, 106,* 13–18.

Cutie J.B., Altman, E., & Lenkel L. (1983).. Compatibility of enteral products with commonly employed drug additives. *Journal of Parenteral and Enteral Nutrition, 7,* 186–191.

Dixon, S. W. (2005). Nutrition care issues in the ambulatory (outpatient) head and neck cancer patient. *Support Line, 27,* 3–10.

Dropkin, M. J. (1997). Coping with disfigurement/dysfunction and length of hospital stay after head and neck cancer surgery. *ORL-Head and Neck Nursing, 15,* 22–26.

Dropkin, M. J., Mogai, C., & Ungar, T. M. (2006). Recovery issues for African Americans following treatment of oral cavity pharynx cancer. *ORL-Head and Neck Nursing, 24,* 6–10 (rev).

Elpern, E. H., Jacobs, E. R., & Bone, R. C. (1987). Incidence of aspiration in tracheally intubated adults. *Heart and Lung, 16,* 527–531.

Hamlet, S., & Nelson, R. L. (1990). Interpreting the sounds of swallowing: Fluid flow through the cricopharyngeus. *Annals of Otology, Rhinology and Laryngology, 99,* 749–752.

Hamlet, S., Penney, D. G., & Formolo, J. (1994). Stethoscope acoustics and cervical auscultation of swallowing. *Dysphagia, 9,* 63–68.

Horner, J., & Massey, E. (1988). Silent aspiration following stroke. *Neurology, 38,* 317–319.

Johnson, J., Reilly, J., & Mallory, G. (1985). Decannulation. In E. Myers, S. Stool, & J. Johnson (Eds.), *Tracheostomy* (Chapter 12). New York: Churchill Livingstone.

Kagan. S. H. (2004). Shifting perspectives: gero-oncology nursing research. *Oncology Nursing Forum, 31,* 293–299.

Lindholm, C. (1985). Choice of tracheostomy tube. In: E. Myers, S. Stool, & J. Johnson (Eds.), *Tracheostomy* (Chapter 8). New York: Churchill Livingstone.

Logemann, J. (1986). Treatment for aspiration related to dysphagia: An overview. *Dysphagia, 1,* 34–38.

Maloney, J. P., Halbower, A. C., Fouty, B. F., Fagan, K. A., Balasubramanian, V., & Pike, A. W., et al. (2000). Systemic absorption of food dye in patients with sepsis [Letter]. *New England Journal of Medicine, 343,* 1047–1048.

McClave, S. A., & Demeo, M. T. (Co-Directors). (2002). North American summit of aspiration in the critically ill patient: Consensus statement. *Journal of Parenteral and Enteral Nutrition, 26*(Suppl. 6), S26–S33.

McGinnis, G. E., Shively, J. G., Patterson, R. L., & Magovern, G. J. (1971). An engineering analysis of intratracheal tube cuffs. *Anesthesia and Analgesia, 50,* 557–564.

Metheny, N. A. (2002). Risk factors for aspiration. *Journal of Parenteral and Enteral Nutrition, 26*(Suppl. 6), S26–S33.

Metheny, N. A., Aud, M. A., & Wunderlich, R. J. (1999). A survey of bedside methods used to detect pulmonary aspiration of enteral formula in intubated tube-fed patients. *American Journal of Critical Care, 8,* 160–169.

Metheny, N. A., Eisenberg, P., & Spies, M. (1986). Aspiration pneumonia in patients fed through nasoenteral tubes. *Heart and Lung, 15,* 256–261.

Munro, C. L., & Grap, M. J. (2004). Oral health and care in the intensive care unit; state of the science. *American Journal of Critical Care, 13,* 65–74.

Sands, J. (1991). Incidence of pulmonary aspiration in intubated patients receiving enteral nutrition through wide- and narrow-bore nasogastric feeding tubes. *Heart and Lung, 20,* 75–80.

Selley, W. G., Ellis, R. E., Flack, F. C., Bayliss, C. R., & Pearce, V. R. (1994). The synchronization of respiration and swallow sounds with videofluoroscopy during swallowing. *Dysphagia, 9,* 162–167.

Sievers, A., Leonard, R., & McKenzie, S. (1992). The safe use of an adaptive early feeding device for impaired patients. *ORL-Head and Neck Nursing, 10,* 17–19.

Splaingard, M., Hutchins, B., Sulton, L., & Chaudhuri, G. (1988). Aspiration in rehabilitation patients: Videofluoroscopy vs. bedside clinical assessment. *Archives of Physical Medicine and Rehabilitation, 69,* 637–640.

Takahashi, K., Groher, M. E., & Michi, K. (1994a). Symmetry and reproducibility of swallowing sounds. *Dysphagia, 9,* 168–173.

Takahashi, K., Groher, M. E., & Michi, K. (1994b). Methodology for detecting swallowing sounds. *Dysphagia, 9,* 54–62.

Trieger, N. (2004). Oral care in the intensive care unit. *American Journal of Critical Care, 13,* 24–33.

van Borkhost–De van de Schueren, M. A., Quak, J. J., von Blomberg-van der Flier, B. M., Kuik, D. J., Langendoen, S. I., Snow, G. B., et al. (2000). Effect of perioperative nutrition, with and without arginine supplementation, on nutritional status, immune function, postoperative morbidity, and survival in severely malnourished head and neck cancer patients. *American Journal of Clinical Nutrition, 73,* 323–332.

White, H. K., & Cohen, H. J. (2006). The older cancer patient. *Medicine Clinics of North America, 90,* 967–982.

Zenner, P. M., Losinski, D. D., & Mills, R. H. (1995). Using cervical auscultation in the clinical dysphagia examination in long-term care. *Dysphagia, 10,* 27–31.

## Recommended Readings

Sievers, A. (In press). Dysphagia and swallowing. In L. Harris & M. Huntoon (Eds.), *Core curriculum.* New Smyrna Beach, FL: Society of Otolaryngology Head and Neck Nurses.

Society of Otorhinolaryngology Head and Neck Nursing Standards of Practice Committee. (1996). *Guidelines for otorhinolaryngology nursing practice.* New Smyrna Beach, FL: Author.

# 8

# *Clinical Swallow Evaluation*

## Susan J. Goodrich
## Alice I. Walker

This chapter addresses the clinical swallow evaluation for adults. The reader is referred to other chapters in this manual for clinical assessment of swallowing problems in the pediatric population. The clinical swallow examination includes a medical and feeding history, clinical examination of oral structures and function, and observational evaluation of swallowing function. Other terms that may be used include "bedside swallowing evaluation."

## DESCRIPTION

The clinical swallow evaluation consists of medical and feeding history review, including current method and schedule of feeding, physical examination of oral-motor anatomy and function, and observation of swallowing. As in any clinical evaluation, the goal is a working hypothesis of the problem. In addition to observations regarding the patient's swallow behaviors, the

clinical swallow evaluation should be concerned with the patient's readiness to undergo more in-depth evaluation, such as a videofluoroscopic or flexible endoscopic evaluation of swallowing (Logemann, 1983). The information obtained in the clinical evaluation also begins the process toward treatment strategy recommendations (Cherney, 1994; Groher, 1984; Logemann, 1983; Steefel, 1981).

## INDICATIONS

A clinical swallow evaluation is indicated in any patient referred for assessment of a suspected swallowing problem. Referral usually takes place when the patient, the family, caregiver, feeder, and/or the physician have concerns regarding the normalcy of eating, when weight loss or nutrition failure occur, and/or when pulmonary history suggests aspiration. Crucial to the assessment process is an understanding of the referral question, so that recommendations may specifically address concerns. For example, the question of whether a person may be therapeutically fed small amounts differs greatly from the question of whether a nonoral source of nutrition may be discontinued. Knowing the concerns of both the healthcare provider and the caregiver, which may be the same or may differ, will enable the assessor to provide more helpful information.

The clinical swallowing evaluation is a first and crucial step toward providing critical information relevant to both the diagnostic and therapeutic processes. It describes and elucidates symptomatology, more thoroughly examines the sensory and motor aspects of the oral mechanism, and helps determine the need and readiness for further diagnostic workup. Clinical assessment of a patient should *always* be performed before any diagnostic swallowing procedure such as videofluoroscopy or flexible endoscopic evaluation of swallowing (FEES).

Clinical assessment also allows the examiner to determine optimal timing if further evaluation is needed. For example, results of videofluoroscopic examination may be affected by days post trauma or crucial event and should, therefore, be performed when the patient will benefit most from the information gathered by the test. Indications for clinical exam may also change and be appropriate at different times during different phases of a patient's treatment. For example, if a patient with a diagnosis of head and neck cancer is undergoing radiation therapy, repeat clinical exams may be appropriate at different intervals throughout the therapy, depending on the patient's progress.

Triage and clinical investigation of radiographic study referrals will also eliminate misguided requests. For example, mix-ups in terminology can result in unnecessary studies, as "barium swallow" and "swallow study" are long accepted names for radiological evaluations of the esophagus.

## LIMITATIONS

The clinical swallowing examination is crucial in any assessment of swallowing function, but it is not all inclusive. It does not allow evaluation of the entire swallowing tract and thus cannot provide certain information regarding oral, pharyngeal, and laryngeal structures and function. Because the pharynx is not visualized, it cannot provide information about timing of the swallow or pharyngeal strength, including ability to constrict or if residue remains after the swallow. Because the larynx is not visualized, it cannot provide definitive information about whether a patient is aspirating or why aspiration is occurring (Linden, Kuhlemeier, & Patterson, 1993; Splaingard, Hutchins, Sulton, & Choudhuri, 1988). It is not meant as a substitute for the current gold standard of dysphagia assessment (i.e., the dynamic swallow study).

Limitations on the clinical swallow evaluation may also be imposed by other factors such as the environment or the patient themselves, allowing only a partial exam. For example, if a patient is for some reason unable to physically cooperate with a full exam, a history may be obtained from other sources such as the patient's chart and the referral source, and a limited physical evaluation performed. If no food is available for oral feeding, a clinician may need to rely on what is available, and limit the exam.

## EQUIPMENT

Basic supplies are a small flashlight and a tongue blade. A lateral view diagram of normal anatomy is useful for explaining normal swallowing to the patient. Other supplies may include the following: small laryngeal mirror (for tactile and/or cold stimulation); feeding apparatus such as a spoon and cup, possibly a syringe and catheter, straw, or pipette; food and liquid such as water, ice chips, thick liquid, puree, cracker, or other similar solid requiring some chewing; emesis basin; washcloth, towel, or paper towels. Suction should be available if problems with airway maintenance are anticipated. Equipment helpful for introducing stimuli without food (and in therapy) includes gauze rolls or gauze to wrap around flexible straws, and lemon juice, sugar water, and saline. A "clinical swallowing kit" containing these items may help the clinician be better prepared for clinical swallowing evaluations. Conversely, if any or all of these items are not available, valuable information will still be gleaned from the clinical evaluation, but may be more limited in scope.

## TASKS/EVALUATION

### Medical History

Gathering of a complete and thorough medical and feeding history is critical. Pertinent medical history should be gleaned from the patient's medical chart and gathered by communication with professionals involved in the patient's care, including the referral source. The patient's primary diagnosis, general medical status, and referral question should be understood and discussed with the referral source and the patient's physician. The specific concerns of the referrer can then be addressed directly in the assessment report and recommendations. Equally important is the patient's complaint or concerns, as they sometimes differ from the concerns of the referral source.

Gathering of case history should follow the model of the standard history and physical interview, beginning with identifying information and patient complaint. The complaint is then elucidated, citing onset time and type, symptoms, precipitating events, and current manifestations and character. Past medical history should cover multiple systems, including cardiac, pulmonary, gastrointestinal, neurological, otolaryngological, and so on. Cardiac problems or illnesses of other types should be noted, as their affect on general patient conditioning and fatigue may prove important (Selnes & McKhann, 2005). Airway status should be understood, with consultation with the patient's physician and/or a pulmonologist or otolaryngologist, if warranted. Pulmonary problems should be recorded, including history and types of pneumonia, as well as any disease process that may contribute to pulmonary compromise and lower tolerance for aspiration. Gastrointestinal information is important, especially a history of gastroesophageal reflux, as problems in this area may directly or indirectly impact laryngeal, pharyngeal, and oral symptoms and problems (Groher, 1984). Neurological problems could impact sensory and/or motor systems for swallowing, and should be recorded. Information from otolaryngological, or head and neck, exam, is crucial in understanding known problems of the oral, pharyngeal, and laryngeal anatomy. Report of mouth care and dental condition is important if available (Langmore et al., 1998; Loeb, Becker, Eady, & Walker-Dilks, 2003). If the vocal folds were observed during motion, their ability to adduct adequately will be important in determining adequate airway protection, as well as laryngeal sensation.

Any other medical problems, hospitalizations, and surgeries should be recorded, including dates of occurrence. Prior voice, speech, or swallowing problems, and intervention given, be it medical, surgical, or radiological, may impact swallowing and thus should be noted. Psychiatric and social history, including independence and availability of support, may impact the diagnostic and/or rehabilitative processes, and should be included, if relevant. A list of medications currently taken is important, as medications may cause xerostomia, drowsiness, or other symptoms relevant to swallowing. The clinician's questions are guided by his or her knowledge of the complaint and history as he or she develops the differential diagnosis.

## Feeding History

### A. Method and Schedule of Feeding or Eating

The current method of nutritional intake is noted (i.e., oral with utensils or syringe, or nonoral feeding tubes, such as nasogastric, gastrostomy, duodenum, or jejunum tubes). Some of these methods may be used in combination, with one supplementing the other (see Chapter 10). Thus it is important to ask the patient or caregiver which feeding method is used at what time and with what substances.

### B. Diet

Note the type, amount, and frequency of food and liquid intake, as well as preferences. Preferences for certain substances may tell you about the patient's comfort level managing certain foods. Has the patient changed his or her eating habits because of the complaint? Does he or she seek out or avoid certain foods or liquids? Ask about changes over the course of a day. For instance, does the person eat more or less at one time of day than another?

### C. Onset of Problem

The time and date of the onset of swallowing problems, and whether gradual or sudden, should be noted. Were problems concurrent with other medical problems, or did they occur following particular incidents?

### D. Description of Problem

Whenever possible, the swallowing problem should be described in detail by the patient. During the interview, it can be important to focus the patient on their symptom descriptions, rather than the perceived diagnosis. Questions should attempt to elicit symptoms, current manifestations and the character of the swallowing problem.

1. *Context:* When do swallow problems occur? Do they occur at particular times of the day or during particular meals, and when during these meals (beginning, middle, end of meals, or after)? Are these meals at home, outside the home, with others, or when alone? (Are distractions such as talking during swallowing occurring?) Do the same or similar problems occur at other times besides eating?

2. *Cough or choke:* Do coughing and/or choking occur, and with what frequency and severity? Is the problem a tickle to which the patient responds or an uncontrollable cough? Has it interfered with breathing? Does it occur during or after swallowing, and/or at other times of the day, when meals are not being taken? Does the food "get stuck?" Ask the patient to point to "sticking" point. Does it eventually go down or need a liquid wash to clear? If the patient regurgitates or coughs, was it uncontrolled or was it done to relieve the sensation of food sticking? Has the patient needed the Heimlich maneuver to dislodge material from the airway?

3. *Weight loss:* Has the patient experienced recent weight change, and has this been because of a change in eating habits? Note the patient's height and present weight compared to past weight.

4. *Localization and characterization:* Are there any other subjective descriptions of the problem? Can the patient point to the area in the mouth, throat, or chest where the problems seem to occur? Does the food "pocket" in certain areas? Is there any pain associated with swallowing? Have appetite changes been experienced? Does the patient experience dry mouth?

5. *Social or emotional impact:* How does the patient feel about the swallowing problem? Is it of concern? Have experiences with swallowing been frightening? Does the patient have a certain eating goal? A checklist may also be employed to record the patient's subjective impression of the swallowing problem on his or her quality of life.

### E. Variability

The variable characteristics of the problem should be described, such as:

1. *Foods:* Do problems occur with certain foods or food types? Note whether problems occur usually with liquids and/or solids, and the texture and consistency of those foods. This information may be used later in trial swallows. Are some foods easier to swallow than others? More difficult? Are liquids difficult to control? Do particular foods get "stuck"? Ask about dental care and problems chewing as this is often overlooked as an important factor with solids.

2. *Temperature:* Is the ease of swallowing affected by the temperature of the food? Are hot or cold foods easier or more difficult to swallow? This information may provide subtle clues or signs of a delayed swallowing response (i.e., if the patient finds cold foods easier to swallow, it may indicate a cold stimulus can facilitate swallow initiation).

3. *Time:* How long does it take to eat a meal? Is this usual for the patient? Longer eating times may indicate more problems are occurring during the meal, or that the patient is eating more slowly to compensate for problems. Again, when does the problem occur during the meal? Does the problem happen outside of meal time?

4. *Secretions:* How is the patient handling secretions? Are there problems with drooling? Are secretions copious, or conversely, is there a lack of saliva? (Xerostomia may occur as a consequence of radiation therapy, and dry mouth outside of eating is a common side effect of some medications.)

### F. Compensations

What has the patient found helpful in dealing with the swallowing problem? Have any particular strategies been useful in helping the patient compensate? Consider the following:

1. *Rate:* Is the patient altering the rate of eating, slower or faster, to better handle food?

2. *Consistency:* Has the consistency of foods eaten been altered? Are certain foods blended or avoided?

3. *Posture:* Are particular body postures or positions (i.e., leaning, tucking the chin) helpful to swallowing? Does the patient think neck extension helps?

4. *Other:* Have any other tactics proven useful? Is food placed in a certain place in the oral cavity to facilitate chewing and/or swallowing? Is a syringe used for food placement, or a straw for drinking? Have the amounts of food attempted on one swallow been altered? Does the patient think coughing or throat-clearing help?

## Clinical Examination or Observation

### A. Overall Conditioning, Including Cognition or Alertness/Endurance

The patient's general overall conditioning, level of awareness, alertness, and cooperation should be noted, along with apparent strength and potential for fatigue. Readiness for a radiographic study may also be assessed at this time: A person should be awake, alert, and able to accept food voluntarily during the study.

### B. Body Tone, Size, Posture, or Positioning

The general body tone and specific oral tone are important to note, as well as the patient's typical sitting position during eating, and whether or not postural support is required. For the radiographic study, the patient must be positioned in a reasonably appropriate posture in the radiology suite, so size and upper body postural support needs may be crucial factors. If special chairs or other accommodations are needed for special positioning, these should be considered, especially if further diagnostic testing is necessary.

### C. Airway

Status of the airway should be noted. If the patient is breathing through a tracheostomy tube, the type and status (cuffed or uncuffed) of the tube should be recorded. Note if breathing appears labored or audible in any way before, during, or after the evaluation.

### D. Following Instructions

How well is the patient able to follow directions? Are verbal or gestural cues needed to elicit desired behaviors? Is demonstration needed for imitation? Does a hearing loss or vision problem impact perception, and can compensation be made for this?

### E. Self-Feeding Potential

Is the patient able to feed independently, and to what degree?

### F. Direct Physical Evaluation

1. Oral phase
   a. *Structure:* The jaw, dentition, lips, tongue, buccal cavity, palate, and velum should all be observed carefully. Tissue condition, including color, configuration, shape, size, symmetry, and any additional findings such as scarring or tethering should be recorded. Observe the presence or absence of tonsil, including size, placement, and condition. Missing teeth, especially molars used for grinding and chewing, are important to note.
   b. *Sensation:* Sensitivity in and around the oral cavity can be assessed by applying light touch to areas of the lips, tongue, buccal cavity, and so on. Areas of reduced or hypersensitivity should be noted, as well as unilateral differences. This information may have im-

plications for bolus management and trigger of the swallow sequence. Noting the area of impaired sensation should provide information about particular cranial nerve involvement. Facial sensation is controlled by cranial nerve (CN) V (Trigeminal). Sensation for the anterior two thirds of the tongue is provided by the lingual nerve, a branch of CN V. (Taste for the anterior two thirds of the tongue is provided by CN VII [Facial].) Sensation and taste for the posterior one third of the tongue and the pharynx is provided by CN IX (Fuller, 1993).

   c. *Reflexes and responses/nonvolitional movements:* Assessment of normal oral reflexes in the adult is usually limited to the gag reflex, as other primitive reflexes are usually not present beyond 6 to 8 months of age. Impairment of reflexes and responses, or presence of primitive or infantile reflexes, such as the bite reflex, may suggest neurological problems (Groher, 1984). Presence or absence of reflexes and responses, and symmetry of movement, are usually noted by tactile stimulation with a tongue blade.
      (1) The gag reflex includes a head and jaw extension, rhythmical tongue protrusions, and pharyngeal contractions in response to stimulation at the posterior part of the oral cavity, usually the faucial pillars or base of the tongue.

(2) The transverse tongue response is a lateral movement of the tongue in response to tactile stimulation at the lateral border.

(3) The bite reflex is clamping of the teeth or up and down movement of the jaw in response to stimulation of the gum, molar, or sometimes other dental surfaces.

d. *Volitional movement:* Volitional movements of the oral-motor mechanism should be assessed in terms of strength, rate, accuracy, and range of motion. Again, noting the area of impairment should provide information about particular cranial nerve involvement.

(1) Jaw: Ability to open and close the jaw, relative ease, and amount of movement should be observed. Jaw opening may actually be measured in millimeters to note any significant trismus, and to compare to normative data. Measurements may be compared to normative data to note limitations (interincisal distance in adults should approximate 40 to 50 mm; if below 20 to 25 mm, it may impact introduction of food into oral cavity) (Gelb, 1985). Ask the patient to clench the teeth, while palpating masseter and temporalis muscles for evidence of contractions. Muscles of motor control of mastication are controlled by CN V (Trigeminal) (Fuller, 1993).

(2) Lips: Labial closure at rest and during swallowing should be observed to note the patient's ability to maintain lip competence and to breathe through the nose during eating. Pursing and retraction of the lips should be noted in isolation and in alternating tasks. Note symmetry of smile and showing of teeth. Muscles of facial expression are controlled by CN VII (Facial) (Fuller, 1993).

(3) Tongue: Anterior lingual movement may be assessed by having the patient extend, lateralize, elevate, and depress the tip, and by having the patient sweep the tongue from the front to the back of the oral cavity along the roof of the mouth. Note symmetry, strength, range of motion, accuracy of movement, and mark inaccurate, weak movements, or searching behaviors. Posterior lingual movement can be observed by having the patient elevate the back of the tongue, as in producing a /k/ sound. Strength can be assessed by asking the patient to push the tongue into the cheek on both sides. Is the cheek pushed outward by this gesture? Lingual movement is controlled by CN XII (Hypoglossal) (Fuller, 1993).

(4) Velum: Movement of the velum, or soft palate, may be assessed by having the

patient open the mouth, and then observing palatal movement during production of a sustained /a/ sound. Amount and vigor of elevation, as well as symmetry, can be noted. Compare to gag movement. Palatal, pharyngeal, and laryngeal movement are controlled by CN IX (Glossopharyngeal) and CN X (Vagus) (Fuller, 1993).

e. *Oral sensorimotor integrity:* In addition to assessing isolated sensory versus oral-motor skills, the integrity of the two working in concert may be important to explore systematically, as the unique interplay of sensation and movement may have implications for bolus manipulation and the oral stage of swallowing. For example, the light touch sensation of a small bolus may not be enough to allow adequate oral manipulation or to trigger a swallow response. A bolus with greater mass or heavier weight, however, may stimulate an adequate motor response.

f. *Secretions:* Oral secretions should be observed, including approximate amount and type, and how the patient manages these during the assessment. The patient may be swallowing, or actively or passively expectorating. Inquiry should be made regarding changes in secretion type, amount or management.

g. *Articulation:* Observation of a patient's articulatory behaviors and patterns may offer much information about oral function. For instance, ability to produce an anterior lingua-alveolar stop /t/ may provide information about anterior lingual movement and control, just as production of /k/ may provide information about posterior lingual movement and control. These sounds should be elicited in diadochokinetic tasks to note agility and speed. Articulation in connected speech may give an indication of the precision of movement of articulatory structures.

h. *Resonance:* Observe resonance during speech for problems with oral-nasal coupling. Be alert to problems with velar function that could impact bolus containment and pressure generation.

2. Pharyngeal and laryngeal evaluation

a. *Vocal quality or changes:* Note changes in vocal quality from the norm, such as hoarseness or breathiness. This could possibly indicate a problem with laryngeal anatomy or function, which may relate to problems with closure to protect the airway. If otolaryngology consultation has not been obtained, problems in this area may indicate a need for it.

b. *Pitch control or range:* The patient should be asked (or this behavior should be elicited through demonstration) to glide up and down his or her pitch range to assess laryngeal agility. This may provide some information about laryngeal control and elevation.

c. *Breathing:* Note any problems with breathing, including stridor or audible breath sounds at rest, which may alert the clinician to respiratory compromise. Note weak vocal intensity or the reported phenomenon of "running out of air" or becoming short of breath, with or without speech.

d. *Volitional cough or throat clear:* Assess the patient's ability to cough or throat-clear on command by simply asking the patient to cough and clear the throat. The behavior may also be demonstrated to obtain an imitative response. Your goal is to assess the ability to volitionally expectorate aspirated material.

e. *Saliva swallow and laryngeal management:* During the clinical examination, before assessing a liquid or food swallow, the examiner should listen carefully to the patient's voice to note any lack of clarity, "wetness," and so on. Note whether the patient coughs or clears the throat during the interview. The patient may be asked to initiate a "dry" swallow of saliva present, and cough and throat-clear, with voice quality noted afterwards.

f. *Liquid and/or food swallow:* Liquid and/or food swallow during clinical evaluation should only be attempted under safe circumstances. Ideally, suction should be available in case problems are encountered with either aspiration or food retrieval. Usually, a small bolus is given to determine management, ability to swallow, and clinical signs of aspiration. However, the patient should not be given any substance that may compromise his or her health. First, note the patient's ability to contain the bolus within the oral cavity. Oral manipulation of the bolus is better observed with purees or solids. Timing and effortfulness of the swallow may be grossly observed, as well as the presence or absence of cough or throat-clear following the attempt. The patient's voice should then be attended to for lack of clarity, "wetness," and so on.

(The form used for bedside evaluation is included in Appendix 8A at the end of this chapter.)

## IMPRESSIONS AND RECOMMENDATIONS

A summary of the clinical findings should contain information relevant to the swallowing problem and provide an impression of factors that may impact and, in fact, dictate further intervention. If the clinical assessment reveals only oral problems or cognitive/behavioral problems, recommendations and therapy usually can be planned without further studies.

If there are indications of problems at the pharyngeal or laryngeal stages of swallowing, further studies may be recommended; for example, a dynamic swallowing study may be indicated to provide information about the safety of continuing oral feeding and/or to determine more specific techniques to manage the swallowing problem. Most obviously, if a person demonstrates coughing or choking during eating, further studies of the swallowing mechanism would be indicated. If inability to maintain nutrition or hydration by mouth has resulted in weight loss or compromised health, further studies may be warranted. If pulmonary health has suffered, imaging of the swallow may provide illumination. And if known problems exist, imaging may guide the development of strategies to improve swallow safety and/or efficiency.

The specific findings of the clinical evaluation will facilitate procedural considerations during the radiographic study. If a patient has posturing or movement limitations, mechanical adjustments may be anticipated and changed. If certain substances are tolerated differently during swallow, by observation or report, they may be used following administration of the standard protocol.

The clinical swallow evaluation may also provide baseline information about swallowing function, making it easier to track and compare a patient's swallowing ability over time. If the patient is not ready for a further workup initially, some aspects of the evaluation may be repeated over time to determine readiness for further workup at a later date.

In summary and reiteration, the clinical swallowing evaluation is a first and crucial step toward providing critical information relevant to both the diagnostic and therapeutic processes. It describes and elucidates symptomatology, more thoroughly examines the sensory and motor aspects of the oral mechanism, and helps determine the need and

readiness for further diagnostic workup. Clinical assessment of a patient should *always* be performed before any diagnostic swallowing procedure such as videofluoroscopy or FEES.

## STUDY QUESTIONS

1. Why are history and physical evaluations necessary before further imaging studies, such as videofluroscopic evaluation?
2. What are some reasons you may not recommend further studies after your clinical evaluation?
3. What are the clinical signs and symptoms of silent aspiration?
4. What are the symptoms of left cranial nerve XII damage and what oral problems would you expect to find during your evaluation?
5. Describe the clinical impact of xerostomia (i.e., what might be the effect on eating and swallowing)?

## REFERENCES

Cherney, L. R. (1994). *Clinical management of dysphagia in adults and children*. Aspen, MD: Aspen.

Fuller, G. (1993). *Neurological examination made easy*. New York: Churchill Livingstone.

Gelb, H. (1985). Patient evaluation. In H. Gelb (Ed.), *Clinical management of head, neck and TMJ pain and dysfunction* (Chap. 3), Philadelphia: W.B. Saunders.

Groher, M. E. (1984). *Dysphagia diagnosis and management*. Stoneham, MA: Butterworth.

Langmore, S. E., Terpenning, M. S., Schork, A., Chen, Y., Murray, J. T., Lopatin, D., et al. (1998). Predictors of aspiration pneumonia: How important is dysphagia? *Dysphagia, 13*, 69–81.

Linden, P., Kuhlemeier, K. V., & Patterson, C. (1993). The probability of correctly predicting subglottic penetration from clinical observations. *Dysphagia, 8*, 170–179.

Loeb, M. B., Becker, M., Eady, A., & Walker-Dilks, C. (2003). Interventions to prevent aspiration pneumonia in older adults: A systematic review. *Journal of American Geriatric Society, 51*, 1018–1022.

Logemann, J. A. (1983). *Evaluation and treatment of swallowing disorders*. Boston: College-Hill Press.

Selnes, O. A., & McKhann, G. M. (2005). Neurocognitive complications after coronary artery bypass surgery. *Annals of Neurology, 57*, 615–621.

Splaingard, M. L., Hutchins, B., Sulton, L. D., & Chaudhuri, G. (1988). Aspiration in rehabilitation patients: Videofluoroscopy vs bedside clinical assessment. *Archives of Physical Medicine and Rehabilitation, 69*, 637–640.

Steefel, J. S. (1981). *Dysphagia rehabilitation for adults*. Springfield, IL: Charles C Thomas.

**Clinical Swallow Evaluation Form**
UNIVERSITY OF CALIFORNIA, DAVIS MEDICAL CENTER
SACRAMENTO, CALIFORNIA

# OPD PROGRESS RECORD

*VOICE, SPEECH AND SWALLOWING CENTER*                    OTOLARYNGOLOGY CLINIC

**PT. NAME:** _____     **UCD ID#:** _____

**BIRTHDATE:** _____     **DATE OF VISIT:** _____

**Diagnosis:** _____     **Referral:** _____

**Concern on referral:** _____

**Related Medical Hx/results of testing:**
*Cardiac:*
*GI:*
*Pulmonary:*
*Neurological:*
*ENT:*
*Other:*
*Dental:*
*Medications:*
*Speech/Voice:*
*Services:*
*Social/Family:*

**Feeding Hx:**
*Method:*
*Schedule:*
*Onset:*
*Variability:*       secretions:                 foods:
                     temperature:                time of day/meal:
*Cough/choke:*       context:                    frequency/severity:
*Compensations:*     rate:
                     consistencies (prep, alternate, avoid):
                     posture:
*Weight:*            present:        usual:      time/loss:

**Clinical Observations:**
*Airway:*            trach:          cuffed/uncuffed:
                     voluntary cough:              breath-hold:

                     <u>labial</u>   <u>lingual</u>   <u>palatal</u>   <u>mandibular</u>   <u>dental</u>
*Oral exam:*         structure:
                     tone:
                     movement:
                     sense:
                     reflexes:
                     secretions:

*continues*

*continued*

|  | labial | lingual | palatal | mandibular | dental |
|---|---|---|---|---|---|
| *Speech:* articulation: | | | | | |
| voice: | | | | | |
| intelligibility: | | | | | |
| resonance: | | | | | |

| *Swallow:* | substance/delivery system | cough/choke | voice | other |
|---|---|---|---|---|
| liquid: | | | | |
| puree/pudding: | | | | |
| cracker/solid: | | | | |

# 9

# *Pediatric Clinical Feeding Assessment*

**Janet Pitcher**
**Margie Crandall**
**Susan J. Goodrich**

Pediatric feeding problems have been recognized in the literature for the past 35 to 40 years (Illingworth, 1969; Logan & Bosma, 1967). Although no comprehensive definition of pediatric feeding problems has been widely accepted, infants and children experiencing feeding difficulties may demonstrate a refusal to eat orally, have difficulty with the act of feeding, or be unable to sustain oral feedings to maintain adequate caloric intake. Feeding problems have been defined by both etiology and function, including categories of food refusal, food selectivity by type or texture, oral-motor delays, or dysphagia (Babbit, Hoch, & Coe, 1994; Field, Garland, & Williams, 2003). In fact, some authors have proposed, and more studies are indicating, that most feeding problems have underlying organic causes (Manikam & Perman, 2000).

Clinically, the health care provider may note that the infant/child is failing to thrive, has impaired oral feeding skills, is potentially aspirating, and/or has difficulty transitioning from enteral to oral feedings. Despite the lack of a universally accepted definition of pediatric feeding problems, numerous articles have identified groups of children who are at risk for feeding problems (Arvedson & Brodsky, 1994; Bier, Ferguson, Cho, Oh, & Vohr, 1993; Case-Smith, Cooper, & Scala, 1989; Herbst, 1981; Imhoff & Wigginton, 1991; Luiselli, 1994; Mercado-Deane et al., 2001; Morris & Klein, 2000; Mueller, 1972; Palmer, Crawley, & Blanco, 1993; Reilly & Skuse, 1992; Reilly, Skuse, Mathisen, & Dieter, 1995; Samour & King, 2005; Stevenson & Allaire, 1991). Table 9–1 lists commonly associated etiologies.

**Table 9-1.** Common Etiologies Associated with Feeding Problems

| |
|---|
| Neurological dysfunction |
| Gastrointestinal diseases or dysfunction |
| Cardiorespiratory compromise |
| Sensory deprivation |
| Structural anomalies |
| Social-behavioral maladaptation |

*Source:* Adapted from "Identifying feeding and swallowing problems in infants and young children." By S. Imhoff and V. Wigginton, 1991, *Clinical Communication Disorders, 1,* 59–67.

More information is now available to provide a basis for assessing feeding problems in children (Arvedson & Brodsky, 1994; Einarsson-Backes, Deitz, Price, Glass, & Hays, 1994; Field et al., 1982; Frappier, Marino, & Shishmanian, 1987; Gisel, 1994; Herbst, 1981; Imhoff & Wigginton, 1991; Measel & Anderson, 1979; Meier & Anderson, 1987; Mueller, 1972; Palmer, Crawley, & Blanco, 1993; Reilly & Skuse, 1992; Reilly et al., 1995; Rogers & Arvedson, 2005; Skuse, Stevenson, Reilly, App, & Mathisen, 1995; Stevenson & Allaire, 1991). Evidence suggests that inadequate nutritional intake is associated with behavioral, developmental, and cognitive impairments (Luiselli, 1994; Oates, Peacock, & Forrest, 1985; Sanders, Patel, LeGrice, & Shepherd, 1993; Singer & Fagan, 1984), and that critical, sensitive periods of feeding development may be influenced by delay of oral feeding or stimulation (Beratis, Kolb, Sperling, & Stein, 1981; Illingworth & Lister, 1964). Therefore, a feeding assessment that provides a framework for early intervention is critical when there is a question whether a child has feeding difficulties.

A clinical feeding assessment is a comprehensive, systematic biopsychosocial approach to the evaluation of a child with feeding difficulties. The assessment can help professionals identify potential or actual feeding problems, including possible etiologies, and develop appropriate interventions. The diagnostic use and value of instrumental procedures including the dynamic swallow study in infants and children is not discussed here (see Chapter 7), but may complement the clinical feeding assessment presented.

A comprehensive feeding assessment includes the medical history, feeding history, developmental history, anatomy and physiology, diet, and psychosocial environment, including a caregiver interview. Assessment involves not only review of a patient's medical chart and direct patient examination, as in the adult patient, but should include a review of the child's educational and therapeutic records. Additionally, in this population, one must consider the complex nature of parent-child interactions and their influence on feeding and swallowing behaviors.

The pediatric feeding assessment is best approached by a multidisciplinary team (Manikam & Perman, 2000). Team members may include the following: physicians, including specialty physicians such as pediatric otolaryngologists, pediatric gastroenterologists, developmental pediatricians, pediatric neurologists, pediatric pulmonologists, pediatric radiologists if radiographic testing is included in the assessment, and pediatric psychiatrists; nurses, including clinical nurse specialists in feeding, neurology, gastroenterology, pulmonology, etc.; speech pathologists and occupational therapists with specialties in dysphagia; nutritionist/dieticians; behavioral psychologists; and social workers.

## PEDIATRIC FEEDING ASSESSMENT

The feeding assessment consists of five parts:

1. Data Collection (obtained before evaluating the child)
2. Nutritional Screening, Feeding History, and Developmental Milestones (obtained from parent or caregiver interview)
3. Physical Assessment
4. Oral Sensory-Motor and Feeding Skills Assessment
5. Psychosocial Interactional Assessment

### 1. Data Collection

Data collection is done before the evaluation of the child. Data collection includes a review of the infant or child's:

- Medical history
- Growth chart
- Current clinical nutritional status

#### Medical History

The medical history review includes evaluating the perinatal and neonatal history, medical diagnosis, previous hospitalizations, and significant illnesses, focusing on organic precursors or causes of feeding problems. The perinatal and neonatal history may provide information detailing any fetal distress, the infant's response during delivery, prematurity, any significant congenital anomalies, and any major illness during the first few months of life. Congenital anomalies, central nervous system insults, or chronic illnesses may affect the child's ability to eat orally. For example, respiratory problems may make it difficult for the infant to breathe comfortably during feeding, cardiac problems may contribute to fatigue during feeding sessions, and/or gastroesophageal reflux may cause association of feeding with discomfort. Neurological problems may prevent the development of normal oral-motor skills as well as interfere with the pharyngeal swallow. Previous hospitalizations and significant illnesses can influence or disrupt the child's developmental skills, including feeding skills. As stated earlier, all or any of these findings can be associated with the infant or child's refusal to eat, oral-motor organization, and/or ability to sustain adequate oral intake. All should be noted when taking a medical history, as well as current health status and medications taken.

#### Growth Chart

It is critical to review the growth chart to determine the child's nutritional status. Prolonged inadequate caloric intake results in an infant or child nutritionally failing to thrive. A child is defined as having failure to thrive when: (1) the weight-to-length ratio is <5% for age and gender, or body mass index (BMI) for children beginning at age 2 years, (2) the weight is <5% for age and gender, or (3) the weight percentage has decreased two standard deviations or more below the norm. In the United States, growth charts were developed by the National Center for Health Statistics in collaboration with the Centers for Disease Control, based on data from national probability samples. The 2000 CDC growth charts represent the revised version of the 1977 NCHS growth charts. These growth charts now have body mass index-for-age charts. They are available through the CDC at www.cdc.gov/growthcharts. However, other growth charts for some specific patient populations, such as Down syndrome and premature infants, are available. An example of a growth chart is provided in Appendix 9-A.

The causes of failure to thrive may be organic (physical cause), nonorganic (psychosocial), or a combination of both. However, not all growth patterns are strictly related to nutrition. The child's medical condition may influence individual patterns of growth. For example, genetic or intrauterine insults (i.e., fetal alcohol syndrome) may result in growth retardation, with the infant's weight, height, weight for height ratio, and head circumference being less than the fifth percentile for age and gender.

### Current Clinical Nutritional Status

A review of the current clinical nutritional status should include laboratory tests and possibly anthropometrics. Laboratory tests can help define nutritional deficiencies. The most readily available screening tests are the complete blood count and a chemistry panel. A complete blood count may reveal concerns such as iron-deficiency anemia or altered immune status. The chemistry panel may reveal electrolyte abnormalities (i.e., sodium and chloride) and protein deficiency (i.e., a low albumin and total protein). Anthropometrics measures triceps skinfold thickness and mid-arm circumference as a serial indicator of body fat and muscle mass (American Academy of Pediatrics, 1985). Anthropometrics may be a preferred measurement of nutritional status compared to growth charts when the infant or child's age is unclear.

## 2. Nutritional Screening, Feeding History, and Developmental Milestones

This information is usually elicited from the parent or caregiver. Feeding history should include past methods and patterns of feeding from birth onward, including transitions to new foods/textures. It is useful to know when the feeding problem began, what medical and social circumstances existed at the time, and the course of progression. The current feeding status needs to include the parent's perception of the feeding problem or difficulty and a thorough description of the child's mealtimes, including the method and schedule of feeding. Information gathered should include type of food, amounts, textures, temperatures, duration of feeding, physical environment including seating and posture, family members usually present, the child's behavior, and any interventions attempted. A 24-hour dietary recall of the child's feeding routine and schedule is helpful to assess individual nutritional patterns. A review of the child's developmental progress with the parent or caregiver helps them to understand what general skills the child has that relate to the child's ability to eat. Normal feeding skills will be discussed later under oral sensory-motor and feeding skills.

## 3. Physical Assessment

An assessment of the child's general physical appearance and findings will provide information about the child's nutritional status. When performing this assessment, one must consider the infant or child's:

- Behavior
- Development
- Physical appearance

### Behavior

When observing the behavioral state, observe how the child acts. Is the child alert, active, irritable, or apathetic? The alert and rested child provides the most realistic information about feeding behaviors. Irritability and apathy are commonly seen with malnutrition.

Observe also the child's apparent response to food presentation and attitude toward eating: is the child hungry, cautious, anxious, relaxed? Is this behavior in direct response to food presentation or to any other stimulus during the feeding?

### Development

The developmental assessment involves observing the child's fine and gross motor skills and muscle tone. Is the child performing tasks at the expected age, or is the child showing some developmental delays? Many children who are developmentally delayed exhibit some alteration in muscle tone,

either hypertonia, hypotonia, or mixed tone. Both the child's motor skills and muscle tone influence his or her ability to eat.

### Physical Appearance

The physical appearance involves assessing the child's:

- Skin
- Hair
- Eyes
- Mouth and oral cavity

**Skin.** First, check the skin for color, bruises, rashes, and turgor. A pale color may indicate iron-deficiency anemia. Bruising may be due to vitamin K deficiency. Essential fatty acids, zinc, or vitamin deficiencies are known to cause skin rashes. When inadequate fluid intake accompanies poor caloric intake, the skin will be dry. Loose skin covering the decreased subcutaneous fat indicates both a calorie and protein inadequacy (marasmus). Excessive fluid retention resulting in edema may be due to insufficient protein intake (kwashiorkor) or electrolyte imbalances.

**Hair.** Check hair for texture, color, and distribution. Hair that is brittle, pale blond colored, and sparsely distributed is seen with protein malnutrition.

**Eyes.** Check eyes for hydration status and infection. Xerophthalmia, or dryness, may be due to vitamin A deficiency. Malnutrition can affect the immune system and cause conjunctivitis (Kleiman & Warman, 1994).

**Mouth and Oral Cavity.** The physical appearance of the mouth and oral cavity portion are checked as part of the oral reflexes and feeding skills evaluation, which is discussed next. Incorporating this aspect of the physical assessment with the evaluation of oral reflexes and feeding skills will diminish additional infant stress and crying associated with oral inspection.

## 4. Oral Sensory-Motor and Feeding Skills Assessment

The infant or child's oral sensory-motor and feeding skills determine the types of foods safely handled. During the first 3 years of life, dramatic oral-motor and developmental feeding skill changes have profound effects on the types of food, textures, and feeding methods the infant or child can safely control. (See Table 9–2 for pediatric feeding skills development.)

The approach recommended for assessing oral sensory-motor and feeding skills is to progress from the least frightening or threatening (external touching of the face and mouth) to the most threatening (internal inspection of the mouth).

Some oral reflexes are common to all ages, but the most rapid oral reflex and feeding skill changes occur in infancy. Therefore, the oral reflexes and feeding skills assessments will be divided into three infant developmental stages covering the first year of life:

- Birth to 4 months
- 5 to 7 months
- 8 to 12 months

It is important to note that, although infants are referred to in this section, the clinician may find similar primitive reflexes still present in an older child with neurological deficits. Reflexes that are common to all age groups will be explained once, during the assessment of the oral reflexes and feeding skills of the infant from birth to 4 months.

### Birth to 4 Months

Developmental feeding skills are affected by the infant's gestational age. For example, preterm infants frequently demonstrate generalized hypotonia and immature development of their suck/swallow/breathing, thus affecting their feeding efficiency. However, somewhere around 33 to 34 weeks gestation, the healthy growing premature infant's oral-motor maturation allows for suck/swallow/breathing coordination and the introduction of oral feedings (Casaer, Delieger, Decock, & Eggermont, 1982; Wolff, 1968). (See Table 9–2, Pediatric Feeding Skills Development; Preterm Infant.)

For term infants and premature infants whose postnatal age is corrected considering their prematurity the following reflexes and responses exist:

- Rooting reflex
- Suck reflex
- Bite reflex
- Gag reflex
- Tongue protrusion reflex
- Swallow reflex
- Lip and jaw closure
- Tongue mobility

When assessing these movements, start with the rooting reflex. Elicit the reflex by gently stroking the infant's cheek. The infant will turn his or her head toward the touch with mouth open. The rooting reflex disappears between 3 and 5 months.

**Table 9–2.** Pediatric Feeding Skills Development

| Age | Positional stability | Reflexes | Feeding skills | Types of food |
|---|---|---|---|---|
| Preterm infants (34–36 wks) | Lower tone<br>More extension<br>Reduced buccal pads<br>Reduced cup shape of tongue | Gag reflex develops usually around 32 weeks gestation<br>Suck reflex functionally mature at 32–34 weeks<br>Rooting reflex elicited at 32 weeks | Coordinated suck/swallow/breathing at 34–37 weeks<br>Feeding readiness: gags with gavage tube insertion, competently swallows oral secretions, demonstrates rhythmic nonnutritive suck | Breast milk or formula |
| Newborn to 3 months (full-term) | Buccal pads present<br>Lip closure<br>Cup-shaped tongue facilitates transfer of liquid to pharynx<br>Oral and pharyngeal structural mobility support both respiration and feeding<br>Limited neck stability | Gag reflex<br>Rooting reflex<br>Tongue protrusion reflex<br>Biting reflex<br>Suck/swallow reflex | Rhythmic sucking pattern (average 1 suck burst/second for nutritive sucking, 2 sucks/sec for nonnutritive suck)<br>Oral-pharyngeal area is shared for feeding and breathing<br>Hand to mouth activity<br>Hand reaching toward bottle | Breast milk or formula |
| 4–6 months | Increasing stability of neck and shoulders<br>Lower lip positions around spoon<br>Tongue fills less space in oral cavity allowing for greater mobility and posterior positional shift | Transitional period—primitive reflexes are disappearing except for gag reflex | Beginning of up-and-down chewing (munching)<br>Lateral tongue movement<br>Lip closure around spoon begins<br>Both hands to hold bottle<br>Cup drinking introduced | Breast milk or formula<br>May begin to introduce solid foods with spoon |

*(continues)*

**Table 9-2.** (continued)

| Age | Positional stability | Reflexes | Feeding skills | Types of food |
|---|---|---|---|---|
| 7–9 months | Teeth eruption (central and lateral incisors) Upper lip more mobility to stabilize spoon feeding | Gag reflex similar to adult | More mature lip movement, mobility, and stabilization Tongue lateralization present Rotary (diagonal) chewing begins Assisting with spoon Beginning to drink from cup held by caregiver | Breast milk or formula Finger foods Crackers, toast Soft fruits and vegetables Strained foods |
| 10–12 months | Molar eruption Corners of lips and cheek are drawn inward during chewing. The cheeks are used to control and move food | Gag reflex | Continued maturation of feeding skills Holding bottle or cup Liquid loss from mouth with cup drinking may be noted Pincer grasp Self-feeding by grasping spoon with whole hand Holds cup with two hands Has 4–5 consecutive swallows | Breast milk or formula Soft table foods |
| 13–18 months | External jaw stabilization begins Full eruption of incisors and molars increases the vertical diameter of oral cavity | Gag reflex | Up-and-down jaw movement stops Rotary chewing becomes more mature Increasing control of liquid during cup drinking Bites down on rim of cup Uses long sequence of drinking at one time Begins to develop controlled bite Chews with lips closed | Whole cow's milk Solid foods Chopped foods |

| Age | Positional stability | Reflexes | Feeding skills | Types of food |
|---|---|---|---|---|
| 19–24 months | | Gag reflex | No longer uses bite to stabilize cup for cup drinking<br>Child cleans lip with tongue<br>May begin to transfer food from one side of mouth to other side<br>Rotary chewing is mature<br>Begin to suck with a straw<br>Skills are refined for independent feeding | Chopped, fine food to regular firmer meats for chewing can be introduced |
| 25–36 months | Anatomic changes continue to place demands on oral sensory-motor agility, and adaptation: continued eruption of molars, inferior-anterior growth of the mandible, and descent of the hyoid and larynx with the hypopharynx. Changes continue through puberty. | Gag reflex is elicited from the posterior third of the tongue (as in adults) and by adulthood can be under some voluntary control. | Skills continue refinement (child develops finer control) as sensory-motor experience continues to shape central representation of feeding. Speech skills and head/neck postural stability develop in parallel with feeding maturation.<br><br>Electromyography suggests mastication coordination is fully mature at 3–6 years. | Regular table food. Concerns re judgment and distractibility may limit foods offered. |

The suck reflex is easily assessed following the rooting reflex. Alert the infant to your finger insertion by progressive touch from cheek to lip, then into the mouth. Gently insert finger with pad side up toward the hard palate. During the sucking reflex, the tongue extends over the gums or lip, with a motion moving from tongue tip to the back of the tongue. A pulling pressure is felt with the inserted finger being pulled to feel the soft palate. The sucking reflex disappears at approximately 6 months.

When assessing the rooting or suck reflexes, oral hypersensitivity may be noted. For example, the infant may demonstrate agitation, facial grimace, arching, and gagging even with gentle touching of the face. Oral hypersensitivity is defined as an aversion to touch or to eating food by mouth and/or food refusal of certain food types or textures. It may occur in children who have experienced prolonged periods of restricted eating or drinking, children who have experienced discomfort associated with feeding or even medical intervention, or children who have impaired oral sensory-motor feeding skills.

When assessing the mouth and oral cavity look at the structure and movement of the mouth and oral cavity, including:

- Gum and mucous membranes
- Palate
- Dentition
- Airway status, including jaw size and presence of tonsils
- Tongue

The gums are checked for hyperplasia (i.e., excessive growth of gum tissue) because of possible side effects of anti-convulsants. Both the gums and mucous membranes are observed for bleeding, sores, and hydration status. The palate is checked for architecture and cleft deformities. If teeth are present, they should be observed for number, caries, grinding, and occlusion. During the oral assessment, the bite reflex is assessed. The bite reflex is demonstrated during infancy by an up-and-down movement of the jaw. Pressure on the anterior and lateral aspects of the gums elicits this response. It usually disappears between 3 and 5 months.

Next assess the gag reflex. The gag reflex is present at birth and throughout our lives. It is elicited by placing a tongue blade on the anterior one third of the tongue and gently "walking back" until the tongue "humps" or elevates. This is one of the signs indicating the child can protect the airway during swallowing. An absent or diminished gag reflex may lead to aspiration. At this point, it is usually necessary to soothe and quiet the infant before proceeding.

Once the infant is quiet, assess the protrusion reflex. The tongue protrusion reflex is present during the first 4 months. This immature tongue movement pushes solid food out of the mouth when it is placed on the anterior part of the tongue. It can be assessed by placing a small quantity of food on the tongue and observing the tongue movement. The tongue protrusion reflex is one of the reasons why infants should not be fed solid foods for the first 4 to 6 months of life.

The swallow reflex can be observed or felt by the upward and forward movement of the cricoid cartilage during the introduction of liquids or solids. Listen for sound change including "wet"-sounding breathing or voice, as well as cough/choke. Coughing or choking may occur with an inadequate swallow, but is not always present during a clinical exam, even if the pharyngeal swallow is incompetent. If an incompetent pharyngeal swallow is suspected, or the child is at risk for pulmonary compromise, pharyngeal imaging may need to be considered (see criteria for Dynamic Swallow Study in other chapters).

Lip and jaw closure and tongue mobility are necessary for eating and swallowing. They can be assessed when observing a feeding or with infants when assessing the suck. Inadequate lip or jaw closure makes eating and swallowing difficult because of an inability to create adequate seal around the bottle, resulting in insufficient negative intraoral pressures. Impaired tongue mobility affects both intraoral pressure and oral transfer of a food bolus before swallow.

### 5 to 7 Months

This is a transitional time for the maturing infant. The infant is:

- Losing the primitive reflexes for rooting, sucking, biting, and tongue protrusion
- Gaining voluntary oral control by alerting with mouth opening at the sight of food, elevating the tongue, and beginning to manipulate food orally
- Starting to initiate self-feeding behaviors

Again assess the structure and movement of the mouth and oral cavity, including:

- Rooting reflex (disappearing at age 3–5 months)
- Suck reflex (disappearing at approximately age 6 months)
- Tongue movements (protrusion reflex disappearing at age 4 months)
- Bite reflex (disappearing at 3–5 months)
- Gag reflex (lifelong)

Besides assessing for previous physical findings, whenever possible, observe for maturing tongue movements. They include tongue elevation (tongue pushes back and touches palate) and lateral (side to side) movements.

To assess voluntary oral control, offer solid pureed food. When the food is first offered, voluntary alerting and mouth opening to accept food are seen in an infant at this stage. The infant may become very active and excited at the sight of food. It may be important to schedule the feeding assessment near or at a regularly scheduled mealtime to assess the infant's genuine response to food at a time normally fed.

If tongue elevation is not noted during the oral assessment, it can be assessed by offering food with a spoon. Tongue elevation clears food from the roof of the mouth and is necessary for the infant to eat and swallow pureed foods. Tongue elevation will be seen when the infant loses the protrusion reflex and gains the ability to manipulate and swallow pureed foods given by spoon. The swallow reflex may be assessed at this time (the same assessment previously described for the younger infant).

Food manipulation or munching involve jaw movements and tongue lateralization, (the ability of the tongue to move side to side). Jaw movements mash the food. Tongue lateralization enables the food to be moved to and from the gums and teeth for swallowing. The beginning stages of food manipulation or chewing start at 5 months of age with voluntary up-and-down jaw movements ("vertical munch"). Tongue lateralization begins at 6 to 7 months of age. The up-and-down jaw movements are followed by lateral jaw movements (and later by mature rotary movements: "rotary grind"). During this initial stage, up-and-down and lateral jaw movement, with tongue lateralization, are normal. Food manipulation can be evaluated by observing the infant's control of food. Jaw movements and tongue lateralization need to be noted. Tongue lateralization, if not observed during oral cavity assessment, can be judged by placing a small quantity of food on the gums, teeth, or in the lateral oral cavity and observing the infant's ability to mash or manipulate the food and then move it to the tongue for swallowing. Inadequate food manipulation or lack of tongue lateralization makes eating textured food difficult or impossible.

Self-feeding is observed during mealtime when food is offered. Self-feeding at this stage is demonstrated by:

- Increasing midline stability to sit independently and begin to hold a bottle or cup.
- The palmar grasp (the infant's ability to pick up large pieces of food between the thumb and palm.)
- Gross motor skills, including voluntary shoulder adduction and abduction, and elbow flexion with supination and pronation.

## 8 to 12 Months

During this stage there is a continued maturing of feeding skills. The important aspects of the feeding assessment are:

- Primitive reflexes disappear
- Food manipulation or chewing skills continue to develop
- Self-feeding skills continue to develop

First assess the mouth and oral cavity, including both structure and function, as mentioned previously. Teeth may be present, most notably, deciduous, or primary central incisors. Lateral incisors may be present or erupting. Voluntary tongue movements may be observed. Assess the gag reflex.

Next, offer the infant food and observe for:

- Voluntary oral control
- Voluntary alerting
- Tongue elevation
- Food manipulation or chewing

The up-and-down and lateral chewing now progresses to the beginning of a mature rotary-type movement. The infant's increasing number of teeth will enable him or her to handle more food textures and larger pieces of food, though true tearing of food may coincide more with eruption of the lateral canines at 16 to 23 months of age, and rotary chewing usually coincides more with eruption of the first molars, from 13 to 19 months of age. The swallow reflex is assessed while the infant is eating.

Self-feeding skills in this age group are demonstrated by:

- Midline stability to sit alone in the chair and to hold a bottle or cup.
- Maturing gross motor control enables easier cup holding with less spillage and smoother control of food from hand to mouth.
- Fine motor skills to self-feed progress from palmer to pincer grasp. The pincer grasp allows the infant to pick up food between his thumb and finger, enabling self-feeding with utensils and the ability to self-feed bite-size pieces of food.
- Independent eating is increasingly occurring as development progresses.

Feeding skills acquired during the first year of life are further refined during the toddler years. These are primarily chewing and further development of fine motor skills and control. See Table 9–2, Pediatric Feeding Skills Development.

## 5. Psychosocial Interactional Feeding Assessment

The relationship and interaction between the infant and parent or caregiver are extremely important. This interaction may have profound effects on the child's nutrition and feeding. For example, parents may be confused and not offer food to their infant if the infant does not provide clear hunger cues (i.e., agitation, crying, and mouth opening). In contrast, the infant who does provide clear cues may not be offered food if caregivers are insensitive to the cues. Therefore the quality of the interaction

between the parent or caregiver and infant may have a significant impact on the amount of food ingested, even if the infant has normal feeding skills. An interactional assessment tool such, as Parent-Child Feeding Scale (NCAST-AVENUW, 2006), provides information about the relationship between the parent and child during the feeding. This information focuses on the parent's sensitivity to the infant's cues, distress, social-emotional and cognitive growth fostering behavior, as well as the infant's clarity of cues and responsiveness to the parent.

In addition to observing interaction patterns, it is critical to note the behavior of the child before, during, and after the mealtime experience. The infant or child's cues of pleasure or distress are fundamental to determining how and where the feeding process is interrupted.

## INTERVENTIONS FOR PEDIATRIC FEEDING DIFFICULTIES

Comrie and Helm (1997) advocate a team approach to the child with feeding problems, stating the individual needs and cues of the child must be read, respected, and responded to, and families must be an integral part of the intervention. The individual infant or child's assessed feeding abilities determine the starting point and plan of interventions. Manikam and Perman (2000) advocate focus on antecedent manipulation (modifying and adapting the environment and caregiver behaviors) rather than relying on management of consequences. Dietician Ellyn Satter (2000) advocates a division of responsibility in successful feeding or eating, with parents being responsible for the what, when, and where of feeding, and children being responsible for how much and whether they eat. This way, the caregiver controls antecedents, yet the child is encouraged and allowed to explore eating at their own comfort and skill level. Common areas of intervention include positioning, control of environmental stimulation, appropriate feeding utensils, appropriate consistencies of food based on the assessed feeding skills level (see Table 9–2), and respect for the infant or child's behavioral cues of acceptance and refusal of food, all based on supporting the natural development of feeding skills.

Refusal to accept oral feedings may be due to a variety of reasons, including organic causes, sensory issues, motor difficulties, and fear due to real or perceived threat of aspiration. Manikam and Perman (2000) have suggested that feeding problems be viewed as on a continuum between organic and psychosocial factors. Therefore, force-feedings are discouraged. The purpose of a feeding evaluation is to determine "why" a child is not feeding appropriately, leading to interventions designed to support a normal developmental feeding sequence, allowing feeding to become both safe and pleasurable.

Infants and children who have feeding difficulties frequently require supplemental nutrition support, such as nasogastric or gastrostomy feedings. Supplemental feedings provide adequate nutrition whereas oral sensory-motor therapy is focused on maintaining and developing the infant or child's feeding skills. Specific stimulation treatments for children with oral-motor impairments are controversial and effi-

cacy is not yet definitively proven. Research is, however, ongoing, and in some instances encouraging (Lamm, DeFelice, & Cargan, 2005).

Interventions relating to feeding difficulties require significant time and investment by family and health care professionals. In addition, infants or children with feeding difficulties may plateau at various oral sensory-motor feeding skill developmental levels. Therefore, some infants or children may require long-term supplemental nutrition to sustain them. In cases where it is unsafe for the infant or child to eat (i.e., because of aspiration risk), the goal of therapy is usually good oral hygiene and dental care, and helping to maximize quality of life through safe patient nutritional intake and pleasurable family interaction.

## CONCLUSION

Various pediatric feeding problems have been identified for over 40 years. One approach to a comprehensive pediatric feeding assessment has been provided, based on normal feeding skills of children from birth to 3 years. This approach provides the practitioner with knowledge to identify potential or actual problems a child may have with eating.

From problem identification, appropriate supportive interventions can be provided to caregivers to help make eating a safe and pleasant experience for their child. Because feeding is a major component of the caregiver's role, information and interventions to help them in providing nutrition to the child will diminish family stress and support their role as caregivers.

## STUDY QUESTIONS

1. Who might be members of a Pediatric Swallowing Team, and what contributions might each make?
2. How might an infant's cardiac problems impact his or her feeding or eating?
3. What are the technical criteria for a diagnosis of "failure to thrive"?
4. What information about the child's feeding method, schedule, or behavior is important to elicit from the family or caregivers when taking a *feeding* history?
5. What is the difference between using antecedent manipulation versus focus on consequences to manage feeding behaviors? What might be advantages and disadvantages of each method?

## REFERENCES

American Academy of Pediatrics, Committee on Nutrition. (1985). In G. B. Forbes & C. W. Woodruff (Eds.), *Pediatric nutrition handbook* (2nd ed.). Elk Grove Village, IL: Author.

Arvedson, J. C., & Brodsky, L. (Eds.) (1994). *Pediatric swallowing and feeding: Assessment and management.* San Diego, CA: Singular.

Babbit, R. L., Hoch, T. A., & Coe, D. A. (1994). Behavioral feeding disorders. In D. N. Tuchman & R. Walters (Eds.), *Pediatric feeding and swallowing disorders: Pathophysiology, diagnosis and treatment* (pp. 77–96). San Diego, CA: Singular.

Beratis, S., Kolb, R., Sperling, E., & Stein, R. (1981). Development of child with long-lasting deprivation of oral feeding. *American Academy of Child Psychiatry, 20,* 53–64.

Bier, J. B., Ferguson, A., Cho, C., Oh, W., & Vohr, B. R. (1993). The oral motor development of low-birth-weight infants who underwent orotracheal intubation during the neonatal period. *American Journal of Diseases of Children, 147,* 858–862.

Casaer, D., Daniels, H., Devlieger, H., Decock, P., & Eggermont, E. (1982) Feeding behavior in preterm neonates. *Early Human Development, 7,* 331–346.

Case-Smith, J., Cooper, P., & Scala, V. (1989). Feeding efficiency of premature neonates. *American Journal of Occupational Therapy, 43,* 245–250.

Centers for Disease Control and Prevention, National Center for Health Statistics. CDC growth charts: United States. Available from: http://www.cdc.gov/growthcharts/ May 30, 2000.

Comrie, J., Helm, J. (1997). Common feeding problems in the intensive care nursery: Maturation, organization, evaluation, and management strategies. *Seminars in Speech and Language, 18,* 239–260.

Einarsson-Backes, L., Deitz, J., Price, R., Glass, R., & Hays, R. (1994). The effect of oral support on sucking efficiency in preterm infants. *American Journal of Occupational Therapy, 48,* 490–498.

Field, D., Garland, M., & Williams, K. (2003). Correlates of specific childhood feeding problems. *Journal of Paediatrics and Child Health, 39,* 299–304.

Field, T., Ignatoff, E., Stringer, S., et al. (1982). Nonnutritive sucking during tube feedings: effects on preterm neonates in an intensive care unit. *Pediatrics, 70,* 381–385.

Frappier, P., Marino, B., & Shishmanian, E. (1987). Nursing assessment of infant feeding problems. *Journal of Pediatric Nursing, 2,* 37–44.

Gisel, E. G. (1994). Oral-motor skills following sensorimotor intervention in the moderately eating-impaired child with cerebral palsy. *Dysphagia, 9,* 180–192.

Herbst, J. (1981). Development of sucking and swallowing. In E. Lebenthal (Ed.),

*Textbook of gastroenterology and nutrition in infancy* (pp. 97–107), New York: Raven.

Illingworth, R. (1969). Sucking and swallowing difficulties in infancy: diagnostic problem of dysphagia. *Archives of Disorders in Children*, 44, 655–665.

Illingworth, R., & Lister, J. (1964). The critical or sensitive period, with special reference to certain feeding preterms in infants and children. *Journal of Pediatrics*, 65, 839–848.

Imhoff, S., & Wigginton, V. (1991). Identifying feeding and swallowing problems in infants and young children. *Clinical Communication Disorders*, 1, 59–67.

Kleiman, R., & Warman, K. (1994). Nutrition in liver disease. In S. Baker, R. Baker, & A. Davis (Eds.), *Pediatric enteral nutrition* (chap. 17). New York: Chapman and Hall.

Lamm, N., DeFelice, A.m & Cargan, A. (2005). Effect of tactile stimulation on lingual motor function in pediatric lingual dysphagia. *Dysphagia*, 20, 311–324.

Logan, W., & Bosma, J. (1967). Oral and pharyngeal dysphagia in infancy. *Pediatric Clinics of North America*, 14, 47–61.

Luiselli, J. K. (1994). Oral feeding treatment of children with chronic food refusal and multiple developmental disabilities. *American Association of Mental Retardation*, 98, 646–655.

Manikam, R., & Perman, J. A. (2000). Pediatric feeding disorders. *Journal of Clinical Gastroenterology*, 30, 34–46.

Measel, C., & Anderson ,G. (1979). Nonnutritive sucking during tube feeding: effect on clinical course in premature infants. *Journal of Obstetrics, Gynecology and Neonatal Nursing*, 8, 265–272.

Meier, P., & Anderson, G. (1987). Responses of small preterm infants to bottle- and breast-feeding. *Maternal and Child Health Nursing*, 12, 97–105.

Mercado-Deane, M., Burton, E., Harlow, S., Glover, A., Deane, D., Guill, M., et al. (2001). Swallowing dysfunction in infants less than 1 year of age. *Pediatric Radiology*, 31, 423–428.

Morris, S., & Klein, M. (2000). *Pre-feeding skills*. Tucson, AZ: Therapy Skill Builders.

Mueller, H. (1972). Facilitating feeding and prespeech. In P. Pearson & C. Williams (Eds.), *Physical therapy services in the developmental disabilities* (pp. 283–310), Springfield, IL: Charles C. Thomas.

NCAST-AVENUW. (2006). Parent Child Interaction (PCI) Program. Retrieved May 15, 2007, from http://www.ncast.org/p-psi.asp

Oates, R., Peacock, A., & Forrest, D. (1985). Long-term effects of nonorganic failure to thrive. *Pediatrics*, 75, 36–40.

Palmer, M., Crawley, K., & Blanco, I. (1993). Neonatal oral-motor assessment scale: a reliability study. *Journal of Perinatology*, 13, 28–35.

Reilly, S., & Skuse, D. (1992). Characteristics and management of feeding problems of young children with cerebral palsy. *Developmental Medicine in Child Neurology*, 34, 379–388.

Reilly, S., Skuse, D., Mathisen, B., & Dieter, W. (1995). The objective rating of oral-motor functions during feeding. *Dysphagia*, 10, 177–191.

Rogers, B., & Arvedson, J. (2005). Assessment of infant oral sensorimotor and swallowing function. *Mental Retardation and Developmental Disabilities Research Reviews*, 11(1), 74–82.

Samour, P. Q., & King, K. (2005). *Handbook of pediatric nutrition* (3rd ed.) .Sudbury, MA: Jones & Bartlett.

Sanders, M., Patel, R., LeGrice, & Shepherd, R. (1993). Children with persistent feeding difficulties: An observational analysis of the feeding interactions of problem and non-problem eaters. *Health Psychology*, 12, 64–73.

Satter, E. (2000). *Child of mine: Feeding with love and good sense*. Palo Alto, CA: Bull.

Singer, L., & Fagan, J. (1984). Cognitive development in failure-to-thrive infant: a three-year longitudinal study. *Journal of Pediatric Psychology*, 9, 363–383.

Skuse, D., Stevenson, J., Reilly, S., App, B., & Mathisen, B. (1995). Schedule for oral-motor assessment (SOMA): Methods of validation. *Dysphagia, 10,* 192–202.

Stevenson, R., & Allaire, J. (1991). The development of normal feeding and swallowing. *Pediatric Clinics of North America, 38,* 1439–1452.

Wolff, P. (1968). The serial organization of sucking in the young infant. *Pediatrics, 42,* 943–956.

# APPENDIX 9-A

## Growth Charts

**Birth to 36 months: Boys**
**Length-for-age and Weight-for-age percentiles**

NAME _____

RECORD # _____

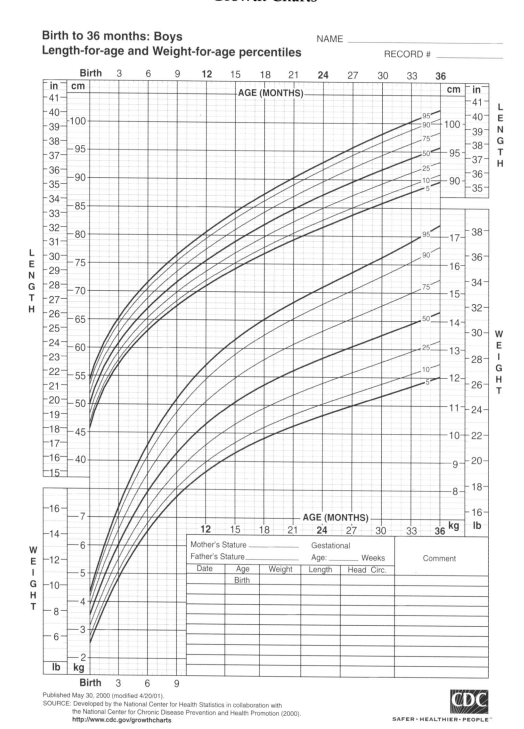

Published May 30, 2000 (modified 4/20/01).
SOURCE: Developed by the National Center for Health Statistics in collaboration with
the National Center for Chronic Disease Prevention and Health Promotion (2000).
http://www.cdc.gov/growthcharts

# APPENDIX 9-A

## Growth Charts (continued)

**2 to 20 years: Boys**
**Body mass index-for-age percentiles**

NAME _____

RECORD # _____

Published May 30, 2000 (modified 10/16/00).

SOURCE: Developed by the National Center for Health Statistics in collaboration with
the National Center for Chronic Disease Prevention and Health Promotion (2000).
http://www.cdc.gov/growthcharts

# Growth Charts (continued)

**2 to 20 years: Boys**
**Stature-for-age and Weight-for-age percentiles**

NAME _____

RECORD # _____

Published May 30, 2000 (modified 11/21/00).
SOURCE: Developed by the National Center for Health Statistics in collaboration with
the National Center for Chronic Disease Prevention and Health Promotion (2000).
http://www.cdc.gov/growthcharts

SAFER · HEALTHIER · PEOPLE™

# 10

# *Nutritional Concerns and Assessment in Dysphagia*

## Beverly Lorens

Successful management of dietary needs in dysphagic patients requires the efforts of all involved caregivers. The particular responsibility of the dietitian is to assess a patient's nutrition and hydration needs, and then to translate these needs into a diet that meets restrictions imposed by the team. These restraints may be unrestricted oral feeding, oral feeding with compensatory safeguards or facilitators, enteral feeding, or combined enteral and oral feeding. As these needs change, the dietitian should be involved to make the transition as effective as possible. Another important responsibility of the dietitian is to make the diet prescribed as appealing and palatable to a patient as possible. Implicit in this obligation is the recognition that eating is not an isolated act of nutrient provision, but is also associated with strong social, cultural, religious, and other influences in patients' lives. To the extent possible, these influences must also be considered in evaluating and treating the dysphagic patient.

Both screening and comprehensive nutritional evaluations require consideration of a patient's *anthropometric characteristics, dietary intake, relevant clinical* and *physical findings*, and *socioeconomic considerations*. Comprehensive assessment will elaborate each of these areas, for example, dietary intake will be assessed in terms of calories, protein, vitamins, minerals, and fluid, and evaluated for adequacy based on the patient's individual needs (Huyck, 1990; Nutrition Assessment, 1992; Nutritional Screening Initiative, 1994; Webber & Splett, 1995 )

## INDICATIONS

Nutritional assessment should be considered when a patient's means of feeding has been altered, when such a change is anticipated, or when there are concerns about the amount and/or nutrition or hydration value of a patient's diet (Wood, 2005).

## Patient Populations at Risk for Nutritional Compromise

Populations considered here are those most likely to benefit from a team evaluation, for example, a patient for whom there is a possibility of safe oral feeding and whose mentation level is judged adequate for at least a minimal level of cooperation with team objectives. The dysphagia may be a result of traumatic accident, surgical or medical event, neuromuscular progressive disease process, or developmental anomaly. Although some patients may be relatively stable in terms of their swallowing ability, others may reflect great variability over time. Many recent-event stroke patients, head trauma patients, and head and neck surgical patients will progress in swallowing during the period of therapeutic intervention. Over time, partial or even full recovery of function may be realized (Goguen et al., 2006). Patients with progressive neurogenic conditions, such as Parkinson's syndrome, demyelinating disease, Huntington's chorea, amyotrophic lateral sclerosis, or multiple sclerosis, may experience periods of stability but, in general, will decline consistent with their disease. Age groupings of patients have additional significance. For example, one can generally expect the CVA (cerebral vascular accident) population to be older, and the head trauma population to be younger. Such differences not only have implications for dietary needs, but also may influence a patient's eligibility for funding sources

that support nutritional needs. Funding resources need to be evaluated early to provide for implementation or exploration of alternatives. Innovative adjustments in formula choice or method of enteral feeding can provide cost savings for the unfunded person.

Other distinctions in patient groups have implications for the timing and frequency of dietary monitoring and/or intervention. In some populations, changes in eating status are *anticipated*, and dietary needs can be addressed before the expected event (Fietkau, Iro, Sailer, & Sauer, 1991; Raykher et al., 2007; Senft, Fietkau, Iro Sailor, & Sauer, 1993). One example of such a change is the intermittent interruption of nutrition because of treatment-related nausea, where the goal may be to maximize nutrition or hydration during nontreatment periods. Additional examples of an expected change are the compromised nutritional intake in the head and neck cancer patient undergoing radiotherapy (Ahmed, Samant, & Vieira, 2005; Fietkau et al., 1991; Senft et al., 1993), or an extended NPO status in a postoperative patient (Koehler & Buhl, 1991). In other populations, the need for nutritional assistance is *acute and unanticipated*. Patients who are apparently well and then experience a sudden insult, that is, CVA or trauma, are examples of this kind of population (Nyswonger & Helmchen, 1992). Other patients may be maintaining adequate nutrition or hydration but have few reserves to cope with new or unexpected problems that compromise their nutritional well being. In such cases, changes in nutrition or hydration status are *not entirely unanticipated*. Careful monitoring to ensure prompt intervention is necessary. For example, a patient with a degenerative disease who has been doing well for a long period of time may begin to fail. Or a patient recovering from surgery may leave the hospital doing well, but experience difficulty later in the postoperative period.

## "Red Flags" for Formal Dietitian Consult

Significant changes in *weight trends* and *hydration* status in a patient signal the need for a comprehensive nutritional evaluation. Guidelines for determining the severity of unintentional weight loss are presented in Table 10–1.

In general, a person losing 10% to 20% of his or her usual weight may sustain moderate impairment, whereas a loss of greater than 20% of usual weight indicates severe impairment (Phinney, 1995). In both situations, thorough elaboration of the cause of weight loss will be required.

Red flags for suboptimal hydration include rapid weight loss (a 48-hour weight loss of 4 pounds can mean a negative fluid balance of 2 liters), com-

plaint of thirst, skin turgor changes, decreased urination, a rising blood urea nitrogen level (BUN) in the absence of other renal indicators, and an increased serum sodium level (hypernatremia). Patients with thin liquid dysphagia may be at particular risk for alterations in hydration status. They will have difficulty augmenting fluid intake to compensate for increased fluid losses because of secondary illness and are also more vulnerable to other fluid-depleting conditions such as fever, diarrhea, or increased perspiration related to heat or physical exertion.

## NUTRITIONAL ASSESSMENT

As noted, careful monitoring of patients' nutritional status can and should be undertaken by members of the dysphagia team and other caregivers. However, expedient referral to the dietitian is indicated when there is any question regarding the patient's ability to safely maintain adequate nutrition or hydration via the current means of food intake. Typically, another member of

**Table 10-1.** Evaluation of Weight Change (%)

| Time | Significant Weight Loss (% of Change) | Severe Weight Loss (% of Change) |
|------|------|------|
| 1 week | 1–2 | >2 |
| 1 month | 5 | >5 |
| 3 months | 7.5 | >7.5 |
| 6 months | 10 | >10 |

*Source.* Reprinted with permission from Blackburn, Bistrian, Maini, Schlamm, & Smith Copyright © 1977, American Society of Parenteral and Enteral Nutrition.

the team has nutritionally screened dysphagic patients and this has triggered a referral to the dietitian for a more comprehensive assessment. Components of the dietitian's examination include the following.

## Anthropometric Data (Nutritional Assessment, 1992; Krystofiak & Mueller, 2007; Pesce-Hammond & Wessel, 2005)

As indicated, a primary cue for dietary referral is weight change. Appropriate weight range is impacted by gender, age, height, and frame. The patient's usual weight, any change in this amount, over what period of time, and whether any change was intentional must be determined (see Table 10–1). If weight loss is too rapid, and in particular if it is associated with inadequate protein intake, it may adversely impact the body's immune function. The ability to resist disease and infection is compromised (Linn, Robinson, & Klimas, 1988). The patient's energy level and ability to participate in the prescribed rehabilitation program may also be affected. Presented in Table 10–2 are

guidelines for interpreting nutritional status based on percent of ideal body weight (IBW) and percent of usual body weight (UBW).

## Laboratory Data (Nutritional Assessment, 1992; Krystofiak & Mueller, 2007; Pesce-Hammond & Wessel, 2005)

Visceral protein status is frequently screened by obtaining a *serum albumin* value (from a blood sample, usually requested as part of a Comprehensive Medical Panel). A value of less than 3.2 (Zeman, 1991, pp. 56, 77) to 3.5 (Nutrition Screening Initiative, 1994, p. 19) is suggestive of the patient being at nutritional risk. Pre-albumin, can provide a more sensitive indicator of current protein status. However, pre-albumin, a negative acute phase protein, may be lowered in the presence of metabolic stressors, inflammation, or infection, irrespective of nutritional state. Therefore, a low pre-albumin value may not, in and by itself, reflect compromised protein or nutrition status. C-reactive protein (CRP), a positive acute phase protein, can be used as an indicator of stress or inflammation (Pesce-Hammond & Wessell,

**Table 10–2.** Evaluation of Nutritional Status Based on a Percentage of Weight

|  | % of Ideal Body Weight | % of Usual Body Weight |
|---|---|---|
| Mild malnutrition | 80–90 | 85–95 |
| Moderate malnutrition | 70–79 | 75–84 |
| Severe malnutrition | 0–69 | 0–74 |

*Source.* Data from Rombeau, Caldwell, Forlaw, & Guenter (1989) p. 43.

2005, p. 19). If CRP is within normal limits, then the pre-albumin can more confidently be accepted to reflect protein status.

Laboratory values that are both commonly available and useful for evaluating hydration status are *serum sodium* and *blood urea nitrogen*. Elevated values are typical in the dehydrated patient. Additionally, albumin will be elevated in dehydration. One needs to remain mindful that hypoalbuminemia may be masked by mild to moderate dehydration causing hemoconcentration and a falsely elevated albumin value. In dehydration, low urine output will occur as the body seeks to conserve fluid (Zeman, 1991, p. 71).

## Nutrition History (Krystofiak & Mueller, 2007; Nutritional Assessment, 1992, pp. 75–77; Nutrition and Your Health, 1995; Pesce-Hammond & Wessell, 2005)

Between the time of referral and the time the patient is evaluated, it is extremely helpful to have obtained a *food diary record* (i.e., a 3-day history up to a 7-day history of dietary intake). The patient or caregiver is instructed to record the time food or drink is consumed, the amount consumed, and a description of the food and how it was prepared, that is, steamed, fried, broiled (Appendix 10–A). The amount of food should be described using standardized measurements. For example, a "glass" of juice might be 4, 8, 12, or even 16 ounces, depending on the size of container and how full it was filled *and* if all was consumed. The patient is also asked to note if this is a typical meal pattern and, if not, what is different. Any nutrient label information concerning calories and protein per serving size should also be included in the report. It is important to appreciate that merely recording one's dietary intake may alter the usual pattern of intake.

Additional measures obtained by the dietitian are a recent (last 24 hours) food intake record as recalled by the patient (referred to as a *24-hour recall*), and a *food frequency list,* which describes how often the patient has had different types of foods over a recent time period.

The history of food intake provided by the patient or caregiver, and the translation of this information in terms of nutrient content are, at best, only approximate. The patient's ability to recall type and quantity of dietary intake may be flawed. In addition, our understanding of the nutrient content of foods and the patient's individual nutrient requirements is not absolute. These limitations notwithstanding, it is still important to make the best interpretation possible from the available information. From all measures considered, the dietitian will compare the patient's dietary intake to standard referents of dietary requirements. For example, the United States Department of Agriculture (USDA) MyPyramid food guidance system (Appendix 10–B) recommendations for daily dietary requirements include:

- 5 to 10 servings of grains, emphasizing whole grains and higher fiber choices
- 1½ to 2½ cups of fruit, eating more in the fresh and natural form

- 2 to 4 cups of vegetables, emphasis on variety and color
- 3 cups from the milk group that also includes fortified soy milk, cheese, yogurt, and tofu
- 5 to 7 ounce equivalents from the meat and bean group (includes poultry, meats, eggs, and nuts)
- 5 to 10 teaspoons from oils (vegetable)
- 130 to 500 calories from discretionary calories group that includes sweets, solid fats, and higher calorie forms of food

It should also be underscored that establishment of nutritional needs is *an estimate* and, as such, simply provides a place to begin. Subsequent monitoring of weight, laboratory values, and the patient's global sense of well-being will assist in fine tuning the nutrition goals.

## Clinical and Physical Findings

Assessment of the patient's oral peripheral structures is addressed at length in other chapters, and will not be reviewed here. Typically, the dysphagia therapist has completed this evaluation before a dietitian consult. It is important to stress that oral cavity structures and their functional integrity impact both how and what type of nutrition a patient may be able to manage. For example, the patient's ability to chew to a ground or puree texture will determine the texture(s) of food that can be offered.

Also important to the nutritional evaluation is the patient's level of physical activity. If activity is very sedentary, the patient's energy need and number of calories required will be low, necessitating the selection of nutri-ent dense food. The goal is to ensure nutritional adequacy of protein, vitamins, and minerals without excess weight gain that would further impact mobility.

Concurrent chronic conditions, such as diabetes, coronary artery disease, renal, and pulmonary impairment that may have pre-existing diet management in place, must also be noted. Pre-existing therapeutic diet modifications may be counterproductive to adequate nutrition or hydration in a patient with newly developed dysphagia. A cardiac patient's low-fat diet may be inappropriate if the patient is unable to consume adequate calories while adhering to the low-fat regimen. The initial priority is to maintain weight. Once this is achieved, a patient may begin incorporating lower fat food choices if the low-fat diet is still indicated. Diabetic diets have undergone significant changes since 1994. The emphasis is on individualizing the diet based on the medical nutrition needs and the results of self-monitoring of blood glucose. Patients may need guidance in adjusting their prior "diabetic" diet within the new constraints of their dysphagia. Additionally, increased reliance on pharmaceutical intervention may be indicated if conditions such as hyperlipidemia or hyperglycemia are not adequately controlled. Chronic medication use, with particular attention to food–drug interactions, must also be evaluated.

Mental health status, and in particular, recent changes in this status, must also be considered. Alterations in cognitive skills, ability to attend, or to speak will affect communication and social interaction. This can have implications for a patient's compliance with treatment objectives. Such changes may also trigger depression or a diminished sense of well being, with resultant decreased appetite and failure to maintain weight.

The social environment a patient is in, or will enter upon leaving the hospital or care facility, is screened as a part of the nutritional evaluation. In particular, adequate funds to purchase food, as well as a living situation that allows food preparation, are important factors to assess. The dysphagic patient will have a greater diet variety if the means to acquire appropriate foods and then prepare them to proper texture and viscosity are available. Also important to the assessment are observations regarding the patient's level of isolation, dependence on others for food procurement or preparation, current or former occupation, cultural background, and other factors that may influence food choices or eating.

## NUTRITIONAL GOALS IN TREATMENT PLANNING

### Establishing Energy, Protein, and Fluid

For purposes of this chapter, the primary nutritional goal for a dysphagic patient is to approximate nutrition needs that will allow achievement or maintenance of healthy body weight. Patients should be monitored closely and the dietitian again consulted if desired outcomes of weight maintenance, gain, or loss are not obtained.

### Energy (Nutritional Assessment, 1992; Recommended Dietary Allowances, 1989, pp. 24–38; American Society of Parenteral and Enteral Nutrition, 1993; Hopkins, 1993; Wooley & Frankenfield, 2007)

**Adults.** Daily energy requirements for adults are based on a calculated reference (ideal) weight for height in kilograms (Table 10–3). A maintenance base is 25 to 35 kcal per kg reference weight per day. Additional allowance must be made for increased activity or metabolic stress. The obese patient may lose weight using his or her "ideal" weight in the calculation and require adjustment of energy goal if weight loss is unacceptable.

**Children.** Daily energy requirements for children must be individualized to age group and weight, activity, spasticity, and also for catch-up growth. Recommended dietary allowances are established for healthy children. These

**Table 10-3.** Calculating Reference Weight (Ideal Body Weight)

| | |
|---|---|
| Adult male (Hamwi method)* | 106 lbs for first 5 feet; 6 lbs for each inch over 5 feet *Example:* 5'9" Reference weight = 160 lbs = 72.7 kg |
| Adult female (Hamwi method)* | 100 lbs for first 5 feet; 5 lbs for each inch over 5 feet *Example:* 5'4" Reference weight = 120 lbs = 54.5 kg |
| Children | Consult standardized growth curves. Some modified growth curves are available for specific conditions, i.e., Down syndrome |

*Source. In Gottschlich, Matarese, & Shronts. (1993), *Nutrition Support Dietetics Core Curriculum* (2nd ed., p. 21).

are used as a base which can be modified for an individual child in a specific situation.

### Protein (Nutritional Assessment, 1992; Recommended Dietary Allowances, 1989, pp. 52–77; Hopkins, 1993, pp. 58–63; Shaw, Wildbore, & Wolfe, 1987; Young, Kearns, & Schoepfel, 2007)

**Adults.** 0.8 gram protein per kilogram reference weight is the recommended daily dietary allowance for an adult. This level is increased or decreased depending on specific disease consideration, level of nutritional debilitation, and metabolic stress (e.g., related to fever or sepsis. For anabolism or during periods of stress, the value is typically increased to between 1.0 and 1.5 grams protein per kilogram reference weight. In burn and trauma patients, protein may be increased to 2.0 g protein/kg.

**Children.** Appropriate daily protein levels for children are highly variable depending on age and metabolic stressors. Infants' and children needs range from 2.2 to 1.0 g /kg with the value decreasing to the adult level of 0.8 g protein/kg at age 15 years for females and age 19 years for males (Recommended Dietary Allowances, 1989).

### Fluid (Nutritional Assessment, 1992; Recommended Dietary Allowances, 1989, pp. 247–250; Hopkins, 1992, p. 63)

**Adults.** There are many accepted formulas to determine appropriate fluid levels for adults. A general guideline is 1 ml fluid per calorie. Another method uses a range: 25 to 40 ml/kg reference weight per day. Fluid needs decrease with age. Influences on fluid require-

ments include amount of total body surface area, illness, activity level, and temperature of the environment. Fluid needs are, in part, proportional to body surface area. The obese person would have increased needs over the person within their ideal weight range.

**Children.** For the first 10 kg of body weight, add 100 ml/kg per day; for the second 10 kg of body weight, add 50 ml/kg per day; for each additional kilogram, add 20 ml/kg per day.

### Vitamins and Minerals (Clark, 2007, pp. 129-159; Nutritional Assessment, 1992; Recommended Dietary Allowances, 1989; Standing Committee on the Scientific Evaluation of Dietary Reference Intakes, Food and Nutrition Board, Institute of Medicine, 1997 and 1998; Hopkins, 1993, pp. 42–51)

Adequacy of the overall diet needs to be assessed for the provision of sufficient vitamins and minerals within the calorie density consumed. In an adult eating orally, a multiple vitamin/mineral supplement is generally indicated if nutritional energy needs are less than 1,500 calories per day. (ADA Reports, 2005; Fletcher & Fairfield, 2002; Fairfield & Fletcher, 2002).

## TRANSLATING ENERGY-PROTEIN-FLUID NEEDS INTO A TREATMENT PLAN

Once the target values for calories, protein, and fluid have been established, the route of nutrient ingestion must be considered. The dysphagia team has typically discussed the available alternatives and decided the best option for the patient. Conventional oral eating, facilitated by strategies as needed, is the most desirable. Oral intake combined with enteral tube feeding may also be recommended. This combination may be used when fatigue or some other limitation may impact the patient's ability to rely totally on oral feeding. Other patients will require enteral feeding for all their nutrition. Whatever method is prescribed, constant re-evaluation is needed to determine if the current option is working or remains appropriate. During these periods, the dietitian provides the team and the physician managing the patient's care with a quantitative analysis of food consumption by reviewing food diaries kept by the patient or caregiver.

## Oral Feeding

If oral feeding is recommended for the patient, the dysphagia therapist will determine what restrictions must be applied to ensure safe oral feeding. The dietitian will help identify foods that both appeal to the patient and meet the safety requirements imposed. In short, the dietitian will translate the team's prescription into everyday foods that the patient can consume in sufficient quantities to meet nutrition or hydration needs.

Textures range over a continuum from pourable liquids with varying viscosities to gel consistencies, to slippery puree foods that deform from shape with gravity, to stiffer purees that hold their shape, to combinations of puree and ground texture, to fine chop. Potentially, texture will be unrestricted, but the length of time required to eat may require selection of nutrient-dense foods. The normal adult swallower enjoys the full range of the texture or viscosity continuum from the least to most viscous. The dysphagic patient may find the tolerable viscosity range restricted, that is, shifted to the low or high end, or compressed from both extremes. The texture continuum in relation to transit ability and airway protection is presented in Table 10–4.

An exercise found useful in our setting was to have members of the dysphagia team meet in the central kitchen. A smorgasbord of food was sampled from our patient tray line. Team members jointly developed a matrix classification of what foods would be considered thick or thin liquids, allowed on puree or ground diet. This process significantly strengthened the complementary relationship the dysphagia therapist and dietitian share in treating the dysphagic patient. The dysphagia therapists gained insights regarding how limited a meal may become given multiple restrictions, and the dietitians gained, among other things, an understanding of how thin a "thick liquid" may be and how broad a range would be acceptable for other characterizations of food used by the therapists. Also emerging from this experience was an appreciation for the *range* of viscosity included in the categories "thick liquid" and "puree" and for the difficulty involved in correlating findings regarding viscosities sampled on the dynamic swallow study with the subjective determination of a tolerable range of viscosities made during the bedside evaluation. Information presented in Appendix 10–C represents the result of the group collaboration. It should be noted that the categories of textures presented are not ironclad. Individualizing dietary restriction to the patient's specific impairment provides maximum variety.

**Table 10–4.** Continuum of Textures or Viscosities. (Susan McKenzie, M.S., and Beverly Lorens, R.D., M.S.)

## TEXTURE OR VISCOSITY CONTINUUM

Places stress on agility of airway closure for swallow but facilitates bolus transfer ⟷ Relieves demands on agility of airway closure and facilitates bolus transfer ⟷ Places stress on oral preparation and oral and pharyngeal transfer competence

| | Thin Liquids | Thick Liquids | Slippery Puree | Puree | Foods requiring mastication in order of ascending difficulty |
|---|---|---|---|---|---|
| E X A M P L E | (Assumed to be at body temperature) apple juice, tomato juice, milk, commercial liquid supplements, fruit ice, sherbet, Jell-O, soft drinks | (Assumed to be at body temperature), juice with thickener added, or commercial juices, water, milk thickened to nectar-like or honey-like viscosity | (Assumed to be at body temperature) pudding, custard, pureed fruit, puree vegetables (not starches) | Mashed potatoes, pureed scrambled eggs, pureed meat | Ground meat, regular scrambled eggs, canned fruit, soft cooked carrots, beets, bread |
| | | | | | Chopped meat, sandwiches (tuna, egg, bologna) |
| | | | | | Unrestricted diet |
| P R O P E R T I E S | Easily deformed, moves very readily in response to gravity and compression. | Less easily deformed than thin liquids, moves fairly readily in response to gravity or compression. | Less easily deformed so may obstruct a narrow passage. Slides in response to gravity or compression. | Less easily deformed, thus can obstruct a narrow passage. Transferred mostly by compression. | As the bolus becomes more viscous, it is less and less easily deformed, less likely to move in response to gravity, more reliant on dental and lingual competence for mastication and transit, sensory competence and judgment of bolus characteristics, adequate salivation, and healthy mucosa. |

| | Thin Liquids | Thick Liquids | Slippery Puree | Puree | Foods requiring mastication in order of ascending difficulty |
|---|---|---|---|---|---|
| **T R A N S I T** | Thin liquids are most likely to move through the upper digestive tract quickly and completely. | Variably likely (depending on the degree of thickness) to move through the digestive tract easily without falling into the airway and to pass fairly well through narrow sites such as strictures. | Slippery purees are more likely to stop at obstacles such as webs and strictures, but may be less likely to "stick." | Purees are likely to stop at obstacles and may not slide easily along dry mucosa. Purees will not move through the pharynx without adequate compression/constriction. Complete transit requires adequate salivary and mucosal health. | Adequate oral and pharyngeal patency and strength of constriction/compression is requisite for safe swallow of high viscosity foods once mastication has transformed the solid into a puree. Adequate transfer requires adequate salivary and mucosal health. |
| **A I R W A Y** | Agility of laryngeal airway closure for swallow is a prerequisite for ingestion of thin liquids. | Swallow of thick liquids requires less laryngeal agility because thick liquids are less easily deformed and move more slowly (speed varies with thickness) in response to gravity or compression. | Slippery purees require less laryngeal agility but more competent oral and pharyngeal constriction. If the bolus is not adequately transferred, residue may fall into the airway after the swallow. The properties of purees present a greater risk of obstructing the airway than liquids. | Because they do not move readily in response to gravity, purees are less likely to fall into the airway quickly. However, if oral and pharyngeal clearing is incomplete because of poor constriction or xerostomia, pharyngeal residue presents a risk to the airway after the swallow has been completed. The properties of purees present a greater risk of obstructing the airway than liquids. | Adequate airway protection during swallow of solids is reliant on adequately complete oral and pharyngeal transit. The airway can be obstructed if penetrated by solid bolus residue, even if mastication is fairly adequate. The properties of solids present a greater risk of obstructing the airway than liquids. |

(continues)

**Table 10-4.** (continued)

| | Thin Liquids | Thick Liquids | Slippery Puree | Puree | Foods requiring mastication in order of ascending difficulty |
|---|---|---|---|---|---|
| P A T I E N T S | Patients with prolonged or incomplete oral, pharyngeal, or esophageal transit because of poor muscular constriction or to narrowing, (e.g., stricture) but who are alert and enjoy good laryngeal function are most likely to achieve adequate intake with liquid consistencies. | Patients with prolonged or incomplete oral, pharyngeal, or esophageal transit because of poor muscular constriction or to narrowing (e.g., stricture) are most likely to achieve adequate intake with liquid consistencies.<br><br>Patients with mild cognitive deficits or who show poor oral bolus control or impaired initiation of swallow gestures may require thickened liquids. | Patients who are slow to initiate swallow gestures, including airway closure, but who are able to apply some compression to accomplish oral and pharyngeal bolus transfer would tolerate slippery purees. | Patients who are able to apply adequate pressures to transfer the bolus through the oral and pharyngeal cavities completely will tolerate puree consistencies. | The goal of mastication is to produce a "swallow safe" bolus, probably one approximating a puree. The ability to tolerate degrees of viscosity in the solid range is dependent on lingual agility and ROM, judgment re: bolus readiness, salivary flow, and dentition. |

148

Subsequently, the National Dysphagia Diet: Standardization for Optimal Care (National Dysphagia Diet Task Force, 2002) was published as a start toward providing a level of consistency in terminology used to describe dysphagia diets and textures, and viscosity standards of liquids.

Our Food and Nutrition Department is in the process of adopting the National Dysphagia Diet groupings while retaining some in-between diet texture stages (McCallum, 2003). We have two modified texture diet series. The first one provides texture changes for those without aspiration risk or cognitive impairment. Typically they are patients that can make modification to the food item to consume it more easily and safely. In contrast to dysphagia diets, rice and bread are included. The second is the Dysphagia Series. The National Dysphagia Diet has Level 1: Dyphagia Pureed; Level 2: Dysphagia Mechanically Altered Characteristics; and Level 3: Dysphagia Advanced. In addition we have inserted "Dyphagia Puree with Ground Meat" between Levels 1 and 2. This level allows oatmeal, fruited yogurt, scrambled egg, and finely ground meat with a side dish of gravy so the patient or caregiver can further moisten the meat or mashed potatoes to needed amounts. All other foods are pureed (see Table 10–4).

## Special Concerns

As previously addressed, the patient with a thin liquid dysphagia may have difficulty maintaining adequate hydration. All fluid intake must be contained in some gradient of thicker liquid to gel-form food. It is helpful that pureed fruit, vegetables, and meat contain a high percent of their weight as water. However, without some form of thick to thickened liquids, a patient will likely consume inadequate fluid. A variety of commercial thickeners are available either by direct order or from local pharmacies. Some common household foods also work well for thickening. Examples of commercial and household products available for this purpose are listed in Appendix 10–D.

If patients are able to consume sufficient fluid in the form of puree foods, gels, and thick liquids, they may find that their total calorie intake is higher than needed. Potentially, most of their fluid will contain calories, in contrast to an individual without thin liquid dysphagia who can consume water for thirst.

Another area of concern is the successful patient who, having mastered weight maintenance with dysphagia to dry foods, has begun to gain excessive weight. This may be a result of the preparation of foods in more sauce or gravy dishes, which increase the moisture and slipperiness of the foods, but also increase the calories. Positive results can be obtained by reducing the caloric value of the food preparation.

## Nonoral Feeding Alternatives

### Total Parenteral Nutrition

When oral feeding is not an option for a patient, other avenues of food intake must be considered. One such alternative is total parenteral nutrition (TPN). Advances in enteral feeding formulas and feeding tubes have made TPN less popular than in the past. TPN is costly, invasive, represents an infection risk, and bypasses the gut, enhancing potential for bacterial translocation (Borzotta et al., 1994; Kudsk, 1994; Kudsk et al., 1994; Minard & Kudsk, 1994; Moore & Moore, 1991). However, TPN must be used when the gut is nonfunctional because of prolonged ileus, or short bowel syndrome, or where there is contraindication to placing a feeding tube for whatever reason. Additionally, there are patients who will not leave the feeding tube in place. This is more likely in a patient with a nasogastric tube before conversion to a gastrostomy or jejunostomy feeding tube.

### Enteral Feeding

A patient's degree of dysphagia may require the placement of a feeding tube if nutrition is to be supplied in a safe and sufficient volume. Access sites of feeding tubes are typically the nose, the stomach, or the jejunum (Figure 10–1). An enteral feeding tube placed nasally may have the tip of the tube located in the stomach (NG), duodenum (ND), or jejunum (NJ). Tubes placed either by percutaneous endoscopic gastrostomy (PEG) method, radiographically, or surgical gastrostomy may have single or dual lumen tubes, accessing the stomach

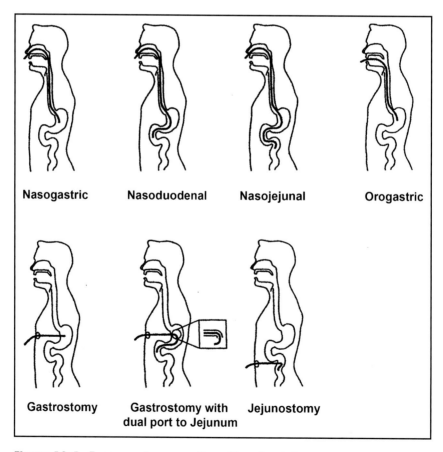

**Figure 10–1.** Types and access sites of feeding tubes.

(GT), or stomach and duodenum (GD) or jejunum (GJ or PEJ, i.e., percutaneous endoscopic jejunostomy). Lastly, the jejunal feeding tube has both its access and end port in the jejunum (JT). Our otolaryngology surgical team places, at the time of surgery, a nasogastric, 14- to 18-Fr. silicone Salem Sump tube (Figure 10–2) that, if needed, can be used for gastric decompression and then for feeding. Its relatively small diameter and pliability make it a reasonably comfortable tube for extended periods of postsurgical feeding. Additionally, the silicone material does not become rigid over time.

Multiple factors are considered concurrently in the decision of what type of feeding tube access will best serve the needs of the patient. These include the following:

- Anticipated duration of enteral feeding (and likelihood of return to oral intake).

**Figure 10–2.** Kendall™ Argyle™ silicone Salem Sump™ tube, 16-Fr., 48" length (Tyco/Healthcare). Dual Lumen. Y-connector with (1) suction drainage lumen/feeding port, (2) suction vent lumen, (3) closed end tip with multiple exit ports.

- Ability to protect the airway, degree of aspiration risk, and pulmonary reserve to withstand aspiration (delivery sites vary in terms of possible airway risk from reflux).
- Presence of impaired gastric emptying may preclude feeding into the stomach (i.e., gastroparesis).
- Types of enteral feeding formula available (i.e., commercial ready-to-feed, name-brand or store brand, or homemade).
- Availability of feeding pump for continuous feeding (gravity drip bolus or syringe bolus recommended only into the stomach).
- Cosmetic considerations (a nasogastric tube is visible, whereas a GT or JT may be concealed behind clothing).
- Patient compliance with location (i.e., an agitated patient can more easily remove a nasogastric tube than a gastrostomy tube that can be concealed behind a dressing or abdominal binder when not in use).
- Availability and condition of organ to be an access site.
- Selection of feeding schedule (*continuous* or *intermittent* feeds can be delivered into stomach, duodenum, or jejunum but only bolus (gravity or syringe) feeds should be administered into the stomach).

*Nasogastric* (NG) feeding is generally selected when the duration of time on tube feeding will be relatively short (may be months), there is an intact gag reflex with normal emptying of the stomach and no evidence of uncontrolled esophageal reflux. Particular advantages of the NG tube are its relatively noninvasive placement and cost effectiveness. (Figures 10–3 and 10–4)

**Figure 10–3.** Kendall™ Kangaroo™, 12 Fr., 36" length, unweighted (Tyco/Healthcare). Y-connector with (1) feeding port, (2) irrigation/medication port, (3) open end tip with exit ports in tubing.

**Figure 10–4.** Kendall™ Entriflex™ Dual Port Feeding Tube without Sylet 12-Fr., 36" length (Tyco/Healthcare). Y-connector with (1) feeding port, (2) irrigation/medication port, (3) exit ports, (4) weighted tip.

*Nasoduodenal* (ND) tubes are appropriate for short-term feeding when gastroesophageal reflux is expected, when there is an increased aspiration risk, or decreased rate of stomach emptying. A continuous feeding rate is employed and commercial formulas are used primarily because these feeding tubes are often smaller in diameter and more prone to plugging. Homemade feedings may not be homogeneous. Also, if they are low enough viscosity to flow, they may be too dilute to deliver an adequate quantity of nutrition. (Figure 10–5).

The *nasojejunal* (NJ) feeding route requires a longer tube (43 inches compared to 36 inches for other tubes). It also requires radiographic confirmation of placement and may need to be placed endoscopically. Its primary advantage is that its extended placement into the GI tract minimizes dislodgment back into the stomach and

**Figure 10–5.** Kendall™ Entriflex™ Dual Port Feeding Tube with FLOW THROUGH™ Stylet, 12-Fr., 43" length (Tyco/Healthcare). Y-connector with (1) feeding port, (2) irrigation/medication port, (3) stylet, (4) exit ports, (5) weighted tip.

feeding can begin shortly after injury. (see Figure 10–5)

*Gastrostomy* (GT) placement is appropriate if nasoenteric route is unavailable, long-term feeding is required, or swallowing dysfunction is permanent. Location of tip placement in stomach, duodenum, or jejunum would follow the same decision tree used with a nasoenterically placed tube. A prime advantage of gastrostomy is cosmetic as the feeding tube is not outwardly visible. (Figures 10–6 and 10–7)

Some dual lumen GTs have a narrow lumen line that serves the duodenum or jejunum (Figure 10–8). This has the advantage of being able to access both the stomach and intestine. Some medications are better absorbed in the stomach. If long-term jejunal feeding is the goal and stomach access is not required, placement directly as a JT may be

**Figure 10–6.** Deutsch Gastrostomy Catheter with AQ® Hydrophilic Coating, 16-Fr., 25 cm long with Cook-Cope type locking loop. (1) Enteral feeding adapter with male Luer lock fitting, (2) Luer lock tube opening, (3) exit ports.

**Figure 10–7.** Kimberly-Clark™ MIC™ Gastrostomy feeding tube, 20-Fr., 7–10 mL balloon (Ballard Medical Products). (1) Feeding port, (2) irrigation/medication port, (3) balloon valve port, (4) external retention disk, (5) balloon, (6) open tip exit port.

**Figure 10–8.** MIC™ Gastro Enteric Feeding Tube, 20 Fr. (Medical Innovations, a Division of Ballard Medical Products). (1) Gastric port, (2) jejunal port, (3) balloon valve, (4) dual lumen tube, (5) Secur-Lok® ring, (6) balloon, (7) tapered gastric exit port, (8) multiple exit ports, (9) weighted tip.

preferred. Tube length will be shorter, possibly less inclined to clogging. As with the PEG, a PEJ can be placed endoscopically and is therefore less costly than a surgical jejunostomy. A JT is indicated in the patient with extensive gastroesophageal surgery or disease.

Rustom, Jebreel, Tayyab, England and Stafford (2006) reviewed 78 head and neck cancer patients for complication rates between three methods of

gastrostomy tube insertion: PEG, radiologically inserted gastrostomy (RIG), and surgically inserted gastrostomy (open or laparoscopic). The PEG group had fewer complications and has become their first choice for head and neck cancer patients. At our facility, the RIG method is more commonly used in our head and neck cancer patients. Consideration for this method is that the gastrostomy is more often placed after the surgical resection of tumor and the dragging of the retention bumper of the PEG tube through the neosurgical site is contraindicated. Additionally, Douglas, Koh, and Laramore (2000) reviewed the literature and found six cases of PEG site metastases occurring in patients with head and neck cancer. A later review sites 29 cases of PEG site metastasis (Mincheff, 2005).

A summary of advantages and disadvantages of each feeding tube is presented in Table 10–5. The dietitian is a key resource in assisting selection of the enteral formula appropriate for each, with consideration given to suitability, availability, tolerance, and cost. Some patients may need to *make* their own tube feeding in lieu of one of the multitude of commercially made formulas. The dietitian is invaluable in such situations. Generally, the cost of formula will be lowest if one retains the ability to feed into the stomach. The stomach acts as a reservoir and hypertonic solutions can be fed; whereas, jejunal feeding usually requires an isotonic formula and a feeding pump. As previously noted, the stomach also allows for an intermittent bolus feeding schedule, which may allow the patient more freedom and more of a feeling of normalcy by engaging in feeding at meal periods.

**Table 10-5.** Advantages and Disadvantages of Feeding Tubes

| Access Site | Advantages | Disadvantages |
|---|---|---|
| Nasogastric | • Minimally invasive, easy placement<br>• Suitable for short-term use<br>• Transitional to bolus feeding<br>• Radiographic confirmation not necessarily required if clinically confirmed placement in stomach | • Cosmetic—feeding tube is visible<br>• Risk of sinusitis<br>• Lack of intact gag reflex may (not necessarily) indicate increased aspiration risk<br>• Stomach must be uninvolved with primary disease |
| Nasoduodenal | • Minimally invasive<br>• Suitable for short-term use<br>• Reduced risk of pulmonary aspiration<br>• Useful in condition of gastroparesis or impaired stomach emptying<br>• Useful if esophageal reflux present<br>• Allows for feeding when bowel sounds are diminished or absent | • Requires radiographic confirmation of placement<br>• Cosmetic—feeding tube is visible<br>• Risk of sinusitis<br>• Bolus feeding is not an option.<br>• Feeding pump is needed, reducing mobility of patient when feeding<br>• 43" length feeding tube is preferred<br>• May not remain placed in duodenum because of tube migration<br>• Typically, smaller diameter tube than NG, more prone to plugging if not properly maintained. Similar to NG size diameter tubes available if specified. |
| Nasojejunal | • Same advantages as nasoduodenal<br>• Placement of tip further down GI tract minimizes dislocation to stomach<br>• 60" length tubes available offering even greater placement security | • Similar disadvantages as nasoduodenal except placement of tip is more secure |
| Gastrostomy | • Suitable for long-term feeding<br>• Cosmetically more appealing than a nasally placed tube<br>• Minimizes risk of tube migration and aspiration because of voluntary or accidental dislocation of nasoenteric tube by patient | • Potential risk of pulmonary aspiration<br>• Lack of intact gag reflex and/or presence of esophageal reflux may indicate increased risk of aspiration<br>• Insertion site care needed<br>• Potential skin excoriation |

*(continues)*

155

**Table 10-5.** *(continued)*

| Access Site | Advantages | Disadvantages |
|---|---|---|
| Gastrostomy *(continued)* | • Percutaneous placement available (PEG)<br>• Some GT have large bore tubes which minimize occlusion from medications and high viscosity formulas<br>• Most suitable of all tubes for use of homemade formula, provided tip is place in stomach and it is a large bore tube | at stoma site from leakage of gastric secretion<br>• Potential fistula at insertion site after GT removal<br>• If GT feeding tip port is place in duodenum, usually a smaller bore tube is used and it is subject to more occlusion risk. |
| Gastrojejunostomy | • Similar advantages to the gastrostomy tube<br>• Dual lumen tube allows access to stomach and duodenum or jejunum, depending on length of enteric portion of tube. | • Similar disadvantages to the gastrostomy tube<br>• Duodenal/jejunal portion of tube may dislodge from initial placement position<br>• Jejunal tube lumen usually is of a small bore diameter and is subject to more occlusion risk |
| Jejunostomy | • Suitable for long-term feeding<br>• Minimizes risk of aspiration<br>• Positive gag reflex need not be present<br>• Useful if esophageal reflux is present<br>• Does not depend on functioning stomach | • Typically smaller bore tube than a GT and at risk for occlusion from medication or viscous formula if not properly maintained<br>• Stoma care needed<br>• Bolus feeding not an option<br>• Feeding pump is needed, reducing mobility of patient when feeding<br>• Potential fistula at stoma site after JT removal |

*Source:* Adapted from Gottschlich, Matarese, & Shronts, *Nutrition Support Dietetics Core Curriculum*, 2nd ed. (1993).

Medications delivered via the feeding tube must be liquid or crushed and sustainable in a slurry. A bolus of water before and after the medication administration will prevent interaction between the medication and feeding that may result in clumping of the feeding which could clog the tube. No sustained release medications can be fed through the feeding tube as crushing will ruin the sustained release property.

## TEAM APPROACH

As stated frequently throughout this text, the benefit of a team approach to dysphagic patients is the opportunity it provides for synergism. The dovetailing of the skills and experience of each individual professional in the assessment and treatment of the patient is an enormous advantage, for both the patient and team members. Members of our team have a healthy regard for the individual skills and backgrounds represented by each participant, and this translates to a broad, comprehensive approach to patient management. The team approach also provides opportunities to reinforce the message of other team members or of the collective "team," while individual specialists deliver their own expertise. The patient benefits from multiple exposure to variations of the same treatment theme and hopefully begins to incorporate successful adaptations for his or her individual condition.

## STUDY QUESTIONS

1. What is the dietitian's role in the treatment of dysphagia?
   a. Nutritional management
   b. Oral and tube feeding recommendations
   c. Weight management
   d. All of the above
   e. a and c
2. What would be some of the indications to place a gastrostomy feeding tube?
   a. Progressive neurologic condition with feeding difficulties leading to compromise of nutrition

b. Head injured patient who is expected to need tube feeding for 2 to 3 months who keeps pulling and removing nasogastric tube
   c. Patient who is expected to regain safe and effective swallow function in 2 to 3 weeks and dislikes how she or he looks with a feeding tube
   d. All of the above
   e. a and b
   f. b and c
3. When evaluating whether percent of weight change is significant or severe, both the length of time over which a person's weight has changed and the amount of weight change is considered. True or False.
4. Specific guidelines define whether a patient's percent of ideal body weight characterizes them as having mild, moderate, or severe malnutrition. True or False.
5. The following elements compose a nutritional assessment:
   a. Anthropometric data
   b. Laboratory data
   c. Nutrition history
   d. Clinical and physical finding
   e. Financial analysis
   f. All of the above
   g. a, b, c, and d.
6. There is clear agreement among dysphagia professionals concerning which food fluids are thin, nectar-like or honey-like and how to describe textural diets. True or False.
7. What would be some of the indications to place a gastrostomy feeding tube?

a. Progressive neurologic condition with feeding difficulties leading to compromise of nutrition

b. Head injured patient who is expected to need tube feeding for 2 to 3 months who keeps pulling and removing nasogastric tube

c. Patient who is expected to regain safe and effective swallow function in 2 to 3 weeks and dislikes how she or he looks with a feeding tube

d. All of the above

e. a and b

f. b and c

8. When evaluating whether percent of weight change is significant or severe, both the length of time over which a person's weight has changed and the amount of weight change is considered. True or False.

9. Specific guidelines define whether a patient's percent of ideal body weight characterizes them as having mild, moderate, or severe malnutrition. True or False.

10. The following elements compose a nutritional assessment:

a. Anthropometric data

b. Laboratory data

c. Nutrition history

d. Clinical and physical finding

e. Financial analysis

f. All of the above

g. a, b, c, and d.

11. There is clear agreement among dysphagia professionals concerning which food fluids are thin, nectar-like or honey-like and how to describe textural diets. True or False.

## REFERENCES

ADA Reports. (2005). Position of the American Dietetic Association: Fortification and nutritional supplements. *Journal of American Dietetic Association, 105,* 1300–1311.

Ahmed, K. A., Samant, S., & Vieira, F., (2005). Gastrostomy tubes in patients with advanced head and neck cancer. *Laryngoscope, 115,* 44–47.

American Society of Parenteral and Enteral Nutrition Board of Directors. Nutrition support for adults with specific diseases and conditions: critical care. (1993). *Journal of Parenteral and Enteral Nutrition, 17*(Suppl.), 20SA–21SA.

Blackburn, G. L., Bistrian, B. R., Maini, B. S., Schlamm, H. T., & Smith, M. F. (1977). Nutritional and metabolic assessment of the hospitalized patient. *Journal of Parenteral and Enteral Nutrition, 1,* 15.

Borzotta A., Pennings J., Papasadero B., Paxton, J., Mardesic, S., Borsotta, R., et al. (1994). Enteral versus parenteral nutrition after severe closed head injury. *Journal of Trauma, 37,* 459–468.

Clark, S. (2007). Vitamins and trace elements. In M. Gottschlich (Ed.), *The A.S.P.E.N. nutrition support core curriculum, a case-based approach—the adult patient* (pp. 129–159). Silver Spring, MD: American Society for Parenteral & Enteral Nutrition.

Douglas, J. G., Koh,W., & Laramore, G. E. (2000). Metastasis to a percutaneous gastrostomy site from head and neck cancer, radiobiologic considerations. *Head and Neck, 22,* 826–830.

Fairfield, K., & Fletcher, R. (2002). Vitamins for chronic disease prevention in adults —scientific review. *Journal of the American Medical Association, 287,* 3116–3126.

Fletcher, R., & Fairfield, K. (2002). Vitamins for chronic disease prevention in adults —clinical applications. *Journal of the American Medical Association, 287,* 3127–3129.

Fietkau, R., Iro, H., Sailer, D., & Sauer, R. (1991). Percutaneous endoscopically guided gastrostomy in patients with head and neck cancer. *Recent Results in Cancer Research, 121,* 209–282.

Goguen, L., Posner, M., Norris, C., Tishler, R., Wirth, L., Annino, D, et al. (2006). Dysphagia after sequential chemoradiation therapy for advanced head and neck cancer. *Otolaryngology-Head Neck Surgery, 134,* 916–922.

Gottschlich, M., Matarese, L., & Shronts, E. (Eds.). (1993). *Nutrition support dietetics core curriculum* (2nd ed.). Silver Spring, MD: American Society for Parenteral and Enteral Nutrition.

Hopkins, B. (1993). Assessment of nutritional status. In M. Gottschlich, L. Matarese & E. Shronts. (Eds.), *Nutrition support dietetics core curriculum* (2nd ed., pp. 15–70). Silver Spring, MD: American Society for Parenteral and Enteral Nutrition.

Huyck, N. I. (1990). Screening: A method to prioritize patient care. *Hospital Food and Nutrition Focus, 6,* 1–3.

Koehler, J., & Buhl, K. (1991). Percutaneous endoscopic gastrostomy for postoperative rehabilitation after maxillofacial tumor surgery. *International Journal of Oral and Maxillofacial Surgery, 20,* 38–39.

Krystofiak Russel, M., & Mueller, C. (2007). Nutrition Screening and Assesment. In M. Gottschlich (Ed.), *The A.S.P.E.N. nutrition support core curriculum, a case-based approach—the adult patient* (pp. 163–186). Silver Spring, MD: American Society for Parenteral and Enteral Nutrition.

Kudsk, K. A. (1994). Gut mucosal nutritional support: Enteral nutrition as primary therapy after multiple system trauma. *Gut, 1*(Suppl.), S52–S54.

Kudsk, K. A., Minard, G., Wojtysiak S. L, Croce, M., Fabian, T., & Brown, R. O. (1994). Visceral protein response to enteral versus parenteral nutrition and sepsis in patients with trauma. *Surgery, 116,* 516–523.

Linn, B. S., Robinson, D. S., & Klimas, N. G. (1988). Effects of age and nutritional status on surgical outcomes in head and neck cancer. *Annals of Surgery, 207,* 267–273.

McCallum, S. (2003). The National Dysphagia Diet: Implementation at a regional rehabilitation center and hospital system. *Journal of the American Dietetic Association, 103,* 381–384.

Minard, G., & Kudsk, K. A. (1994). Effect of route of feeding on the incidence of septic complications in critically ill patients. *Seminars in Respiratory Infections, 9,* 228–231.

Mincheff, T. (2005). Metastatic spread to a percutaneous gastrostomy site from head and neck cancer: Case report and literature review. *Journal of the Society of Laparoendoscopic Surgeons, 9,* 466–471.

Moore, E. E., & Moore, F. A. (1991). Immediate enteral nutrition following multi-system trauma: A decade perspective. *Journal of the American College of Nutrition, 10,* 633–648.

National Dysphagia Diet Task Force. (2002). *National Dysphagia Diet: Standardization for Optimal Care.* Chicago, IL: American Dietetic Association.

*Nutrition and Your Health: Dietary Guidelines for Americans* (4th ed.). (1995). Washington, DC: US Dept of Agriculture, US Dept of Health and Human Services.

Nutritional Assessment. (1992). In: American Dietetic Association. *Handbook of clinical dietetics* (2nd ed., chap. 1). New Haven, CT: Yale University Press.

Nutrition Screening Initiative. (1994). *Incorporating nutrition screening and interventions into medical practice.* Washington, DC: Author.

Nyswonger, G. D., & Helmchen, R. H. (1992). Early enteral nutrition and length of stay in stroke patients. *Journal of Neuroscience Nursing, 24,* 220–223.

Pesce-Hammond, K., & Wessel, J. (2005). Nutrition assessment and decision making. In R. Merritt (Ed.), *The A.S.P.E.N. nutriton support practice manual* (2nd ed., pp. 3–26). Silver Spring, MD: American Society for Parenteral and Enteral Nutrition.

Phinney, S. D. (1995). Advances in diagnosing malnutrition in hospitalized patients. *Nutrition in Clinical Practice.* Conference Syllabus. Sponsored by UC Davis Division of Clinical Nutrition and Metabolism, Department of Internal Medicine and the Office of Continuing Medical Education; April 8, 1995.

Raykher, A., Russo, L., Schattner, M., Schwartz, L., Scott, B., & Shike, M. (2007). Enteral nutrition support of head and neck cancer patients—Invited review. *Nutrition in Clinical Practice, 22,* 68–73.

*Recommended dietary allowances / Subcommittee on the Tenth Edition of the RDAs, Food and Nutrition Board, Commission on Life Sciences, National Research Council* (10th ed.) (1989). Washington, DC: National Academy.

Rombeau, J. L., Caldwell, M. D., Forlaw, L., & Guenter, P. A. (Eds.). (1989). *Atlas of nutritional support techniques.* Boston: Little, Brown.

Rustom, I., Jebreel, A., Tayyab, M., England, R., & Stafford, N. (2006). Percutaneous endoscopic, radiological and surgical gastrostomy tubes: A comparison study in head and neck cancer patients. *Journal of Laryngology and Otology, 120,* 463–466.

Senft, M., Fietkau, R., Iro, H., Sailer, D., & Sauer, R. (1993). The influence of supportive nutritional therapy via percutaneous endoscopically guided gastrostomy on the quality of life of cancer patients. *Supportive Care in Cancer, 1,* 272–275.

Shaw, J. H. F., Wildbore, M. & Wolfe, R. R. (1987). Whole body protein kinetics in severely septic patients: The response to glucose infusion and total parenteral nutrition. *Annals of Surgery, 205,* 288–294.

Standing Committee on the Scientific Evaluation of Dietary Reference Intakes, Food and Nutrition Board, Institute of Medicine. (1997 and 1998). *Dietary reference intakes.* Washington, DC: National Academy Press.

Young, S., Kearns, L., & Schoepfel, S. (2007). Protein. In M. Gottschlich (Ed.), *The A.S.P.E.N. nutrition support core curriculum, a case-based approach—the adult patient* (pp. 71–87). Silver Spring, MD: American Society for Parenteral and Enteral Nutrition.

Webber, C. B., & Splett, P. L. (1995). Nutrition risk factors in a home health population. *Home Health Care Services Quarterly, 15,* 97–110.

Wood, K. (2005). Audit of nutritional guidelines for head and neck cancer patients undergoing radiotherapy. *Journal of Human Nutrition and Diet, 18,* 343–351.

Wooley, J., & Frankenfield, D. (2007). Energy. In M. Gottschlich (Ed.), *The A.S.P.E.N. nutrition support core curriculum, a case-based approach—the adult patient* (pp. 19–32). Silver Spring, MD: American Society for Parenteral and Enteral Nutrition.

Zeman, F. J. (1991). *Clinical nutrition and dietetics* (2nd ed.). New York: Macmillan.

# APPENDIX 10-A

## Recording Food Intakes

Patient Name _____ DOB _____
UCD MR# _____
Telephone _____
Clinic/Service _____
Ht. _____ Wt. _____

### Directions for Recording Your Food Intake:

It is essential that food intake records be filled out as accurately and completely as possible. Each day list all of the foods and beverages you have eaten for any meal and snack. Along with the type of food eaten, record the amount of food and how it was prepared. For example, was it fried? baked? Were bacon drippings or butter added?

### Record portion sizes or the amount of food eaten as follows:

tablespoon – Tbsp.  Cup – C
teaspoon – tsp.  slice – sl.
ounce – oz.

The more details you include, the better we can analyze the diet. For combination dishes and sandwiches, list ingredients: 2 sl. wheat bread, 1 oz. cheese, 1 tsp. mustard.

Carry your daily record with you and fill out the record after you have eaten. Please include times food was eaten.

### Equivalent Measures

3 teaspoons = 1 tablespoon
16 tablespoons = 1 cup
1 ounce = 2 tablespoons
8 ounces = 1 cup
16 ounces = 1 pound
32 fluid ounces = 1 quart

---

## SAMPLE PAGE

Date _Tuesday, 4/20_

Vitamin/Mineral Supplements: _50 mg. Vitamin C_

| Time | Food/Drink | Amount | Method of Preparation |
|---|---|---|---|
| 8:00 | eggs | 1 | soft cooked |
|  | orange juice | 1/2 C. |  |
|  | toast | 1/2 sl. | plain |
| 10:00 | vanilla wafers | 6 |  |
| 12:00 | turkey sandwich | 1 |  |
|  | whole wheat bread | 2 sl. | with 1 tsp. mayonnaise |
|  | turkey | 2 sl. |  |
|  | low fat milk | 4 oz. |  |
| 3:00 | fresh apple | 1/2 | (medium size) |
| 5:30 | baked fish | 1 | 3 inches x 1/2 inch thick |
|  | mashed potatoes | 1/2 C. | made with low fat milk |
|  | spinach | 1/2 C. |  |
|  | low fat milk | 6 oz. |  |
|  | salad, tossed | 1 C. | w/1 Tbsp. french dressing |
| 8:00 | frozen yogurt | 1/2 C. |  |
|  |  |  |  |
|  |  |  |  |

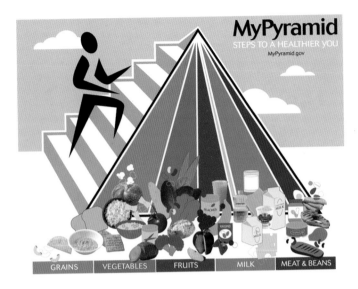

**Grains    Eat 6 oz. every day\***
Eat at least 3 ounces of whole grain cereals, breads, crackers, rice, or pasta every day.

1 ounce is about 1 slice of bread, 1 cup of breakfast cereal, or 1/2 cup of cooked rice, cereal or pasta.

**Vegetables    Eat 2½ cups every day\***
Eat more dark-green veggies like broccoli, spinach, and other dark leafy greens.
Eat more orange vegetables like carrots and sweet potatoes.
Eat more dry beans and peas like pinto beans, kidney beans, and lentils

**Fruits    Eat 2 cups every day\***
Eat a variety of fruit.
Choose fresh, frozen, canned, or dried fruit.
Go easy on fruit juices.
3/4 cup of fruit juice.

*\*This is the amount from each food group to provide a 2000 Calorie diet. Find individual calorie levels at **www.MyPyramid.gov***

**Milk    Get 3 cups every day\***
Go low-fat or fat-free when you choose milk, yogurt, and other milk products.
If you don't or can't consume milk, choose lactose-free products or other calcium sources such as fortified foods and beverages.

**Meat and Beans    Eat 5½ oz. every day\***
Choose low-fat or lean meats and poultry.
Bake it, broil it, or grill it.
Vary your protein routine—choose more fish, beans, peas, nuts, and seeds.

**Know the limits on fats, sugars, and salt (sodium)**
Make most of your fat sources from fish, nuts, and vegetable oils.
Limit solid fats like butter, stick margarine, shortening, and lard, as well as foods that contain these.
Check the Nutrition Facts label to keep saturated fats, *trans* fats, and sodium low.
Choose food and beverages low in added sugars. Added sugars contribute calories with few, if any, nutrients.

Some foods fit into more than one group. Dry beans, peas, and lentils can be counted as servings in either the meat and beans group or vegetable group. These crossover foods can be counted as servings from either one or the other group, but not both. (U.S. Department of Agriculture Center for Nutrition Policy and Promotion, April 2005. www.MyPyramid.gov)

## APPENDIX 10-C

## Food Texture Continuum Matrix

| Thin Liquid ↔ | Thick Liquid ↔ | Slippery Puree ↔ | Puree ↔ | Puree Foods ± Ground Meat ↔ | Soft Foods ± Ground Meat ↔ | Soft Foods ± Chopped Meat |
|---|---|---|---|---|---|---|
| water | NECTAR-LIKE | thin cream of wheat | cooked cream of wheat | cooked oatmeal regular | eggs, all types | *cereal dry |
| coffee, tea | 4 oz. juice + ~1 Tbsp commercial thickener | baby puree meat | pureed scrambled eggs | scrambled eggs | ham, ground sausage, ground Canadian | bacon sausage |
| broth | | | | ham, ground sausage, ground Canadian | bacon, ground | biscuit |
| juice: | Commercially made nectar-like: | custard | pregelled, slurried breads on French toast | bacon, ground | pancakes | bread |
| apple | juices | pudding | | | muffins | crackers |
| cranberry | milk | pureed fruit | entrée meat, pureed | pregelled, slurried breads or French toast | | toast |
| grape | water | | | | roast beef, ground | waffle |
| orange | | | | entrée meat, ground | roast pork, ground | chicken, chopped |
| tomato juice | | | mashed potatoes, yams | | meatloaf | fish |
| nectar | | | | mashed potatoes, yams | Salisbury steak | hamburger patty |
| soft drinks | | | mashed winter squash | mashed winter squash | stew, pieces <½ inch | hot dog |
| milk: | | | pureed cooked vegetables | | | roasts, chopped |
| nonfat | | | | pureed cooked vegetables | noodles | rice |
| lowfat | | | soups, blended smooth | | potatoes | |
| whole | | | | | pasta entrees | |
| chocolate | | | | | | |
| buttermilk | | | | | | |

*(continues)*

163

| Thin Liquid ↔ | Thick Liquid ↔ | Slippery Puree ↔ | Puree ↔ | Puree Foods ± Ground Meat ↔ | Soft Foods ± Ground Meat ↔ | Soft Foods ± Chopped Meat |
|---|---|---|---|---|---|---|
| Instant Breakfast | HONEY-LIKE Generally, 4 oz. thin liquids + ~2 Tbsp commercial thickener | pureed cooked vegetables (no potatoes, yams) | pudding | soups, blended smooth | soups | sandwiches: tuna, egg, bologna, chicken salad, cheese |
| commercial supplement | | | custard | pudding | canned beets | |
| fruit ice | | | yogurt, smooth (no fruit pieces) | custard | soft cooked vegetables: | cooked vegetables: |
| sherbet | | | pureed fruit | yogurt with fruit pieces | carrot coins, peas, spinach, zucchini | broccoli, cauliflower, green beans |
| ice cream | | | | pureed fruit | | tomato, fresh sliced |
| Jello | | | | cottage cheese, small curd | canned fruit, no pineapple, fruit, fresh: banana, strawberries, kiwi | green lettuce salad |
| | | | | | cake | fruit, fresh: banana, melon (cut up), orange (sectioned), pear |
| | | | | | pie, bottom crust only | graham crackers |
| | | | | | | vanilla wafers |
| | | | | | | cookies, no nuts |

# APPENDIX 10-D

## Thickeners

Patients who need to restrict liquids to a thicker consistency will find that the use of either commercial thickening products or the addition of certain foods will allow them to increase the variety of liquids and foods that they are able to eat.

The amount of thickener added will allow control of thickening from nectar-like to honey-like, to an even stiffer spoon-thick consistency. Thickeners can be used to stiffen a pureed food item that may be too thin. Some products work better in hot liquids. Others are supplemented with vitamins and minerals. It is important to compare the amount of product needed to achieve the desired consistency—some products have greater thickening power and, as a result, require less product. Manufactures recommend different amounts of their product to obtain a nectar-like, honey-like, or spoon-thick consistency. The amount of product needed also may differ depending on the temperature, acidity (pH) and amount of sugars and other solids present in solution. Individual product Web sites provide information on product use and recipes.

Following is a list of commercial products and "kitchen cupboard" foods useful as thickeners. Prices vary depending on where purchased and amount ordered. Some companies provide mail order shipping directly to the consumer. Hospital-based speech departments may be able to order through their Food Service Department thereby accessing commercial venders. The local drug store usually stocks a thickening product. If not found on the shelves, or behind the counter, the pharmacy can order it.

Thick-It®
   Powder added to foods

Thick-It® 2
   Concentrated formula for
   maximum thickening

Thick-It® Purees
   Shelf-stable pureed foods,
   "heat and serve" convenience
   and/or for emergency needs.

Precision Foods, Inc.
   (800) 333-0003

www.Precisionfoods.com/retail/branded_
solutions.cfm

Select: "Thick-It®"

Ultra THIXX®
   Mixes easily without a
   blender

THIXX All Purpose Thickener®

Bernard Foods
   For Consumer orders:
   eDietShop
   P.O.Box 1037
   Evanston, IL 60204-1397
   (800) 325-5409
   www.edietshop.com/onlinestore/items.
   asp?CurrentDepartmentNumber=5&
   DEPARTMENT_ID=50
      or, Internet search "THIXX"

Thick & Easy®
  Thickening powder
  Thickened juices
  Thickened water
  Thickened dairy/milk

Hormel Health Labs
http://www.HormelHealthLabs.com
  Order from:
  http://www.HomeCareNutrition.com

NutraThick™
  contains 19 vitamins
  and minerals

Shape & Serve® Thickener for
Shaping and Texture

Hydra Aid
  A non-powder thickening
  agent for hot or cold
  beverages

Links Medical Products, Inc
330 Goddard
Irvine, CA 92618

http://www.linsmed.com
http://info@linksmed.com

KITCHEN CUPBOARD RESOURCES:

Dehydrated potato flakes
Baby instant rice cereal
Pureed vegetables and fruits
Dehydrated baby food
Bread crumbs
Unflavored gelatin—powder needs to be put into solution, then cooled

# 11

# *Endoscopy in Assessing and Treating Dysphagia*

## Rebecca Leonard

Endoscopy is a valuable instrument in both the assessment and treatment of dysphagic patients. The intent of this chapter is to describe both uses of this tool in our clinic. Video clips of evaluations and treatment sessions incorporating endoscopy are included on the DVD-ROM accompanying this text. They can be found in the in the materials folder for Chapter 11.

## FLEXIBLE ENDOSCOPY AS AN ASSESSMENT TOOL

### Description of Flexible Endoscopic Evaluation of Swallowing Safety (FEES)

Flexible endoscopic evaluation of swallowing safety (FEESS) was first described by Langmore, Schatz, and Olsen in 1988, and has been elaborated on frequently in the intervening period by these and other authors (Kidder, Lang-more, & Martin, 1994; Langmore & McCullough, 1997; Langmore, Schatz, & Olsen, 1991). The original "FEESS" procedure is now popularly referred to as "FEES." It has also been referred to as a videoendoscopic evaluation of dysphagia (VEED) (Bastian, 1991). In 1993, Aviv, Martin, Keen, Debell, and Blitzer described flexible endoscopy with sensory testing, referred to as "FEEST." The goal of the latter is to assess laryngeal sensation, but it may also involve an endoscopic assessment of swallowing.

A particular advantage of endoscopy is that it can be performed at bedside or in the clinic, ideally with the patient seated in an upright position. Although not trivial, particularly for inpatients, being able to keep the back straight while bending forward slightly from the waist is helpful. An anesthetic may also optimize the procedure. In our setting, a topical anesthetic agent (lidocaine, 4%), usually combined with neosynephrine (0.25%) is introduced to one nasal passage, the most open if there is a difference from left to right. A gel form of the anesthetic can be applied to the tip of the scope and inserted slowly into the nostril and held in a stable position until it takes effect. Alternatively, the anesthetic can be delivered in spray form. In our experience, the topical anesthetic agent allows the patient to accommodate the procedure more comfortably, but the examiner must take care not to interrupt sensory input to structures of interest. Some clinicians have, in fact, refrained from using an anesthetic agent because of this concern. However, in a double-blind crossover study, Johnson, Belafsky, and Postma (2003) reported no differences in laryngopharyngeal sensory testing in patients who underwent multiple exams with different anesthetic agents and a saline sham, respectively. These authors used two sprays in each nostril, and each spray was 1 second in duration. As noted, we typically apply the agent used to only one nostril. If no anesthetic is used, a small amount of lubricating jelly on the scope may allow more comfortable insertion. The tip of the scope can be dipped into an antifogging agent, as well. All food materials to be used have been previously prepared and are readily at hand.

When these preparations are complete, the scope is inserted into the nares, usually along the floor of the nose. If there is some question about velar function, or about the degree of closure of the velopharyngeal port during swallow, the scope may be inserted between the inferior and middle turbinates to ensure a viewing position that will enable simultaneous visualization of the velum, and lateral and posterior pharyngeal walls. For observation of other structures during swallow, the scope is inserted along the floor of the nose. Observation of oropharyngeal structures is completed with the tip of the scope in the oropharynx, typically at or just below where the inferior soft palate would be at rest during quiet breathing (mouth closed), with the tongue base, pyriform sinuses, posterior pharyngeal wall, postcricoid area, and laryngeal structures in view. Laryngeal structures are better viewed with the scope tip lower, at about the epiglottis, with the full length of the true vocal folds visible. With the scope appropriately placed, the patient is asked to engage in tasks directed to evaluating the integrity of swallowing structures, and the safety or efficiency of swallowing. Ideally, a videocamera attached to the flexible nasopharyngoscope and a videocassette recorder (VCR) or digital recorder (DVR) are used to record the study for later review. A monitor permits not only the examiner but others present, including the patient, to view the study. There are some situations, for example, when subtle silent aspiration is suspected, in which we may also use a rigid oral endoscope (typically used in stroboscopic imaging of the larynx). Although this scope is not in place during swallow, it can provide a large, very bright view of the larynx and other structures postswallow. Using a rigid scope, we have sometimes identified small amounts of bolus material on the vocal folds, or even in the subglottic airway, that were not observed with the flexible scope.

## Indications for FEES

Evaluation of swallowing function with FEES does not provide the same information as a dynamic videofluoroscopic study (DSS) of swallow; rather, the two studies are probably best viewed as complementary to each other. Recent studies have demonstrated that the two exams may be equivalent in diagnosing dysphagia and implementing treatment strategies to facilitate safe and effective swallowing (Leder & Karas, 2000; Rees, 2006). Both exams have also been reported to be equally sensitive in identifying delayed initiation of swallow, penetration, aspiration, and post-swallow residue (Langmore, Shatz, & Olson, 1991; Leder, Sasaki, & Burrell, 1998). Aviv (2000) reported further that, whether dysphagic patients had their dietary and behavioral management directed by fluoroscopy or FEES with sensory testing, their outcomes with respect to the incidence of pneumonia or pneumonia-free time interval were essentially the same. In our view, there are a number of indications for FEES, some related to information provided by FEES but not videofluoroscopy, and others related to the exigencies of an endoscopic exam as opposed to a radiographic study.

Indications for FEES related to the unique type of information provided by the procedure include:

- Concerns about alterations in nasopharyngeal, oropharyngeal, or laryngeal anatomy that may not be apparent on videofluoroscopy. Certainly, the larynx and true vocal folds are better evaluated with endoscopy.

- Concerns about sensory integrity of pharyngeal and/or laryngeal structures.
- Concerns about the patient's ability to initiate and maintain airway protection over a given period of time.
- High risk of aspiration, where it is desirable to assess swallow function without food or liquid.
- Repeated swallows are of interest, as when there is a question of the patient fatiguing over time.
- It is desirable to assess symmetry of pharyngeal constriction, that is, differences from right to left. This can be done to some extent with fluoroscopy (in the anterior-posterior view), but endoscopy provides insights into the simultaneous contributions to constriction from both tongue and pharynx that are not possible with other techniques.
- It is desirable to provide "on-line" visual feedback to the patient or others.
- It is desirable to assess effects of various strategies, that is, head turning, breath holding, in a repeated fashion over time.

Indications related to the exigencies of the exam include the following:

- Patient cannot be transported to the site of a radiographic study.
- There are concerns about repeated exposure to radiation associated with videofluoroscopy, as when a patient's condition is changing rapidly over a brief period of time.

■ Information is needed more quickly than scheduling a radiographic exam will permit.

## Limitations of FEES

As noted, FEES cannot provide the examiner with all the same information that can be obtained from videofluoroscopy. For example, FEES does not allow evaluation of bolus management in the oral cavity. The patient's ability to form and hold a bolus in the mouth, transfer it from anterior to posterior oral cavity, and deliver it into the pharynx are better observed with fluoroscopy. Another limitation of FEES is that, during the moment of swallow, approximation of tongue and pharynx often precludes visualization of pertinent events. In addition, information regarding *degree* of pharyngeal constriction, opening of the upper esophageal sphincter, and hyoid/laryngeal elevation during the swallow is not available. This is important because the integrity of these gestures often explains the mechanics of dysphagia in an individual patient. Similarly, penetration or aspiration of the bolus, which occurs at, or in close proximity to, the time of swallow, may not be visualized, although it may be inferred after the swallow from inspection of laryngeal structures. Some clinicians would argue that FEES and fluoroscopy provide comparable information regarding subtle aspiration. In our experience, this depends on the quality of a FEES exam. We would suggest that, given comparable levels of exam quality and clinician skill, subtle aspiration is likely to be identified more often with fluo-

roscopy than with endoscopy. This may be particularly true when aspirated material is noted only below the vocal folds. In addition, most quantitative measures of timing and displacement, which can be obtained from radiographic studies, are not possible with FEES. Some clinicians have noted that endoscopy provides better information than fluoroscopy about the presence of secretions in the airway. In our experience, however, if secretions are sufficiently copious, they may preclude endoscopic visualization of important structures. In such situations, fluoroscopy may be more useful.

## Assessment Tasks

Specific tasks included in FEES will depend on a number of factors, including *how much the patient is able to tolerate without fatigue, and the direction the exam takes based on preliminary findings.* In addition, some tasks may be included to address specific questions posed by the referring professional. Tasks designed to assess particular structures or functions are summarized below. In some instances, it may be both possible and desirable to perform all or most of them. But, as noted, the particular tasks included in the exam are very much dependent on the individual patient. What is reasonable in an outpatient who is recovering nicely from some incident or illness may be very different from what is possible in an inpatient who has been NPO (nothing by mouth) for days or weeks and is just being considered for limited oral eating. In all cases, the exam is begun when the patient is appropriately positioned, the scope has been inserted, and the structures of interest are in view. If the exam is being videotaped and there is a need to provide feedback to the patient, the monitor should be placed so that both examiner and patient can easily refer to it. If the study is being performed by a sole examiner, it is imperative to have all materials previously prepared and easily available.

### Assessment of Valves and Chambers

One way to consider the structures of the upper airway is as a series of valves and chambers. Chambers, including the oral cavity, oropharynx, and hypopharynx, first expand to accommodate bolus material, and then compress. With compression, a gradient in favor of flow (from a region of higher pressure to a region of lower pressure) is established and bolus material is propelled and then cleared from the chamber. Failure of a chamber may thus impair both propulsion and clearing of bolus material. Valves, including the linguavelar, velopharyneal, laryngeal (including arytenoids and epiglottis, false vocal folds, and true vocal folds), and the pharyngoesopohageal segment (PES) regulate bolus flow from one chamber to the next. In doing so, they either appropriately permit or prevent bolus material from moving from chamber to chamber. Impairment in a valve may lead to early loss of the bolus, inappropriate entrance or reflux of bolus into a chamber and and/or ineffective bolus transmission. The first objective of FEES is to evaluate the integrity of these valves and chambers. Tasks for doing this are described next.

**Tasks for Assessment of Velopharyngeal Valving.** In a normal swallow, the velum first lowers, acting with the tongue to contain bolus material in the oral cavity. As the bolus is moved into the pharynx, the velum must then elevate to form another valve with the posterior and lateral pharyngeal walls. The rapid elevation of the velum may help to propel the bolus, and its valving action with the pharynx prevents bolus material from entering the nose. During speech, the area of the velopharyngeal orifice is typically less than 20 $mm^2$ for nonnasal sounds. At rest, this area is thought to be much larger; during speech, for example, areas greater than 100 $mm^2$ have been associated with the perception of extreme nasality (Warren & Mackler, 1968). During swallow, the area approximates zero (Figure 11–1). The tasks described here should allow the examiner to assess the valving function of the velum and corresponding lateral and posterior pharyngeal walls. (See "VPPORT" in Chapter 11 materials folder.)

- With the nasopharyngoscope between inferior and middle turbinates, the patient is asked to produce a sustained vowel sound, then a sustained /s/, and, if possible, a sentence that contains no nasal sounds ("Is Sassy sick?"). Elevation of the velum and constriction of the lateral and posterior pharyngeal walls are observed. Collectively, these structures contribute to closure of the velopharyngeal port during speech and swallow.
- Symmetry and contributions of each structure to closure are

**Figure 11-1.** On left, velopharyngeal port is shown during production of /n/ (velum is at bottom, posterior pharyngeal wall at top, and lateral pharyngeal walls on right and left, respectively); on right, port is shown during closure for vowel /i/.

noted. Typically, one should see tighter closure for /s/ than for a vowel, and closure that is maintained for the duration of the sentence. Closure during a dry swallow can then be observed, and may be noted to be somewhat different from the closure for speech, for example, contact of structures may be lower. Following these tasks, the patient can be asked to swallow a small liquid bolus (1–3 cc). The velopharyngeal port is observed for any leakage of material into the nose. Alternatively, the examiner may elect to include this task in the evaluation of swallow function.

**Tasks for Assessment of Pharyngeal Chamber and Valve.** The walls of the pharynx can constrict several millimeters in going from a relaxed to maximally constricted position. Normative data from our laboratory, in fact, sug- gest that mean pharyngeal area in a pseudorest position, measured in the lateral view from videofluoroscopic studies and thus representing only two of three dimensions of the pharynx (anterior-posterior and superior-inferior, but not lateral or left-right), is 6.5 cm$^2$ in female adults under 65 years of age, and 7.9 cm$^2$ in male adults of compara- ble age (8.1 cm$^2$ and 11.4 cm$^2$ in normal females and males, respectively, over 65 years of age). At the point of maxi- mum constriction and shortening dur- ing swallow, this value approximates zero. (These measures are discussed at length in Chapters 16 and 17.) During swallow, sequential changes in both size and shape of the pharynx help to propel the bolus from mouth to esophagus. The tasks described here should allow the examiner to observe the patient's potential for effecting appropriate pharyngeal dynamics. (The reader is encouraged to view the video clips "OROPHX" and "HYPOPHX" included in the Chapter 11 materials folder while reviewing these tasks.)

■ Scope is advanced along the floor of nose into the oropharynx, being sure to find a placement that will allow pharyngeal structures to be observed when the soft palate elevates. The patient is asked to produce /a/, pronounced "ah," and to then retract or move the tongue posteriorly in an attempt to produce pharyngeal frication, that is, fricative-like sound produced by forcing air across a constriction of posterior tongue to pharynx. Contact between tongue base and posterior pharynx is observed. Not all patients will be able to perform this task, but if they are able to attempt it, the information is very useful (Figures 11–2, 11–3, 11–4, 11–5).

**Figure 11-2.** Oropharynx expanded (*left*) and then compressed (*right*) as subject moves tongue (*at arrows*) posteriorly. Scope is just above oropharynx, at about the velum.

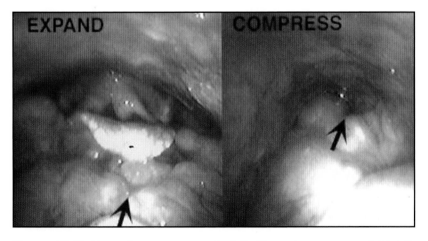

**Figure 11-3.** Hypopharynx expanded (*left*) and compressed (*right*); scope tip is below velum.

**Figure 11–6.** Thin secretions in right pyriform sinus; thick secretions appear as folds in left piriform sinus and postcricoid area.

**Figure 11–4.** Scope tip is just above epiglottis. Pharynx is expanded.

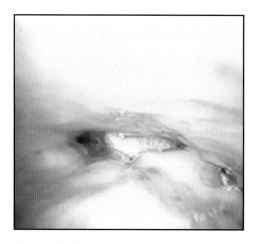

**Figure 11–5.** Scope tip above epiglottis; pharynx compressed (not a swallow). Upper portion of epiglottis can be seen between tongue base and posterior pharyngeal wall.

■ Pyriform sinuses, valleculae, pharyngeal walls, base of tongue, and postcricoid area are examined for evidence of pooled secretions (Figure 11–6). At sites of pooling, examiner may want to lightly touch the tissue with the scope tip and

ask the patient to respond when the stimulus is felt. In the normal case, there should be no or minimal secretions at these sites, perhaps only a few bubbles, and even light touch with the scope tip should elicit a response. The presence of pooling may indicate poor sensation, or poor ability to clear tissues. If pooled secretions clear well with swallow, sensation may be implicated. Secretions that do not clear with swallow, on the other hand, may suggest incomplete or ineffective movements of structures. In some patients, sensory and motor functions may both be impaired.

■ Ask patient to elevate vocal pitch to as high a level as possible. Observe pharyngeal constriction. Note presence or absence, and whether there is a difference from one side to the other. Typically, the pharynx does constrict during this task. The maneuver is sometimes described as a surrogate measure of pharyngeal strength, but this has yet to be documented. However, intact pharyngeal squeeze has been associated with a reduced risk of aspiration on pureed foods, independent of laryngopharyngeal sensation (Perlman et al., 2004).

- Ask patient to hold the nose and bear down. Observe piriform sinuses for maximal opening. Have patient relax and observe return of sinuses to rest.
- Ask patient to turn head from one side to the other. Observe closure of piriform sinuses (Figure 11–7). Note, in particular, asymmetries from right to left that may suggest weakness.

**Tasks for Assessment of Laryngeal Chamber and Valves.** Typically, the larynx acts to protect the airway and assist in opening of the PES during swallow. The tasks described here allow the examiner to assess the ability of the larynx to close, thereby protecting the airway, and to elevate, further protecting the airway and facilitating opening of the PES. The tasks also

**Figure 11-7.** Piriform sinus on right is compressed with head turned to right.

consider the ability of the larynx to respond to bolus materials that may come in contact with its structures.

- With the scope lowered to approximately the epiglottis, ask the patient to sustain a vowel sound for several seconds (a high, front vowel sound, such as "ee," typically causes the larynx to elevate, and facilitates visualization of laryngeal structures). If good visualization of the larynx is difficult because of elevation of the soft palate, a nasal sound, such as a sustained "mmm," may be used for this task. Observe the mobility of the true vocal folds, the completeness of closure of the true vocal folds along their anterior to posterior dimension, and the length of time they remain in an adducted position (patients with impaired swallow may need to protect the airway for several seconds). Note the quality of the voice produced. Incomplete closure, inability to maintain closure, and weak, breathy voice quality may be indicative of vocal fold dysfunction and compromised ability to protect the airway.
- With the scope held in as constant position as possible, ask the patient to produce a vowel at a low vocal pitch, and to then shift to as high a pitch as possible. Note changes in length of vocal folds, any elevation of laryngeal structures, and patient's ability to raise pitch

**Figure 11–8.** With scope held in place at patient's nostril, patient is asked to alternate between low- (*on left*) and high-pitched (*on right*) /i/s. True folds elongate and also appear to elevate on high-pitched production (note enlarged size of superior arytenoid cartilages, as well as of true folds).

(Figure 11–8). Typically, raising pitch (fundamental frequency) is associated with the larynx elevating, as well. An inability to alter pitch in this way may indicate some dysfunction of the superior laryngeal nerve, or cricothyroid muscle, or of the suprahyoid muscles of the larynx.

■ Observe patient's ability to produce a series of brief /i/ sounds ("i" is pronounced as the vowel in "P<u>e</u>te"), each of which is followed by inspiration (preferably, through the nose). Instructing the patient to sniff after vocalization may

facilitate the task. Watch for obvious or subtle asymmetries in abduction and adduction of the true vocal folds that could indicate a paralysis or paresis of one fold.

■ Ask the patient to hold his or her breath (Figure 11–9). Observe degree of adduction of true folds, as well as any constriction/medialization of the false folds, and/or approximation of the arytenoids to the epiglottis. Typically, the false folds are closed during breath holding. With tight breath holding, the larynx may appear sphincteric, with the false folds

**Figure 11-9.** During tight breath holding, true vocal folds close, then false folds constrict, followed by approximation of arytenoids to epiglottis.

constricted and arytenoids approximating the epiglottis. This task is a good way to evaluate all the valves of the larynx. In Figure 11–10, a patient has gagged and the larynx has rocked forward, opening the PES. This rocking action of the larynx is also associated with opening of the PES valve during swallow, which is not typically observed during FEES.

■ Observe effectiveness of true fold adduction for throat clearing and cough.

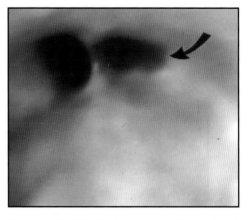

**Figure 11-10.** During gag, the cricoid can be seen to rock forward, and the PES opens (*at arrow*).

## Tasks for Assessment of Swallow Function

Requirements for normal swallow include the transfer of a bolus quickly and safely from the oral cavity through the pharynx to the upper esophagus. The tasks described here allow the examiner to assess several events before and after swallow that are critical to this process.

With the scope positioned back in the oropharynx, bolus materials are introduced, starting with a small amount of liquid that has been colored green with food coloring (i.e., edible vegetable dyes). In our clinic, the standard exam is begun with a 1-cc liquid bolus, or a small amount of ice chips. Ice chips may be particularly helpful in patients who have not been eating orally for a period of time (Rees, 2006). With the scope positioned appropriately for observing relevant structures, the patient is asked to perform the following:

- Hold the bolus in the mouth until the examiner counts to three, then swallow. Any early loss of the bolus into the valleculae or pyriform sinuses, or any penetration or aspiration of bolus material prior to the swallow, is noted.
- Following the swallow, sites previously examined (i.e., nose, valleculae, piriform sinuses, tongue base, pharyngeal walls, postcricoid area, true and false vocal folds) are examined for evidence of residue. Sites and sidedness of residue material, and estimate (if possible) of how much of bolus introduced appears as residue, are noted.

- If residue is observed, evidence of repeat swallow is noted. If none is observed, the patient is asked to repeat the swallow. Any clearing that takes place during the repetition is noted.
- If residue is present on the vocal folds, cough or throat-clearing responses are noted. If no response is noted, the patient is asked to cough and then repeat the swallow. Effectiveness in clearing residue is assessed.
- If the swallow approximates normal, the examiner is unlikely to actually observe the instant of swallow because constriction of tongue and pharynx obscures visualization. In patients with weak tongue–pharynx constriction, however, it may be possible to obtain more information.

Following swallow of a 1-cc bolus, the patient repeats the tasks with a 3-cc liquid bolus, and then a larger self-selected bolus in a cup. For the latter task, the patient selects how much of the bolus material he or she wants to attempt. These tasks are repeated for the larger liquid boluses if it appears safe to do so, and with pudding if difficulties are encountered on any of the liquid swallows. If the liquid swallows are managed without incident, the pudding bolus is replaced with a paste bolus (e.g., peanut butter).

These assessment tasks represent similar tasks, in the same order, as those used in videofluoroscopic studies at our institution. Bolus materials used for FEES typically do not contain radiopaque material, but they do represent similar consistencies and a similar order of presentation. The reason for this is twofold. If you anticipate following a patient over time, the ability to repeat at least some of the same tasks from exam to exam permits more uniform assessment of progress or deterioration over time. Furthermore, if both fluoroscopy and endoscopy studies are performed on a patient, completion of a portion of the same or very similar tasks on both provides some basis of comparison across evaluation techniques.

When these protocol swallows are complete, specific foods that have been identified as causing particular difficulty for a patient can be tried. Or, if the objective is to determine if a patient's diet needs to be altered, either advanced or restricted, the exam can be tailored to answer these questions. In following patients serially, it is important to maintain a balance between identifying changes in integrity of structures and functions, and changes in swallowing capabilities. Attempting to adhere to a protocol, that is, some uniformity in tasks and task order across exams, can in our opinion usually be accomplished even with patients whose tolerance for the exam is quite limited.

## Implications of Findings

By the completion of the FEES evaluation, the examiner should have good insights into the integrity of oropharyngeal and laryngeal structures and functions for food management and swallowing. For example, the patient's ability to effect lingua-velar, velopharyngeal, lingua-pharyngeal and laryngeal *valving actions* necessary for safe and effective swallowing should be well

understood. Impressions gained will lead to therapeutic strategies directed at improving, bypassing, or compensating for any deficits identified. Similarly, indications of *diminshed sensation* identified during the examination will require consideration of strategies that may enhance sensory stimulation, as by manipulating bolus characteristics or redirecting bolus materials to a more intact side or site. In like manner, the patient's *ability to compensate* for the early loss of bolus material, or residue remaining after an attempted swallow, will have been sampled across bolus materials, and in terms of both sites and amounts of loss or residue noted. The resulting observations will enter into decisions regarding whether oral feeding is safe, or under what conditions it can be made safer.

As noted, a particular appeal of FEES is the opportunity it provides for assessing the likely benefit of behavioral strategies via *therapeutic probes* (including the effects of positional changes, voluntary maneuvers, bolus manipulation, etc.) The length of the examination is constrained by the patient's comfort and attention levels, but not greatly by concerns about hazards associated with the examination technique, itself. Trial probes performed with both examiner and patient observing the consequences on the video monitor are particularly useful. The ability to make *observations over time* is another feature of FEES that adds to its value. Evidence of fatigue in valving functions, consequences of collective swallows, or residue buildup, over precise periods of time, are examples of the kinds of time-delay observations that can have implications for treatment planning and can be explored more thoroughly with endoscopic evaluation than with other assessment techniques.

## FLEXIBLE ENDOSCOPY AS A THERAPEUTIC TOOL

Endoscopy is an extremely valuable assessment tool, and an equally useful tool in the management of dysphagic patients. Very often in our setting, patients who have undergone fluoroscopy studies, and for whom particular strategies have been identified as potentially useful, are brought in for at least one therapy session to explore in depth the strategies previously identified. During these sessions, the emphasis is on assessing the effects of strategies, and on providing clinician, patient and other caregivers with feedback regarding these techniques. The conduct of these sessions is different from an assessment with FEES, particularly if they occur in close proximity to the fluoroscopy evaluation and there is no evidence of significant change in the patient's capabilities.

Noted below are therapeutic swallowing strategies, that is, strategies designed to facilitate safe swallowing. Visual feedback provided to the patient during their performance may be useful in teaching their effectiveness and in improving the patient's control of volitional gestures involved. (The reader is directed to the "FEESPT1" clip in the Chapter 11 materials folder for an example. The patient in this clip has undergone base of tongue/pharynx resection for head and neck cancer).

- Tongue–pharynx constriction: Ask the patient to produce "ah" or "uh," and to then move the tongue posteriorly until pharyngeal frication can be produced.
- Pharyngeal constriction by producing high-pitched vocalization.
- Laryngeal elevation by raising pitch, or rapid alternation of high and low pitches.
- Breath holding, with true vocal folds, and with sphincteric closure involving true and false vocal folds, and arytenoid to epiglottis approximation.
- Effects of postural changes, such as head turning or side-lying. Note changes in voice and breath holding, but also any closing off of piriform sinuses.

Equally important in attempting strategies that have been identified as potentially helpful to safe or effective swallow is the determination of any *aversive* consequences of these strategies. For example, the reader is directed to video clip "FEESPT2" in the Chapter 11 materials folder. In this clip, a patient for whom airway protection has been determined to be impaired is counseled to hold his breath during swallow. Because his transit times have been determined (via dynamic fluoroscopic swallow study) to be prolonged, he is encouraged to hold his breath tightly for several seconds, thereby protecting his airway throughout the swallow. With the patient complying with this instruction, that is, "Hold your breath, tighter ... tighter ... " for a few seconds, a massive reflux event occurs that imperils his airway. This was not observed on fluoroscopy and, had we not scheduled the endoscopic follow-up to assess the effectiveness and safety of our recommendations, the strategy would have been recommended to the patient with no recognition of the potential aversive consequences it posed to his safe swallowing. **We view this type of postevaluation appraisal of any behavioral strategies recommended as a necessary and valuable part of our management plan for a patient.**

## ISSUES OR CONCERNS

Major issues associated with endoscopic examination include the examiner(s), the setting in which the exam is performed, the use of a topical anesthetic, and other risks posed by the procedure. The examiner, whether physician or speech pathologist, should be skilled in the use of flexible endoscopy, and, of course, knowledgeable about both head and neck anatomy, and the particular physiology of swallowing. The setting or settings in which the exam is performed should have both staff and equipment resources to respond appropriately to a medical emergency. Some states, including California, require that speech–language pathologists complete a certification program beyond licensure in order to perform endoscopy procedures (details are specified in California Senate Bills 1379 and 1285). Specific requirements (in California) include the speech pathologist's mentoring by an otolaryngologist during the completion of 25 flexible endoscopic procedures. The physician must then document the speech-language pathologist's competency to perform the exam. Beyond this requirement, settings in which the procedure can be performed must meet certain require-

ments regarding the availability of medical professionals and resources for the management of a medical emergency.

Potential risks associated with the procedure include vasovagal responses, nose bleed, and a reaction to the topical anesthetic (if used). Much can be done to minimize the likelihood of any of these risks, for example, by taking pains to put the patient at ease before proceeding with the exam, careful insertion of the scope, limitation of the anesthetic agent to the nasal mucosa (and away from the larynx), or performing the exam without an anesthetic. Precautions for cleaning and maintaining equipment must be observed strictly, as well. Even with careful adherence to these guidelines, however, the potential risks associated with the procedure require that it be undertaken, in our opinion, in a setting with resources available for handling any emergencies that might arise. In our setting, all patients who are undergoing bedside, clinical, radiographic, or endoscopic evaluations for dysphagia are followed by a team of professionals, all of whom share in the evaluation of diagnostic studies and treatment planning for each patient. Similarly, specific guidelines for use of topical anesthetic agents, responses to medical emergencies, and cleaning and maintenance of equipment have been developed by our institution. Beyond this, our team has invested considerable time and energy in continuing education activities, both formal and didactic, to ensure that specialists who are performing endoscopic examinations are well-qualified to do so. Depending on individual specialists, patient populations, and settings, different approaches to endoscopic swallow studies may be applicable and appropriate. However, in our opinion, any approach must maximize the patient's safety and ensure the most accurate information possible.

## Details of Instrumentation

Basic equipment includes a nasopharyngoscope and portable light source, the total cost of which may approximate several thousand dollars. Newer videoendoscopes, which house a camera chip in the tip of the scope (and thus, much closer to structures) are excellent, but also more expensive than traditional nasopharyngoscopes that use a camera attached to the eyepiece. The next major expense is for a video camera. Miniature video CCD cameras used for most endoscopic procedures, with low lux levels and good resolution, currently start at about $3500, plus costs for appropriate lenses and cables. A good quality, medical-commercial grade videocassette or digital recorder (VCR or DVR) may begin at about $2500. TV or computer monitors may be purchased for a few hundred dollars, but increase in cost with improved resolution. Many home-use recorders and monitors may be adequate, if they meet electrical standards governing the use of such appliances in medical settings. A microphone attached to the VCR or DVD recorder permits an audio record of the exam, which is extremely helpful.

Timing information can be added to the videotape with the use of a timing generator, for example, the Horita Time-Code Generator, TG-50 or Video Stopwatch VS-50 (Horita, Mission Viejo, California). Timing instrumentation can currently be purchased for about $350 to 450. Although timing of specific events, that is, pharyngeal transit, hyoid elevation, typically extracted from the dynamic swallow study cannot be obtained from FEES, timing information of other types, that is, time required to clear residue with repeat swallows, time vocal folds can be maintained in adducted position, may be obtainable and of interest

## STUDY QUESTIONS

1. What is the difference between FEES and FEEST?
2. What are the concerns about using a topical anesthetic agent in assessing dysphagic patients with FEES? What other risks are associated with FEES?
3. What aspects of swallowing typically *cannot* be observed during FEES that can be observed with fluoroscopy?
4. Name five indications for using FEES rather than the MBS/DSS.
5. Name the physiologic "valves" and "chambers" involved in swallowing. What tasks might you use to assess the integrity of each with endoscopy?
6. How might you use endoscopy to implement information about a patient's swallow learned from a fluoroscopic study?
7. What is the advantage of using a standard protocol when assessing dysphagia with FEES?

## REFERENCES

Aviv, J. (2000). Prospective, randomized outcome study of endoscopy versus modified barium swallow in patients with dysphagia. *Laryngoscope*, 110, 563–574.

Aviv, J. E., Martin, J. H., Keen, M. S., Debell, M., & Blitzer, A. (1993). Air pulse quantification of supraglottica and pharyngeal sensation: A new technique. *Annals of Otology Rhinology and Laryngology*, 102, 777–780.

Bastian, R. W.(1993). The videoendoscopic swallowing study: An alternative and partner to the videofluoroscopic swallowing study. *Dysphagia*, 8, 359–367.

Johnson, P. E., Belafsky, P. C., & Postma, G. N. (2003). Topical nasal anesthesia for transnasal fiberoptic laryngoscopy: A prospective, double-blind, cross-over study. *Otolaryngology-Head and Neck Surgery*, 128, 452–254.

Kidder, T. M., Langmore, S. E., & Martin, B. J. (1994). Indications and techniques of endoscopy in evaluation of cervical dysphagia: Comparison with radiographic techniques. *Dysphagia*, 9, 256–261.

Langmore, S. E., & McCulloch, T. M. (1997). Examination of the pharynx and larynx and endoscopic examination of pharyngeal swallowing. In A. Perlman & K. Schulze-Delrieu, (Eds.), *Deglutition and its disorders* (pp. 201–226). San Diego, CA: Singular.

Langmore, S. E., Schatz, K., & Olson, N. (1988). Fiberoptic endoscopic evaluation of swallowing safety: A new procedure. *Dysphagia*, 2, 216–219.

Langmore, S. E., Schatz, K., & Olson, N. (1991). Endoscopic and videofluoroscopic evaluations of swallowing and aspiration. *Annals of Otology and Rhinology*, 100, 678–681

Leder, S. B., & Karas, D. E. (2000). Fiberoptic endoscopic evaluation of swallowing in the pediatric population. *Laryngoscope*, 110, 1132–1136.

Leder, S. B., Sasaki, C. T., & Burrell, M. I. (1998). Fiberoptic endoscopic examination to identify silent aspiration. *Dysphagia*, 13, 19–21.

Perlman, P. W., Cohen, M. A., Setzen, M., Belafsky, P. C., Guss, J., Mattucci, K. F. et al. (2004). The risk of aspiration of pureed food as determined by flexible endoscopic evaluation of swallowing with sensory testing. *Otolaryngology-Head and Neck Surgery*, 130, 80–83.

Rees, C. (2006). Flexible endoscopic evaluation of swallowing with sensory testing. *Current Opinion in Otolaryngology-Head and Neck Surgery*, 14, 425–430.

Setzen, M., Cohen, M. A., Perlman, P. W., Belafsky, P. C., Guss, J., Mattucci, K. F., et al. (2003). The association between laryngopharyngeal sensory deficits, pharyngeal motor function, and the prevalence of aspiration with thin liquids. *Otolaryngology-Head and Neck Surgery*, 128, 99–102.

Warren, D., & Mackler, S. B. (1968). Duration of oral port constriction in normal and cleft palate speech. *Journal of Speech and Hearing Research*, 11, 391–401.

# 12

# *Radiographic Evaluation of the Pharynx and Esophagus*

## C. John Rosenquist

Radiographic evaluation of the pharynx and esophagus is usually considered as two separate examinations that may be performed either separately or together for evaluation of a specific clinical problem (Logemann, 1983, 1986). Radiographic examination of the pharynx is typically referred to as a dynamic swallowing study, and is accomplished by videofluoroscopy, or video radiography. Other radiographic methods that can be used for examination of the pharynx include cineradiography and rapid sequence digital radiography. Recently, dynamic magnetic resonance imaging techniques (cine-MRI), which are noninvasive, have been described (Hartl, Kolb, Bretagne, Marandas, & Sigal, 2006; Kitano, Asada, Hayashi, Inoue, & Kitajima, 2002). However, technical limitations (i.e., poor temporal resolution, supine positioning) have, to date, limited their wide application. Radiographic examination of the esophagus is termed barium swallow or esophagram. This study is often combined with examination of the stomach and duodenum. To obtain optimal information from the examination and minimize radiation exposure, it is important to have an understanding of the indications and technique for each of these examinations.

## DESCRIPTION OF EQUIPMENT

Examination of the pharynx and esophagus is generally done in a standard radiographic and fluoroscopic x-ray room that is equipped with some type of system for rapid sequence filming. The rapid sequence recording is necessary because the process of swallowing occurs quickly, and in order to analyze the swallowing process, this capability must be available. During the early years of development of these examinations, cineradiography, which is essentially a recording of the amplified fluoroscopic image on film, was used for rapid sequence filming. The major advantage of this system was the high spatial resolution of the images and the ability to easily analyze individual frames; the major disadvantage was greater radiation exposure than with other methods, as well as difficulties related to processing and analysis of the film. Cineradiography is no longer available in most facilities and has been replaced by videofluoroscopy, which is a recording of the fluoroscopic image by a television monitor and magnetic tape or digital disk. Although spatial resolution is less than with cineradiography, it is generally adequate for most studies. It has the advantages of less radiation exposure, easier manipulation of the images, and the ability to record sound. More recently rapid sequence digital radiography which is capable of rapid sequence filming of up to six frames per second has become available. Advantages of this system include excellent spatial resolution, easy manipulation of the images, including brightness and contrast changes, and relatively low radiation exposures. The chief disadvantages are too few frames per second for some studies, and its lack of availability in many departments.

Exposure to radiation occurs with examination of both the pharynx and esophagus. For this reason, patients should be carefully evaluated before these studies are done to determine with certainty that the examination is indicated. This is of particular concern with younger patients. The referring physician, radiologist, and speech pathologist should all be involved in the decision. In addition, individuals conducting the examination should have knowledge of radiation exposure and use appropriate protection from radiation, for both the patient and the individuals conducting the examination. Radiation exposure to the patient can be measured in several ways, including skin exposure, gonadal dose, and total body exposure. Of additional concern in examination of the pharynx and upper esophagus is radiation exposure of the thyroid. Radiation exposure of the lens of the eye is also an important issue when the head and neck are exposed to radiation. A comparison of radiation exposure for the techniques used for radiographic swallowing studies is seen in Table 12–1. Factors affecting radiation dose include: kilovolt peak (kVp), which is the peak voltage across the x-ray tube; milliampere seconds (mAs), which is the tube current multiplied by exposure time; image field size; source to skin distance; source to detector distance; and use of a grid.

**Table 12-1.** Radiation Dose Rate During Videofluoroscopic Swallowing Study (mGy/min)*

| Projection | Skin | Thyroid |
|---|---|---|
| Posterior–anterior | 9.5 | .27 |
| Lateral | 7.7 | .99 |

*Exposure factors include: Automatic brightness control with 65 kVp, 1.1 ma, 8:1 grid, source to skin distance, 46 cm; source to detector distance, 86 cm; 9" field of view.

## INDICATIONS

Radiographic study of the pharynx and esophagus is an essential part of the examination for a variety of clinical problems, including dysphagia, odynophagia, aspiration, chronic cough, substernal pain, epigastric pain, and postoperative evaluation following various surgical procedures (Ekberg & Nylander, 1983). Because of the complexity, cost, and radiation exposure that result from radiographic examination of the pharynx and esophagus, it is important that a physician and the speech pathologist evaluate the patient before the examination. This is necessary to determine that the examination is indicated and to tailor the study to the specific clinical problem. Contraindications to esophageal examination with standard barium swallow and esophagram include inability of the patient to swallow, obstruction of the pharynx or esophagus, and a strong likelihood of aspiration. These problems are minimized with the dynamic swallow study.

## EXAMINATION TECHNIQUE

Because of its general availability and ability to demonstrate motion, videofluoroscopy is the method most often used for swallowing studies and other examinations of the pharynx. The examination is done in the standing or sitting position using a standard fluoroscopy table in the upright position. For patients who are unable to support themselves, chairs that provide support for the patient's head and neck have been developed. The examination is usually done first in the lateral position. The patient takes a bolus of barium (about 60% weight/volume) into the mouth and is instructed to swallow while a recording is made from the oropharynx to the cervical esophagus. Structures that are visualized include the base of the tongue, valleculae, epiglottis, piriform sinuses, cricopharyngeus muscle, and cervical esophagus (Figure 12–1) (Dodds, 1989; Dodds, Stewart, & Logemann, 1990). In the normal person, the passage of a bolus of barium from the mouth to the cervical esophagus takes approximately one second. A similar recording of a swallow is then done in the frontal projection (Figures 12–2 and 12–3). The valleculae and pyriform sinuses are usually better seen in this projection, whereas the epiglottis and cricopharyngeus muscle are less well visualized. Some pathologies, such as Zenker's diverticulum, may be bet-

**Figure 12-1.** Lateral view of the pharynx. The base of the tongue and uvula are indicated by arrows. The pharyngoesophageal segment is completely relaxed and therefore not seen.

**Figure 12–2.** Anterior posterior view of the pharynx. Residue is noted in the valleculae.

**Figure 12–3.** Slight narrowing in anterior posterior view reflects location of cricopharyngeus m.

ter viewed from this position, as well (Figure 12–4). Asymmetries reflecting unilateral weakness, for example, of the pharynx, are also likely to be better appreciated in the frontal view. In both projections recordings are made while the patient swallows several different quantities and consistencies of barium, and in some cases, swallowing is evaluated with a bolus of food mixed with barium.

The esophagus is generally examined by fluoroscopy and spot films, which can be obtained either by standard films or digital recording of individual frames. Because it is possible for an abnormality in the esophagus to cause dysphagia or odynophagia, in most cases this organ should be evaluated along with the pharynx. This examination is also done by observing a bolus of barium as it passes through the esophagus from the level of the cricopharyngeus to the stomach. The examination is performed in the frontal, lateral, and oblique projections, and observations are

**Figure 12–4.** Zenker's diverticulum (at arrow) is filled with barium in anterior posterior view.

made both in the upright and recumbent positions.

The esophagus is a tubular structure that measures approximately 23 to 25 cm in length and 1 to 2 cm in diameter. The upper border of the esophagus is the cricopharyngeus muscle and the lower border is the cardiac orifice where the esophagus joins the stomach. The aorta causes an indentation on the left side of the mid-portion (Figure 12–5), and just below this level, there is often an indentation caused by the left main-stem bronchus. The anatomy of the distal esophagus is somewhat complex but important to understand when evaluating clinical problems. In the distal esophagus there is an area of increased pressure known as the lower esophageal sphincter (LES). The increased pressure in this area can be measured by intraluminal manometry and an area of intermittent narrowing is often seen during barium studies. Approximately 2 cm below the LES a second ring is often visualized, which is the junction of the esophageal mucosa and the gastric mucosa. This mucosal indentation is named Schatzki's ring. If this ring is above the diaphragm, an esophageal hiatus hernia is present. The anatomy of this region is seen in Figure 12–6.

Radiologic examination of the esophagus is done by fluoroscopic observation of a series of swallows of barium, both in the upright and recumbent positions. The esophagus is observed in the frontal, lateral, and oblique positions, and any abnormality is recorded either by digitized imaging or standard x-ray spot films. In addition to evaluation of the esophageal anatomy, peristalsis is observed in the prone position. The types of peristalsis that are seen include the primary wave (initiated by swallowing), secondary peristalsis (initiated by retained barium in the esophagus), and tertiary contractions (nonpropulsive contractions of the distal third of the esophagus) (Laufer, 1994; Megibow, 1994).

**Figure 12–5.** Barium in esophagus; arrow indicates indentation of aortic arch on left.

**Figure 12–6.** Anatomy of the distal esophagus demonstrated by barium swallow. Schatzki's ring is well demonstrated (*at arrow*).

An important part of this examination is the evaluation for possible reflux of barium from the stomach into the esophagus. Reflux of stomach contents into the esophagus is a very common condition that usually causes pain in the epigastric or substernal regions, but occasionally produces dysphagia or odynophagia. In addition, reflux into the hypopharynx may result in aspiration, hoarseness, and cough. The examination is done in the supine position after the patient has consumed about 300 to 400 mL of barium solution. While the examiner observes the gastroesophageal junction fluoroscopically, the patient is asked to cough, do a Valsalva maneuver, and raise both legs above the x-ray table. All of these techniques increase intra-abdominal pressure and thus may produce reflux. Some radiologists advocate using the "water siphon test," which consists of observation for reflux with the patient in the Trendelenburg position while drinking water. Although this test is more likely to induce reflux, the argument against its use is that it is highly unphysiologic and no one would be likely to eat or drink in this position. Thus, this maneuver results in more false positive results.

Common abnormalities that may be seen during the examination of the esophagus include hiatal hernia, with or without reflux; evidence of esophagitis; and motility disorders of the distal esophagus. Less common abnormalities include benign and malignant tumors, strictures, and achalasia. When abnormalities are seen on the esophagram, the findings must be correlated with the findings of the dynamic swallowing study and the patient's clinical symptoms to determine the clinical significance. These patients are often referred to a gastroenterologist for further evaluation, including possible endoscopy, and treatment.

## STUDY QUESTIONS

1. How is radiation exposure to a patient measured?
2. What five factors affect radiation dose?
3. What are some contraindications for a barium esophagram?
4. What structures, and pathologies, may be better viewed from a frontal (A/P) projection than a lateral projection?
5. What are the typical dimensions of the esophagus?
6. Can the aorta be appreciated on an esohpagram?
7. If a Schatzki's ring is identified, where is its location?
8. What is the difference between primary and secondary peristalsis in the esophagus?
9. What techniques are used to test for reflux?
10. How much radiation exposure occurs with a typical DSS?

## REFERENCES

Dodds, W. J. (1989). The physiology of swallowing. *Dysphagia*, 3, 171–178.

Dodds, W. J., Stewart, E. T., & Logemann, J. A. (1990). Physiology and radiology of the normal oral and pharyngeal phases of swallowing. *American Journal of Roentgenology*, 154, 953–963.

Ekberg, O., & Nylander, G. (1983). Pharyngeal dysfunction after treatment for pharyngeal cancer with radiotherapy. *Gastrointestinal Radiology*, 8, 97–104.

Hartl, D. M., Kolb, F. Bretagne, E., Marandas, P., & Sigal, R. (2006). Cine magnetic resonance imaging with single-shot fast spin echo for evaluation of dysphagia and aspiration. *Dysphagia*, 21, 156–162.

Jones, B., Kramer, S. S., & Donner, M .W. (1985). Dynamic imaging of the pharynx. *Gastrointestinal Radiology, 10,* 213–224.

Kitano, H., Asada, Y., Hayashi, K., Hiroshi, I., & Kitajima, K. (2002). The evaluation of dysphagia following radical oral and pharyngeal carcinomas by cine-magnetic resonance imaging (Cine-MRI). *Dysphagia, 17,* 187–191.

Laufer, E. I. (1994).Barium studies: Principles of double contrast diagnosis. In R. M. Gore, M. S. Levine, & E. I. Laufer (Eds.), *Textbook of gastrointestinal radiology* (chap. 4). Philadelphia: W. B. Saunders.

Levine, M. S., &. Rubesin, S. E. (1990). Radiologic investigation of dysphagia. *American Journal of Roentgenology, 154,* 1157–1163.

Logemann, J. A. (1983). *Evaluation and treatment of swallowing disorders.* San Diego, CA: College-Hill Press.

Logemann, J. A. (1986). *Manual for the videofluoroscopic evaluation of swallowing.* San Diego, CA: College-Hill Press.

Megibow, A. J. (1994).Computed tomography of the gastrointestinal tract: Techniques and principles of interpretation. In R. M. Gore, M. S. Levine, & E. I. Laufer (Eds.), *Textbook of gastrointestinal radiology* (chap. 8). Philadelphia: W. B. Saunders.

# 13

# Emerging Technology in Dysphagia Assessment

Peter C. Belafsky
Catherine J. Rees

Technological developments over the past 10 years have greatly enhanced our ability to diagnose and subsequently care for individuals with swallowing disorders. In order to provide comprehensive treatment for individuals with dysphagia, a broad understanding of these emerging diagnostic modalities is necessary.

## AMBULATORY REFLUX TESTING

Reflux disease is a major contributor to pharyngeal and esophageal phase swallowing disorders. Extraesophageal or laryngopharyngeal reflux (LPR) has been implicated in symptoms such as intermittent dysphonia, chronic cough, excessive throat mucus and throat clearing, otitis media, chronic sinusitis, and postnasal drip (Koufman, 2002).

LPR has been causally linked to cricopharyngeal dysfunction and Zenker's diverticulum (Sasaki, Ross, & Hundal, 2003). The ability to accurately diagnose reflux disease is essential to the care of persons with dysphagia. Many consider ambulatory pH testing to be the gold standard for the diagnosis of reflux. The diagnosis of gastroesophageal reflux disease (GERD) and LPR on pH testing differs.

In order to diagnose GERD on pH testing the pH sensor must be placed 5 cm above the upper border of the lower esophageal sphincter (LES). The location of the LES may be determined by endoscopy or manometry. The distal sensor may be hard-wired to a transnasal catheter or may be wireless. Hard-wired reflux testing can be uncomfortable and unsightly, and it has been shown to cause dysphagia and decrease reflux-provoking behavior. Wireless pH testing is more comfortable and has the advantage of routinely collecting 48 hours of data (Belafsky, Allen, Castro-Del Rosario, et al., 2004). A wireless pH telemetry capsule is placed 5 cm above the LES or 6 cm above the endoscopic determination of the esophagogastric junction (Figures 13–1A and 13–1B). The wireless capsule transmits to a data receiver worn on the belt or kept in a purse. The capsule falls off spontaneously in 7 to 10 days and is then passed harmlessly through the gastrointestinal (GI) tract.

In order to diagnose extraesophageal reflux or LPR, a pH sensor must be placed outside of the esophagus 1 to 2 cm above the upper esophageal sphincter (UES) in the hypopharynx (Merati, Lim, Ulualp, & Toohill, 2005). The wireless pH sensor cannot be safely placed in the hypopharynx. Therefore, in order to accurately diagnose LPR on reflux testing, a hardwired pH catheter must be used. Most pH labs that use dual-probe pH testing

place a distal sensor 5 cm above the LES and a proximal sensor 10 or 15 cm cephalad. This places the proximal sensor somewhere in the mid or upper esophagus. In order to diagnose extraesophageal reflux, however, a sensor must be outside of the esophagus in the hypopharynx. The reason most pH labs do not place the upper sensor above the UES is that it is technically more difficult to do so. It requires a large inventory of catheters with different interprobe differences to accommodate individuals of different sizes. In addition, it also requires the manometry technician to perform manometry on the UES to accurately place the extraesophageal sensor. This adds more time to an already lengthy procedure. Figure 13–2 displays the appropriate placement of the dual probe pH catheter.

We all reflux. Up to 46 reflux episodes per day can be considered normal. This "normal" amount of reflux is referred to as physiologic reflux. The normal pH of the esophagus approaches 7.

A.

B.

**Figure 13-1.** Wireless pH telemetry capsule. **A.** Capsule with introducer. **B.** Endoscopic view of capsule in the esophagus.

**Figure 13-2.** Endoscopic view of the proximal sensor (1–2 cm above the upper esophageal sphincter) in dual probe pH testing.

A reflux episode on pH testing is registered when the pH drops below 4. Normative reflux data have been established for GERD based on a pH sensor 5 cm above the LES. Normative data for LPR based on hypopharyngeal pH values suggest that some "acid" in the hypopharynx is normal. Although controversial, most clinicians consider a pH test for LPR to be abnormal when there is more than one reflux episode in the hypopharynx.

New technologies have recently emerged for reflux testing, and further research is needed to define their role in LPR. A nasopharyngeal pH catheter that measures pH in the gaseous form (Respiratory Technology Corporation, San Diego, CA) may provide improved sensitivity for reflux events in the laryngopharynx. Furthermore, there is increasing evidence to suggest that the most injurious component of gastric refluxate is the activated gastric enzyme pepsin (Johnston, Knight, Dettmar, Lively, & Koufman, 2004; Roh & Yoon,

2006). In the near future, it may be possible to detect pepsin levels in saliva to diagnose LPR.

## MULTICHANNEL INTRALUMINAL IMPEDANCE

Not all symptoms of reflux are caused by damage from acid and pepsin. Regurgitated pH neutral gastric contents (nonacid reflux) can still cause symptoms in the upper aerodigestive tract. Nonacid reflux has been implicated in chronic cough and aspiration, dysphagia, throat clearing, and globus. Standard pH testing cannot measure nonacid reflux. Combined multichannel intraluminal impedance and pH (MII-pH) testing is a novel method of reflux testing that can quantify acid and nonacid reflux. Impedance measures resistance to current flow. Intraesophageal content with high ionic concentrations (food or refluxate) have a low resistance (high conductivity). When food from the pharynx or refluxate from the stomach enters the esophagus, impedance drops. Thus MII provides a measure of antegrade or retrograde bolus transit within the esophagus. MII can be coupled with manometry or ambulatory pH testing. MII-pH has been particularly helpful in evaluating persons with persistent reflux symptoms on acid-suppressive therapy. Of individuals on reflux medication with persistent symptoms, 20% will have symptoms from persistent acid reflux, 40% will have symptoms from nonacid reflux, and 40% will have symptoms not related to reflux (Tutuian & Castell, 2005). Figure 13–3 displays a MII tracing of a nonacid reflux event.

**Figure 13–3.** Multichannel intraluminal impedance (MII) tracing of a nonacid reflux event. In this trace, time is represented along the horizontal axis, and information from each of six sensors is represented along the vertical axis. Vertical lines (*at arrows*) in the traces represent changes in impedance recorded by the respective sensors as material passes over them. It can be seen that the first set of lines (at impedance drops), on the left, precede in time (*left to right*) from the lowest to the highest, indicating material moving in a direction consistent with retrograde flow. In contrast, impedance changes that precede in time from top to bottom are consistent with swallow.

## TRANSNASAL ESOPHAGOSCOPY

Distal chip videoscopes are now available that can provide high-resolution images of the esophagus through ultrathin transnasal endoscopes. Typical esophagoscopy is performed through the mouth with a rigid or flexible scope in a sedated individual. Transnasal esophagoscopy (TNE) may now be performed reliably and comfortably through the nose without sedation. We introduced TNE in 2000. Since that time we have reported our experience of over 700 cases (Postma et al., 2005). The most frequent indications for TNE were esophageal screening in persons with reflux, globus, and dysphagia. Only 17 procedures had to be aborted because of a tight nasal vault. The most serious complication has been self-limited epistaxis (<2%). In our practice, TNE has replaced radiographic imaging of the esophagus in patients with reflux, globus, and dysphagia. It has greatly enhanced our ability to diagnose esophageal pathology in persons with dysphagia. The most common findings encountered on TNE in persons with dysphagia are peptic esophagitis, hiatal hernia, Schatzki's ring, *Candida* esophagitis, Barrett's metaplasia, and carcinoma. Patients are not very accurate at localizing the site of their swallowing problem. Approximately one third of individuals who localize the site of their dysphagia above the clavicle will have an esophageal etiology to their symptom. Therefore evaluation of the esophagus is a critical component of a comprehensive dysphagia evaluation.

## GUIDED OBSERVATION OF SWALLOWING IN THE ESOPHAGUS

The fiberoptic endoscopic evaluation of swallowing (FEES) is a tool to endoscopically evaluate the oropharyngeal phase of deglutition. Because TNE is performed in an unsedated, upright individual, we now have the ability to endoscopically evaluate the esophageal phase of swallowing. The guided observation of swallowing in the esophagus (GOOSE) is the esophageal counterpart to the FEES (see videoclip of GOOSE in materials folder for Chapter 5. In the

clip, patient is given applesauce and its passage through the esophagus is observed. In the last portion of the clip, the scope is inserted through the lower esophageal sphincter and retroverted to watch a pill exit the esophagus into the stomach). The ultrathin endoscope is passed through the nose and placed at the level of the soft palate approximately 3 cm above the tip of the epiglottis. FEES is performed as per a previously established protocol (see Chapter 11). If an obvious source of the patient's swallowing problem is encountered during the FEES, the GOOSE may be deferred. If the FEES is normal and no oral or pharyngeal disorder responsible for the patient's dysphagia is encountered, or a comorbid esophageal disorder is suspected, the endoscope is passed through the upper esophageal sphincter into the cervical esophagus. Normal esophageal transit time is less than 13 seconds. Any residue from the previously performed FEES in the esophagus suggests delayed esophageal transit. With the scope in the esophagus the patient is first given a 15-cc bolus of thin liquid impregnated with blue or green food coloring. Esophageal peristalsis is visualized as the liquid passes. The lumen of the esophagus should obliterate around the endoscope as the liquid is transported through. The esophagoscope is promptly advanced to follow the food bolus as it moves through the entire length of the esophagus. The bolus is visualized until it passes into the stomach. If the liquid traverses the esophagus without difficulty the person is fed a puree (applesauce) and then a solid (marshmallow, cracker, or bagel) consistency. If the patient has a problem with pills or any particular food, they are administered as well. At the end of the examination a retroflexed view of the gastric cardia is obtained from within the stomach. The patient is given a 15-cc bolus of thin liquid and the timing from the initiation of the swallow to the entry of the bolus into the stomach is noted. A transit time of more than 15 seconds suggests an esophageal transit problem.

## PHARYNGEAL AND ESOPHAGEAL MANOMETRY

In an individual with profound dysphagia, it is often difficult to distinguish between pharyngeal weakness, poor pharyngeal or cricopharyngeal coordination, and incomplete upper esophageal sphincter (UES) relaxation. Simultaneous pharyngeal and UES manometry provide valuable information about pharyngeal strength, UES resting pressure and relaxation, and pharyngeal-UES coordination.

Solid state pharyngeal-UES manometry is performed with a 4.5-mm-diameter catheter that has two circumferential solid-state pressure sensors spaced 3 cm apart and a third directional sensor placed 2 cm above the proximal circumferential sensor (Sandhill Scientific Inc., Highlands Ranch, CO). This places one sensor at the level of the UES, one in the hypopharynx, and one in the pharynx (Figures 13–4A and 13–4B). The catheter is inserted transnasally into the esophagus just below the UES. Baseline intraesophageal and pharyngeal pressures are then established. The UES pressure is determined by a 0.5-cm station pull-through technique. A smaller 2.1-mm-diameter catheter is also available for pharyngeal manometry (Gaeltak, Hackensack, NJ) (Hiss & Huckabee, 2005).

Esophageal manometry is typically performed with a 4.5-mm-diameter catheter that has two circumferential solid-state pressure sensors at 5 and 10 cm from the tip and three unidirectional pressure sensors at 15, 20, and 25 cm. This places four sensors in the esophagus and one in the LES. High resolution manometry (HRM) has recently been introduced (Sierra Scientific Instruments, Los Angeles, CA). In comparison to only 5 solid-state sensors with traditional manometry, HRM incorporates 36 circumferential sensors at 1-cm spacing to provide a unique high fidelity measurement of pharyngeal, sphincteric, and esophageal body physiology and pathophysiology. The role of HRM in the diagnosis and management of swallowing disorders is currently being defined (Ghosh et al., 2006).

## STUDY QUESTIONS

1. What is the advantage of impedance testing as compared to traditional manometry?
2. Does wireless pH testing measure proximal reflux, distal reflux, or both?
3. What is considered a "normal" esophageal transit time in the supine position?
4. In true dual-probe pH testing, sensors are located where?
5. What percentage of patients who localize their site of dysphagia to the area above the clavicle will actually have an esophageal etiology to their symptoms?

**Figure 13–4. A.** Fluoroscopic image indicating the correct positioning of the sensors for pharyngeal or upper esophageal sphincter manometry. **B.** Normal manometric tracing in the pharynx and upper esophageal sphincter.

**A.**

**B.**

## REFERENCES

Belafsky, P. C., Allen, K., Castro-Del Rosario, L., & Roseman, D. (2004). Wireless pH testing as an adjunct to unsedated transnasal esophagoscopy: The safety and efficacy of transnasal telemetry capsule placement. *Otolaryngology-Head and Neck Surgery, 131,* 26–28.

Ghosh, S. K., Pandolfino, J. E., Zhang, Q., Jarosz, A., Shah, N., & Kahrilas, P. J. (2006). Quantifying esophageal peristalsis with high-resolution manometry: A study of 75 asymptomatic volunteers. *American Journal of Physiology: Gastrointestinal and Liver Physiology, 290,* G988–G997.

Hiss, S. G., & Huckabee, M. L. (2005). Timing of pharyngeal and upper esophageal sphincter pressures as a function of normal and effortful swallowing in young healthy adults. *Dysphagia, 20,* 149–156.

Johnston, N., Knight, J., Dettmar, P. W., Lively, M. O., & Koufman, J. (2004). Pepsin and carbonic anhydrase isoenzyme III as diagnostic markers for laryngopharyngeal reflux disease. *Laryngoscope, 114,* 2129–2134.

Koufman, J. A. (2002). Laryngopharyngeal reflux 2002: A new paradigm of airway disease. *Ear Nose and Throat Journal, 81*(Suppl 2), 2–6.

Merati, A. L., Lim, H. J., Ulualp, S. O., & Toohill, R. J. (2005). Meta-analysis of upper probe measurements in normal subjects and patients with laryngopharyngeal reflux. *Annals of Otology, Rhinology and Laryngology, 114,* 177–182.

Postma, G. N., Cohen, J. T., Belafsky, P. C., Halum, S. L., Gupta, S. K., & Bach, K. K. (2005). Transnasal esophagoscopy: Revisited (over 700 consecutive cases). *Laryngoscope, 115,* 321–323.

Roh, J. L, & Yoon, Y. H. (2006). Effect of acid and pepsin on glottic wound healing: A simulated reflux model. *Archives of Otolaryngology Head and Neck Surgery, 132,* 995–1000.

Sasaki, C. T., Ross, D. A., & Hundal, J. (2003). Association between Zenker diverticulum and gastroesophageal reflux disease: Development of a working hypothesis. *American Journal of Medicine, 115*(Suppl 3A), 169S–171S.

Tutuian, R., & Castell, D. O. (2005). Reflux monitoring: Role of combined multichannel intraluminal impedance and pH. *Gastrointestinal Endoscopy Clinics of North America, 2,* 361–371.

# 14

# DSS: Swallow Evaluation with Videofluoroscopy

## Susan McKenzie
## Rebecca Leonard

Known in our center as the dynamic swallow study and in others as the modified barium swallow, this well-known procedure was initially described by Logemann, Boshes, Blonsky, and Fisher (1977). When we began doing these studies in 1982, we chose the name dynamic swallow study (DSS) to reduce confusion with other barium swallow studies and to indicate our focus on oral, pharyngeal, and laryngeal movements during the swallow, as well as on anatomy. Recording and imaging technologies have evolved since we began DSSs. Digital recording is now supplanting videotaping and, like videotaped fluoroscopy, offers relatively low radiation exposure (see Chapter 12) as long as fluoroscopy time is restricted.

## INDICATIONS

Patients whose complaints, signs or symptoms and/or histories suggest oral, pharyngeal, laryngeal, or pharyngoesophageal segment dysfunction are referred for DSS. All will have undergone evaluation, at least by their primary physician, and perhaps treatment for underlying diseases, most frequently directed by a gastroenterologist, neurologist, or otolaryngologist. In our practice, which includes both out- and inpatients, the dysphagia may be acute or chronic, obvious or subtle, severe or mild. The DSS is undertaken to identify risks to respiratory, pulmonary, nutrition or hydration health, and to target behavioral, surgical or medical intervention more precisely and effectively.

Because standard protocols and objective measures are used, repeated DSS can be used to assess changes in dysphagia related to surgical, medical, or behavioral treatment, or to deterioration or progression of disease or condition. DSS is not indicated in situations where performance status might fluctuate rapidly because of expected improvement or deterioration in health or when moving the patient is dangerous.

## FOCUS

Fluoroscopy studies of this type are intended to identify swallowing disorders that threaten pulmonary, respiratory, nutrition or hydration health. The perfoming clinician seeks not only to identify aspiration (which can be done during other barium swallows) but to clarify the reasons for aspiration to direct treatment (Logemann, 1983).

DSS differs from other fluoroscopic swallow studies in that it is not considered a "feeding evaluation," but a protocol of standard tasks testing a range of swallow capabilities that can be compared to performance by normal swallowers. While under some circumstances, real food and drink (mixed with contrast) is included in the study, in all cases the DSS begins with a standard protocol of swallow tasks, with standard instructions.

## LIMITATIONS

Use of fluoroscopy in dysphagia assessment and management must be limited because of its invasive nature. In our facility, fluoroscopy time is limited to 3 minutes or less. Thorough knowledge of individual patient history and clinical assessment help to obtain as much information as possible within that time. Review of the recorded DSS after the study is completed also helps to retrieve maximum information from a limited period of observation. Frequency of repetition is similarly limited because of the risks of radiation exposure.

A fluoroscopic swallow study is further limited by its audiovisual nature. That is, other important biomechanical aspects of swallow (such as pharyngeal pressures) are not directly assessed (although studies can be combined, as in manofluoroscopy). Other aspectscan be inferred, however, sometimes very accurately (Leonard, Belafsky, & Rees, 2006).

Finally, the conditions of a fluoroscopic swallow study, including the setting, the use of bolus material, and time and positioning constraints, can have an effect on swallow performance, rendering the study only faintly similar to real life eating or drinking. Additionally, young children and others who require and are used to being held or otherwise supported physically during feeding are usually denied this because of radiation exposure concerns. These dissimilarities reduce the power of generalizations from the fluoroscopy study to eating or drinking in other settings.

## BALANCING ASPIRATION RISK WITH FULL ASSESSMENT

The dysphagia evaluation, including the DSS, is an attempt to

- determine potential for threat to the subglottic respiratory system during eating or drinking;

- clarify and characterize behaviors that lead to such risks, and
- modify them, if possible.

As is stated throughout this text, because fluoroscopy is an invasive tool, the obligation to extract information fully is greater. Yet the need for complete assessment must be balanced with the risks to respiratory health associated with aspiration. Each step of the dysphagia exam is a way of collecting information that defines aspiration (and other) risk for an individual patient. During parts of the clinical evaluation and throughout the DSS, the clinician must decide, following swallow of each bolus, whether to proceed with the exam, or to discontinue the DSS because of excessive risk and be satisfied with less information.

Ability to make risk assessments during the DSS is based in part on prior knowledge regarding:

- medical, especially respiratory, fragility or tolerance;
- performance on clinical evaluation of oral, pharyngeal, and laryngeal tasks;
- effects of diseases and/or their interventions on swallow; and
- cognitive or behavioral conditions that interfere with instruction or self-control.

In addition to the above, the ability to make risk assessments during DSS is also, obviously, based on the examiner's ability to identify evidence of patient awareness of any failure and the vigor of compensatory or protective responses to this failure.

Clearly, because the above conditions and behaviors will be different for each patient, the DSS is not a pass or fail (or does not/does aspirate) exam. If the swallow is not fully assessed because historical or clinical information is unknown beforehand, if all the above factors are not taken into account, if feeding decisions are based only on presence or absence of aspiration during fluoroscopy, then risks to respiratory and nutrition or hydration health can be over- or understated with obvious consequences to the patient.

## THE DYNAMIC SWALLOW STUDY

### Standard DSS Protocol

In light of the accumulating reports regarding factors that affect swallow performance, it is reasonable to control as many variables as possible by developing a standard protocol. Developing and following a standard protocol during the DSS also facilitates comparisons of a patient

- over time or treatment,
- to other patients or patient populations, and
- to normative data.

All DSSs for adults and older children (infant DSSs follow a different protocol) begin with this protocol, very similar to that initially proposed by Logemann (1983), and continue until the protocol is completed or must be abandoned because of the clinician's judgment of excessive risk. At that point, systematic diagnostic probes, including mixing particular foods with the contrast, can be explored.

## Participants

Currently, in our setting (an ENT clinic), the dysphagia or speech pathologist conducts the DSS assisted by a radiology technologist who is supervised by a medical doctor licensed to conduct fluoroscopy exams. Because the invasive nature of the exam imposes additional responsibilities beyond dysphagia assessment, a physician familiar with head or neck anatomy should review the images for pathology of the anatomy. If triage, clinical evaluation, or events during the DSS indicate, the evaluation is extended to include a full esophagram. Because of known relationships between oral–pharyngeal and esophageal dysfunction (Triadafilopoulos, Hallstone, Nelson-Abbott, & Bedinger, 1992), most DSSs include at least a screening observation of the esophagus. The esophageal portion of the fluoroscopic exam is read and reported separately by the physician. If additional documentation of aspiration is desired, a chest film taken by the technologist is read by the physician.

## Image Views and Fluoroscopy Time

The DSS routinely includes observation in both lateral and anterior–posterior (A/P) views. The use of other views is dictated by the questions that arise during study. Optimally, in the lateral view, the fluoroscopy field includes the lips anteriorly, the palate superiorly (including enough of the nasopharynx to account for palatal knuckling), and the cervical spine from the atlas to the cervical esophagus posteriorly and inferiorly. Current fluoroscopy tech-

nology permits for imaging of all these various densities without "burn out" of the larynx. In the A/P view, the field includes the nasopharynx superiorly to the cervical esophagus inferiorly, and the walls of the pharynx laterally.

Our protocol includes a 3-minute limitation on total fluoroscopy time. The technologist or radiologist warns the clinician when the time limit approaches.

### Positioning

Care in establishing and maintaining the standard position should be part of any swallow assessment protocol. The patient is seated upright with head or neck and upper body as symmetrically within the fluoroscopy planes as possible and with neither flexion nor extension of the neck. If the patient is unable to maintain position, external support is provided. If the patient is unable to achieve good lateral position, this must be taken into account during analysis and interpretation of the results. In addition to reducing the strength of the observations, failure to control patient head or neck and upper-body position changes biomechanics of the swallow. Even slight head or upper-body leaning or rotation or neck extension affects the biomechanics of the swallow (Castell, Castell, Schultz, & Georgeson, 1993; Ohmae, Ogura, Kitahara, Karaho, & Inouye, 1993), complicating interpretation and diagnostic probing if the effects of position on biomechanics are to be systematically explored.

## Calibration and Timing

A metal ring of known diameter placed on the midline under the chin is used in calibration for spatial measures obtained after the study. If the relationship between the patient and the fluoroscopy arm is changed during the study, the image must be recalibrated. Timing information is also superimposed on the monitor, and recorded, so that pertinent timing measures can be obtained poststudy (Kendall, McKenzie, Leonard, Gonsalves, & Walker, 2000).

## Contrast: Bolus Sizes and Consistencies

Since 1983 (for most tasks), we have followed this standard protocol for adults:

> *In the lateral view:*
> Two, 1-cc boluses of liquid contrast
> One, 3-cc liquid contrast
> One, 3-cc paste contrast
> One, ¼ Lorna Doone cookie coated with paste contrast
> One, 20-cc liquid contrast
> One, 60-cc liquid contrast by straw-drinking (added in 1998)
>
> *In the A/P view:*
> One, 1-cc liquid contrast
> One, 3-cc paste contrast
> One, 20-cc liquid contrast

The standard protocol for infants is as follows:

Normative information regarding swallow performance of normal infants on fluoroscopy is scant. The protocol we use is similar to the adult protocol in that it follows a sequence of maximum caution to maximum challenge.

The focus is on pharyngeal, particularly hypopharyngeal, performance.

| | |
|---|---|
| Position: | swaddled, head stabilized, reclining only adequate for head stability. |
| Bolus: | see below |
| First task: | trace contrast on nipple or pacifier |
| Second task: | undiluted liquid contrast from a bottle; sustained suck-swallow sequence |
| Third task: | ½ sterile water-½ contrast; sustained suck-swallow sequence |

For both age groups, if oral transit is inadequate delivery is modified to achieve

- stable preswallow position in adults;
- bolus control in both infants and adults while
- either provoking or instructing posterior oral bolus control behaviors as much as possible. In adults, if this is not possible, instructing preswallow laryngeal closure is important.

## Instruction (Adults and Children)

The bolus is offered by spoon, cup, or straw by the clinician. The patient is instructed to hold the bolus on the tongue (or the straw at the lips) and wait. When a stable baseline or hold position is established, the patient is instructed to "swallow all at once." If a stable hold position is not achieved the patient can be reinstructed or support strategies to achieve a stable position can be introduced.

As long as swallow performance is adequate on a given bolus, the exam proceeds to the next step in the protocol. Instructions are repeated each time a bolus is offered. Otherwise, feedback, except for general encouragement (e.g., "you're doing great," "do your best") should be avoided because it can change behavior. Similarly, the monitor should be positioned out of the patient's field of view unless instruction regarding feedback is intended. If the swallow is not successful because of biomechanical failure but does not threaten airway safety for the next bolus step, then the protocol should proceed without changes in instruction.

- Instructions for liquid, pudding, and paste boluses from spoon or cup: "Put this in your mouth, hold it in your mouth (or the front of your mouth) and, when I tell you to, swallow it all at once."
- Instructions for solid boluses: "Chew this and swallow when you are ready."
- Instructions for straw-drinking: "Put the straw in your mouth and, when I tell you, drink this as fast as you can."

Oral, pharyngeal, or laryngeal failure that results in aspiration during the DSS justifies systematic alteration of the protocol. Compensations to avoid aspiration can be instructed so that the swallow can be evaluated as completely as possible. Because all compensations change swallow biomechanics, they must be taken into account during interpretation of objective and subjective observations.

## DIAGNOSTIC AND THERAPEUTIC PROBES

### Replicate the Symptoms

All DSSs begin with the standard protocol, which is followed as far as the patient can tolerate. Whether or not the standard protocol appears to reveal biomechanical failure, an attempt may be made to replicate the complaint. For example, if dysphagia symptoms indicate dysphagia is bolus-specific, swallow of the problem bolus (including capsules or tablets) can be observed. Similarly, if dysphagia symptoms vary with position, this can be systematically observed during fluoroscopy.

### Tasks Not Requiring Additional Contrast

If introduction of additional boluses appears too risky, swallow and non-swallow behaviors that do not require contrast can be observed. For example, speech tasks targeting behaviors important to swallow can be observed (i.e., "k" repetition to assess posterior linguapalatal valving, sustained sibilants and repeated plosive+vowel syllables (ka, pa) to assess velopharyngeal valving). Nonspeech tasks might include effectiveness of hawk-spit to clear the pharynx, or cough to see if material in the larynx or trachea can be cleared. In the A/P view, tasks requiring blowing against resistance can reveal asymmetry in lateral wall tone, if unilateral weakness is suspected.

## COMPENSATION OR FACILITATION BY CHAMBERS AND VALVES

### General Principles

If abnormalities in timing, clearing, and/or valving have been detected during the standardized protocol, compensatory strategies targeting the specific impairment are systematically explored. The ability of the clinician to apply compensations or facilitations during the DSS is dependent on ongoing interpretation of swallow biomechanics, and identification of effective and defective components (see Chapter 15). Compensation and facilitation strategies are aimed at maximizing intact components and minimizing or avoiding failures. Strategies include:

- changing the size and relationships of pharyngeal spaces and structures;
- changing the effects of gravity on bolus flow; or
- increasing effort to increase range, timing, or vigor of swallow gestures.

The effectiveness of the strategy should always be compared to the performance on the task where failure is noted. For example, if head turning is used to reduce residue, the success of the compensation can only be compared if the head is returned to the original position, and the swallow repeated. Addi-

tionally, the effectiveness of the strategy can only be assessed if the goal of the strategy is clear. For example, the goal of head rotation may be to clear hypopharyngeal residue, avoid it in the first place, or both.

The compensatory tasks or strategies available to a given patient depend on cognition; upper aerodigestive tract sensory integrity; head or neck oral, pharyngeal, and laryngeal anatomy and range of motion, control, and strength; respiratory health or resilience; and upper-body postural stability and control. Again, because progression through both the standard protocol and exploration of strategies involves constant risk assessment, this information must be compiled *before the DSS*.

### Compensations of Oral Chambers and Valves

Because many observations of the mouth can be made without fluoroscopy, the DSS is most valuable in assessing the competence of the posterior oral cavity (OC.) Nevertheless, inadequate oral bolus management has implications for airway safety; all observations are thus valuable in combination with clinical findings. In the OC, a bolus is prepared, created, and maintained as it is transferred toward the pharynx. These competencies are dependent on lingual shaping and agility of a muscular floor within a hard-walled chamber of bone and, usually, teeth. Successful oral transit also requires sensation for judgment (bolus readiness in consistency and size) and mucosal wetness.

When ability to control and propel the bolus in the oral cavity is poor, compensatory tasks or "tools" available to the therapist include *bolus consistency, bolus placement,* and *gravity.* Site of placement of the bolus on the tongue and/or head or neck flexion and/or extension may be used to manipulate bolus position and flow. If necessary, the OC can be bypassed by using a syringe with a short catheter to deliver the bolus to the posterior tongue (an example of this strategy is included in the materials folder for Chapter 18). If oral transit must be bypassed in this manner, competent bolus control is less likely and the patient should be instructed for preswallow breath-holding to prevent the uncontrolled bolus from entering the airway before glottic closure for swallow. Very lateral bolus placement and side-lying may also reduce the likelihood of aspiration during this maneuver. It should be remembered that the decision to undertake manipulation of OC events that facilitate oral transit is dependent on the competence of events in the pharynx. That is, oral transit impairments cannot be fully assessed if pharyngeal transit and laryngeal airway protection are intractably incompetent.

### Observation of Nonswallow Tasks

When the amount of contrast must be very limited because of airway threat, speech and other oral nonswallow tasks may provide insight. Speech tasks require different but perhaps no more demanding range of motion and agility than oral deglutitive tasks, especially mastication of hard solids. Observations of speech tasks can be helpful in clarifying subtle limitation in the lingual and palatal range for movement.

Our standard protocol includes repetition of vowel extremes (/i/ as in "heat," /a/ as in"hot," and /u/ as in "hoot") as well as consonants whose production requires lingual tip (/t/, /d/) or posterior palatal contact and palatal closure (/k/, /g/). If historical or clinical findings leave questions regarding posterior lingual or palatal competence, additional tasks can be added to the DSS without adding much more time to the study. Techniques to measure palatal anatomy and competence using multiview fluoroscopy have long been available and aid in differentiating between anatomic and movement failures when valving for swallow is incompetent.

### The Linguapalatal Valve

The anatomy and physiology of the oral and pharyngeal chambers are linked by the linguapalatal valve (or retro-oral portal [Bosma, 1956]), which is created by posterior tongue elevation against the bony palate or against the tensed and lowered soft palate. This valve acts alternately to contain the bolus within the oral cavity and then release it into the pharynx.

The linguapalatal valve differs from other pharyngeal valves in the complexity of its relationship with oral preparatory and oral transit components of deglutition, and because it is central in the relationship between the initiations of swallow gestures and initiation of pharyngeal transit. During swallow of liquids, especially boluses larger than 1 cc, failure to coordinate onset of bolus transit with swallow gestures is likely to result in nasal reflux, aspiration, or regurgitation. In swallows of other consistencies and perhaps very small liquid boluses, particularly those associated with mastication, the linguapalatal valve may open repeatedly to allow small amounts of the bolus into the pharynx some time before swallow gestures are initiated. Because of this normal variability, interpretation of linguapalatal valving failure can only be made if instructions are clearly understood and the patient is able and attempting to comply.

Failure of lingualpalatal valving may result in absent pharyngeal transit or in discoordination of onset of pharyngeal transit with initiation of the sequence of swallow gestures.

If linguapalatal valving failure results in bolus entry into the pharynx before initiation of swallow gestures, strategies that can delay or prolong bolus flow or employ pharyngeal anatomy and gravity to deflect the bolus from the airway are useful. Such strategies include *head or neck flexion and/or rotation, upper-body reclining on one side or the other (the degree depending on the impact desired), increasing bolus viscosity (the degree depending on the need),* and *limiting bolus size to the capacity of the valleculae and piriform sinus.* Alternatively or additionally, *voluntary preswallow laryngeal closure* can protect the airway until pharyngeal transit is complete. Strategies believed to facilitate timely initiation of pharyngeal gestures by enhancing sensory information are widely used and involve manipulation of the characteristics of the bolus (size, temperature, texture, taste) or presenting other stimulation (e.g., cold touch to the fauces) just before offering the bolus (see Chapter 18 for discussion of the effects of various stimuli on swallow).

When failure of linguapalatal valving results in initiation of pharyngeal transit after initiation of swallow gestures, the bolus will fall into the pharynx partway through the sequence of swallow gestures, or after they have been completed. Depending on the impairment, strategies may be aimed at slowing or deflecting the bolus, or at facilitating bolus flow. Strategies to slow or deflect the bolus include limiting the amount of the bolus falling into the piriform sinuses (side-leaning and head rotation) until repeated swallow gestures can complete pharyngeal transit. Strategies to facilitate bolus flow include head or neck extension with voluntary preswallow airway closure followed by flexion and head (not upper body) tilting or rotation.

## Compensations of Pharyngeal Chambers and Valves

The pharynx switches from respiratory to deglutitive physiology by altering the shape of its chamber and the configuration of its valves. Most of the time, the pharynx is an airway: the linguapalatal valve may be open or closed, the velopharyngeal valve is open, the laryngeal valve is open and pharyngoesophageal valve is closed. Failure of any of these valves and/or failure to maintain pharyngeal patency for respiration can at least disturb respiration and negatively impact deglutition.

During normal swallow, the switch from respiratory to deglutitive valving begins immediately, often before, the bolus is delivered to the oropharynx (see Chapter 1). During pharyngeal transit the pharyngeal airspace first expands and then is obliterated (completely in young normal swallowers). In the oropharynx, expansion to accommodate the bolus is achieved by forward movement of the tongue base and flexibility of the lateral walls and obliteration by medial movement of these structures. In the hypopharynx, expansion is accomplished by forward movement of the hyolaryngeal complex and lateral wall, including the flexible pharyngoesophageal segment. At the same time, elevation or foreshortening of these structures helps to engulf the bolus and draw it into the esophagus (Kennedy & Kent, 1985).

### Pharyngeal Valves

**The Velopharyngeal Valve.** Failure of velopharyngeal valve timing or extent of *closure* results in leakage of the bolus (or of air) into the nasopharynx and diminished ability to generate adequate oropharyngeal pressures to propel the bolus through the oropharynx for swallow (or to divert air through the mouth for speech). Observation of velopharyngeal function during speech (plosives and fricatives) may yield insights into velopharyngeal function for swallow. Strategies to compensate for or improve velopharyngeal valve closure include *head or neck rotation* and *manipulation of bolus size and/or viscosity*. When compensatory strategies fail, other therapies, either prosthetic or behavioral, can be guided by findings of the dynamic swallow study.

Failure of timing or extent of velopharyngeal valve *opening* results in competition between respiration and deglutition, particularly during mastication. This can slow meals and decrease the comfort and ease of eating or drinking. Strategies to compensate for diminished velopharyngeal airway are those that increase the time allowed for respiration between swallows. Techniques that accomplish this objective include *limiting the size and viscosity of the bolus, the rate of bolus presentation,* and *the total number of boluses given.*

**The Laryngeal Valves.** Dysphagia related to structural or sensorimotor laryngeal valve dysfunction may be poorly amenable to behavioral compensations during the DSS. This is, after all, the last line of defense against aspiration. If the patient's history or clinical evaluation suggests laryngeal dysfunction contributes to dysphagia or breathing problems, the dysphagia evaluation must include an otolaryngology exam.

Failure of timing or extent of supraglottic and glottic laryngeal valve *closure* results in leakage into the trachea and in decreased ability to generate adequate hypopharyngeal pressure to propel the bolus through the pharyngoesophageal segment (PES) and into the esophagus. Strategies available to compensate for ineffective laryngeal closure will depend on the etiology (i.e., sensation, movement, structure). These strategies aim to deflect bolus flow around the larynx and/or optimize laryngeal elevation and closure. These potentially include *head or neck flexion and/or rotation, upper body side-reclining* and *increased effort and prolongation of laryngeal closure* and/or *elevation.*

Failure of timing or extent of supraglottic and glottic laryngeal valve *opening* may or may not be obvious during quiet breathing and swallowing small boluses. In other cases, stridor may be present even in these situations. However, even subtle laryngeal airway obstruction, like other conditions that result in air hunger, can result in intolerance for the obligatory respiratory pause during swallow, thus interfering with adequate nutrition and the subtle relationships between deglutition and respiration (Hiss, Strauss, Treole, Stuart, & Boutilier, 2003).

**The Pharyngoesophageal Valve** (Pharyngoesophageal Segment or PES). Failure of extent or timing of PES opening (expansion) because of changes in the PES valve structure itself may be a consequence of neuromuscular impairment or decreased tissue compliance (fibrosis). Inadequate opening limits the amount of food or liquid entering the esophagus per swallow.

Strategies to compensate for decreased PES patency aim at prolonging maximum opening or increasing the number of swallows per bolus, and protecting the laryngeal airway from residue after or between swallows. Strategies include *repeated swallows per bolus on a single respiration, increased and prolonged maximum hyoid-laryngeal elevation and closure, head or neck rotation, flexion or extension, or upper body reclining.*

When the PES never closes completely, the pharynx and larynx are vulnerable to reflux of just-swallowed material in the esophagus or to gastroesophageal reflux (GER). Compensatory strategies are aimed at maximizing the effects of gravity on the bolus to keep it in the esophagus. These include *slowing the rate of bolus presentation*, and *adhering to behavioral precautions* (i.e., postprandial maintenance of upright posture and caution in the ingestion of substances that may reduce lower esophageal sphincter [LES] pressures or otherwise increase the likelihood of GER). Like the laryngeal valve, the PES valve is less amenable to behavioral compensation. The finding of PES valve dysfunction requires teaming with ear, nose, and throat (ENT) and gastrointestinal medicine (GI) physicians.

### Pharyngeal Chamber

Failure of pharyngeal chamber obliteration results in contrast residue that falls into the available distal pocket (valleculae or piriform sinuses) after or between swallows. Selection of strategies depends on identification of site of incompetence. Strategies to compensate for incomplete pharyngeal clearing can be aimed at diversion of the bolus away from the failure site, increased effort (extent or duration) of pharyngeal constriction or of PES opening, and prevention of aspiration when clearing takes longer to achieve. These strategies may include *head or neck rotation or flexion, prolonged and increased laryngeal elevation, repeated swallows, postswallow voluntary laryngeal clearing, and upper-body reclining.*

Failure of pharyngeal expansion related to pharyngeal wall stiffness reduces the size of the bolus that can be accommodated. If wall stiffness affects the size or presence of essential pharyngeal spaces (the "gutters" lateral to the epiglottis and the piriform sinuses) the bolus is diverted into, rather than around the larynx. Compensation for these structural changes includes *effort strategies aimed at early, prolonged, and vigorous laryngeal closure.* Observation of the pharynx during vocal pitch change and other speech and nonspeech aerodynamic tasks may offer insight into pharyngeal tone and movement range.

## TEAMWORK

The upper aerodigestive tract is remarkable for the number of professionals whose patients can be profoundly affected by dysphagia, and who have their own particular and nuanced insights into diagnosis and management of dysphagia (the dysphagia therapist, the radiologist, the laryngologist, the physiatrist and neurologist, the gastroenterologist, and the pulmonologist). We believe that the fluoroscopic swallow study should contribute to diagnosis and management of dysphagia beyond the bailiwick of the behavioral therapist.

## STUDY QUESTIONS

1. What aspects of the DSS make it "standardized"?
2. Can you name three benefits of using a protocol when conducting a DSS?
3. Ideally, what structures would you like to visualize in lateral view fluoroscopy?
4. What strategies might you try with a patient who has difficulty getting bolus material out of the oral cavity? What concerns would you have about using these?
5. Can speech tasks be helpful in understanding swallowing deficits?
6. What strategies might you use to facilitate initiation of pharyngeal gestures?
7. Why would poor velopharyngeal *opening* interfere with swallowing?
8. What strategies may be helpful in deflecting bolus flow around the larynx? In optimizing laryngeal elevation and closure?
9. What techniques might facilitate decreased PES opening?
10. What might you try in a patient with poor pharyngeal clearing?

## REFERENCES

Bosma, J. F. (1956). Myology of the pharynx of cat, dog, and monkey with interpretation of the mechanism of swallowing. *Annals of Otology, Rhinology and Laryngology, 65*, 981–992.

Castell, J. A., Castell, D. O., Schultz, A. R., & Georgeson, S. (1993). Effect of head position on the dynamics of the upper esophageal sphincter and pharynx. *Dysphagia, 8*, 1–6.

Hiss, S. G., Strauss, M., Treole, K., Stuart, A., & Boutilier, S. (2003). Swallowing apnea as a function of airway closure. *Dysphagia, 18*, 293–300.

Kendall, K. A., McKenzie, S., Leonard, R. J., Gonsalves, M. I., & Walker, A. (2000). Timing of events in normal swallowing: A videofluoroscopic study. *Dysphagia, 15*, 74–83.

Kennedy, J., & Kent, R. D. (1985). Anatomy and physiology of deglutition and related functions. *Seminars in Speech and Language, 6*, 257–272.

Leonard, R., Belafsky, P. C., & Rees, C. J. (2006). Relationship between fluoroscopic and manometric measures of pharyngeal constriction: The pharyngeal constriction ratio. *Annals of Otology, Rhinology and Laryngology, 115*, 897–901.

Logemann, J. (1983). *Evaluation and treatment of swallowing disorders*. San Diego, CA: College-Hill Press.

Logemann, J. A., Boshes, B., Blonsky, E. R., & Fisher, H. B. (1977). Speech and swallowing evaluation in the differential diagnosis of neurologic disease. *Neurologia, Neurocirugia, and Psiquiatria, 18*(2–3 Suppl), 71–78.

Ohmae, Y., Ogura, M., Kitahara, S., Karaho, T., & Inouye, T. (1993). Effects of head rotation on pharyngeal function during normal swallow. *Annals of Otology, Rhinology and Laryngology, 107,* 344–348.

Triadafilopoulos, G., Hallstone, A., Nelson-Abbott, H., & Bedinger, K. (1992). Oropharyngeal and esophageal interrelationships in patients with nonobstructive dysphagia. *Digestive Diseases and Sciences, 37,* 51–57.

# 15

# DSS Analysis and Interpretation

## A Systematic Approach for the Clinician

### Susan McKenzie

The normal oral-pharyngeal-laryngeal swallow, observed fluoroscopically or otherwise, is one smoothly coordinated, highly skilled event (Martin-Harris, Michel, & Castell, 2005). Nevertheless, assessment of the dysphagic patient involves analysis to determine (1) whether one or more of the many oral, pharyngeal or laryngeal events required to accomplish a swallow are abnormal; and (2) the implications of that abnormality for a patient with a unique pattern of medical, surgical, neurological and social histories. The more narrowly and accurately abnormalities can be described and interpreted, the more likely treatment will be successful.

The number of swallow events and their requisite speed, normal variability, and adaptability are obstacles to specifying and interpreting abnormalities on fluoroscopic swallow studies. For this reason, we have adopted a standard approach to directing, analyzing and interpreting fluoroscopic swallow studies (for us, the Dynamic Swallow Study) described earlier. This approach aims to control many of the conditions that affect swallow performance, facilitating analysis and interpretation.

Analysis of the swallow observed fluoroscopically aims at systematic objective and subjective description of critical aspects of swallow. Observations are organized by chamber (oral, oropharyngeal, and hypopharyngeal) and kinetic categories including timing, movement of critical structures, and valve competence. Events that are measured can be compared to the performance of normal swallowers on the same task, making determinations of normal versus abnormal possible even for less experienced clinicians. Events for which DSS does not provide normative data may be rated on a 5-point scale as a supplement to subjective description. If objective comparisons of between swallows by the same patient are desired, normative data are not needed for measurements to be informative.

Interpretation of fluoroscopic observations, whether an abnormality is detected or not, involves correlation of the observed performance to a complex array of contexts. The first correlation might be with other swallows observed (clinically or fluoroscopically) or with the patient's complaint; for example, does the patient complaint predict performance on fluoroscopy? Or, does performance change with the swallow task? When detailed analysis such as DSS can be made, correlation of individual events within the same or different swallows has implications for swallow safety (e.g., pharyngoesophageal [PES] opening time with laryngeal closure). Correlation of different swallowing tasks within the same fluoroscopy session can reveal conditions that provoke decompensation. Correlation with broader contexts, including the nutritional, medical, surgical, and neurological histories and the social/cultural history reveal consistencies or inconsistencies with implications for prognosis and medical/surgical management. For a given patient, additional contexts might be relevant. Thus, interpretation of fluoroscopic swallow studies determines consistency or "fit": is the observed behavior predictable based on what is known about the patient? For

example, if fluoroscopy demonstrates nasopharyngeal incompetence, what evidence in the complaint, the clinical observation, behavioral history, surgical history, and so on would predict that finding? If the observation is not explained by what it known about the patient, further investigation (fluoroscopic, clinical, or historical probing) may be warranted.

Clearly, accurate interpretation of fluoroscopy findings is dependent not only on accurate analysis but also on appreciation of the wide variety of conditions and variables that might affect swallow performance of a given patient. Although thorough discussion of these is beyond the scope of this chapter, some important variables are listed below.

Interpretation of swallow events must take into account factors that might facilitate or complicate swallow performance. Several examples follow.

## BIOMECHANICAL INTERRELATIONSHIPS

Although only kinematic (movement) observations can be made from fluoroscopy, other biomechanical elements (e.g., kinetics [force] and friction) can be inferred. Such inferences can be strengthened by studies that assess these elements directly, such as manometry. (Leonard, Belafsky, & Rees, 2006)

Distinguishing primary or causal from secondary swallow events depends on knowledge of kinematic interrelationships. For example, absence of epiglottic retroversion can be related to failure of timing or range of movements that constrict the oropharynx, or movements that foreshorten the hypopharynx, or both. On the other hand, a primary event such as incomplete PES opening can be associated with multiple secondary observations within an individual swallow, such as incomplete pharyngeal clearing and velopharyngeal valve failure.

## Position

Position of the torso, the head and neck, and the oral, pharyngeal, and laryngeal structures within the head and neck influence swallow performance by altering the effects of gravity on the bolus, the relationships of structures, and shapes of the oral, pharyngeal, and laryngeal chambers.

Position of the torso changes the swallow task in the head/neck. For example, oral transit in a patient with kyphosis can be more or less against gravity and bolus flow through the pharynx is biased toward the larynx.

Position of the head/neck affects the shape of the pharyngeal chamber and structural relationships. Well-recognized examples include rotation of the head to increase or decrease the size of the pyriform sinus spaces or neck flexion aimed at changing the shape of the vallecular space. Another example is head/neck extension (as in the kyphotic patient trying to look forward) where the relationship between hyoid movement direction and the PES is altered.

Dysphagic patients may decompensate when head/neck position changes. For example, a patient with tenuous velopharyngeal valving may experience reflux into the velopharynx when leaning over to drink from a fountain or extending the neck to take the last drops from a cup.

## Posture Stability and Flexibility

Fine movements such as those associated with swallow depend on a stable support structure. In patients with neurological conditions, the effectiveness of external postural support is widely appreciated. In the case of swallow, postural stability of the pharyngeal (including nasopharyngeal) and laryngeal airways is essential. Difficulty in achieving an adequate pharyngeal and laryngeal airway might preclude swallow without respiratory alternatives such as tracheostomy.

Often applied postural compensatory strategies such as side-reclining, neck flexion, and head/neck rotation are dependent on the flexibility of the upper body, the head/neck, and component structures. The importance of flexibility for adaptive strategies is seen in patients fitted with stabilizing appliances whose mild dysphagia is exaggerated by reduced flexibility.

## Respiratory Sufficiency

It hardly needs to be said that immediate respiratory needs trump swallow, but this condition is sometimes overlooked when assessment is confined to the fluoroscopic suite.

## Stamina and Endurance

Similarly, when assessment is focused on the events of swallow themselves (as happens during fluoroscopy) the effects of poor stamina and endurance associated with some neurological conditions or with prolonged illness can be overlooked.

## Lubrication

The health of oral, pharyngeal, laryngeal, and esophageal mucosa and the presence and condition of saliva is not assessed directly by fluoroscopy, but can have dramatic effects on swallow timing and clearing performance (see Chapter 2).

## Bolus Characteristics

In addition to size and thickness, multiple variations of bolus taste, texture, viscosity, and temperature facilitate or complicate timing, valving, and clearing performances during swallow. The potential for variation should be considered when interpreting swallowing performance. Normative data on performance during a standard set of swallow tasks is valuable because fluoroscopy time constraints prevent exploration of the infinite combinations of food, drink, and saliva that a dysphagic patient may face. (See Chapter 18 for a discussion of the therapeutic use of these types of variables in dysphagia management.)

## COMPETING BEHAVIORS AND STATES

Multiple behaviors and state share with, or affect responses of, the oral, pharyngeal, and laryngeal structures during swallow: Gagging, sneezing, hiccupping, laughing, crying, speech, startle, fear—essentially any distraction—can affect swallow performance. Clinician direction during the fluoroscopy studies should take this into account.

## Environmental Variables

Some environmental circumstances, even the presence of pictures (Maeda, Ono, Otsuka, Ishiwata, & Kuroda, 2004), promote interest in eating or drinking but others do not. The fluoroscopy suite likely represents the latter category for most people. The influence of environment is one of the many reasons why we do not consider the fluoroscopic swallow study a feeding assessment.

## Adaptability

In view of the number and complexity of variables affecting swallow, adaptability must be a signature characteristic of the normal swallow. Indeed, when a swallower's ability to adapt is overwhelmed or unavailable, dysphagia results. Evidence of spontaneous adaptability is one of the most important pieces of information available on fluoroscopic swallow studies. Clues to patient awareness of real or potential swallow failures can be inferred from behaviors that could be called precautionary, protective, or adaptive. Cough in response to aspiration or supraglottic penetration is the most recognized protective response, but there are spontaneous preventative behaviors less appreciated (e.g., early lingual retraction and early laryngeal closure among them). Spontaneous compensations have been observed for many years (Bosma, 1957a, 1957b) and more recently encouraged. Observations of older nondysphagic patients who demonstrate change in swallow performance with age support the idea that adaptability of swallow movements is essential

(Kendall & Leonard, 2002; Leonard, Kendall, & McKenzie, 2004a, 2004b).

Conversely, recognition of a patient's maladaptive or excessive responses during fluoroscopy, leads to more appropriate intervention. With evidence of good adaptability in a dysphagic patient, both swallow assessment and therapeusis can be more aggressive.

## CHAMBERS DIVIDED BY VALVES—A PERSPECTIVE FOR ANALYSIS

Analysis of the oral, pharyngeal, and laryngeal spaces as a series of mutable chambers (tubes or cavities) and valves is an accepted tool for the analysis of speech or voice (Fant, 1970, 1980; Flanagan, 1972). Kennedy and Kent (1985) proposed a similar model of tubes and valves for description of swallow. They divided the oral and pharyngeal chambers based on spatial orientation (horizontal and vertical), the differences in their function, and on the presence of a functional valve between them, the posterior linguapalatal or retro-oral valve (Bosma, 1957a, 1957b). We have found this model to be valuable in approaching analysis and interpretation.

During analysis of fluoroscopic studies, we have also found it insightful to further subdivide the pharynx into the oropharynx (mesopharynx) and the hypopharynx (laryngopharynx). In our experience conducting and analyzing fluoroscopic swallow studies, this division has become apparent to us in the following ways:

- Airway threat escalates significantly as the bolus passes from one chamber to another. Contrast retained in the oral cavity is least likely to be aspirated and most easily expelled. Contrast retained in the oropharynx is more threatening, but can be expelled by hawk-spit or suctioned fairly easily. Contrast retained in the hypopharynx cannot be voluntarily expelled unless it is at the entry to or in the larynx (and cough is effective) and it is very difficult to suction. Awareness of the progression of risk is helpful when directing the swallow study.

- The oropharynx and hypopharynx differ in their actions for swallow. Bolus flow through the oropharynx is normally midline propelled by the retracting tongue and the medializing constrictors. In the hypopharynx, bolus flow is deflected around the larynx, primarily laterally, by the epiglottis as the pharynx foreshortens to engulf and draw the bolus distally.

- Finally, in our experience, patients appear to use the midpharyngeal deflecting structures, the valleculae/epiglottis as a functional valve, the opening and closing of which can be controlled, if need be. Certainly, patients lacking the means to control, even stop, the bolus at that point are severely impaired.

In any case, as noted, we have found the perspective of the oral, pharyngeal, and laryngeal spaces as a series of chambers and valves a useful model in our analysis and interpretation of the fluoroscopic swallow study. What follows is a discussion of our approach to analysis and interpretation using this model.

## DSS Analysis: Bolus Transit Time Versus Swallow Gesture Times

The goal of swallow gestures (movements of the chamber and valve structures) is to move the bolus quickly and completely from the mouth, through the pharynx, and into the esophagus, without leaks into the trachea or nasopharynx (or backflow into the mouth from the pharynx or into the pharynx from the esophagus). DSS analysis considers swallow gestures separately from their effects. In this case, timing of swallow gestures is considered separately from timing of bolus transit through the pharynx. (See detailed discussion in Chapters 16 and 17.)

Comparing timing of swallow gestures with timing of bolus positions reveals breakdowns in sequence that are associated with increased aspiration risk, for example, arrival of the bolus in the PES more than 0.10 sec before completion of supraglottic closure (Kendall, Leonard, & McKenzie, 2004a, 2004b; Leonard, unpublished data). Gestures timing versus bolus transit timing highlights competent, as well as failed, performance. An excellent example of this is a swallow in which the bolus moves no further than the oropharynx (i.e., remains in the valleculae), while hypopharyngeal swallow gestures (including hyoid and laryngeal displacement and PES opening and closing) continue on in a timely manner. Although it is true in this case that the swallow has failed to be effective (in transferring the bolus to the esophagus), it must be said that a swallow sequence was completed. The distinction between gestures and their effects helps to specify incompetent gestures while appreciating competencies: information that is valuable in planning treatment and developing prognoses.

## DSS Analysis: Displacement

DSS analysis offers tools to determine whether range of motion (apart from time) of some critical swallow gestures is normal for age and gender. Distinction between range of movement and timing of movement clarifies whether failure of a component is due to poor movement, or to lack of coordination of movements with each other or with position of the bolus as it moves through the pharynx. Movements chosen to be measured (e.g., hyoid and laryngeal displacement, opening of the pharyngoesophageal segment [PES]), pharyngeal space obliteration, are difficult to judge subjectively, but readily lend themselves to objective measurement. Measures of hyoid and laryngeal displacement target individual structures. PES opening and pharyngeal clearing measures are comprised of movement of multiple structures with a single goal (i.e., expansion of the PES and obliteration of the pharyngeal chamber space).

## DSS Analysis: Discussion by Chamber and Valve

As noted earlier, DSS analysis begins by describing each chamber in terms of timing, clearing, and valving. If one of these functions has failed, components of that chamber that would normally contribute to successful timing, valving, or clearing are inspected. For example, if oropharyngeal clearing is incomplete, lingual or pharyngeal wall medialization, velopharyngeal, and/or epiglottic valving may have failed. Each component is judged objectively or subjectively, with the goal of determining relative contribution to the clearing failure. Not infrequently, in our experience, designation of incompetence or competence cannot be made with confidence without objective measurement of both timing and displacement. (Detailed descriptions of measures developed by our team, and how to make them, are presented in Chapters 16 and 17.)

The following is a discussion of our approach to systematic analysis of chambers and valves in the mouth to esophagus sequence associated with swallow.

### Oral Cavity: Oral Chamber, Linguapalatal Valve

As noted in Chapter 14, fluoroscopic observations are most valuable for assessment of the posterior oral chamber, especially linguapalatal valving, since that is least available to clinical observation. Other observations (e.g., bolus creation, containment [including labial] and control), the nature of searching or groping lingual behaviors and so forth are helpful in correlation with clinical oral motor and speech evaluations and the particular history (medical, surgical, neurological, etc.) of the individual patient.

### Oral Preparation and Transit Time

*Analysis:* DSS analysis does not provide norms for timing of oral preparation or transit. Subjective observations are recorded for comparison to input from other evaluations.

*Interpretation:* Oral transit time is especially subject to wide normal variation in response to a wide range of variables (see discussion of variables affecting swallow). Performance on fluoroscopy has meaning only when correlated with clinical evaluations and relevant histories as noted above.

### Oral Clearing

*Analysis:* Similarly, DSS analysis does not provide norms for measurement of oral clearing. Subjective descriptions should include rating of severity, location, and variation in performance with changes in bolus characteristics. Clearing of the oral chamber is probably less normally variable than transit time.

During some DSS tasks (i.e., swallow of 1 and 3 boluses of liquid), the bolus should be almost completely transferred to the pharynx on one swallow, as instructed. A slight to mild amount of residue, especially for larger or thicker boluses would not be considered abnormal but should prompt spontaneous, immediate repeated swallow.

When oral clearing is incomplete, the site of residue is more likely to be related to the site of impairment than it is in the pharynx where analysis can be clouded by the effects of gravity. Components to inspect when oral clearing is incomplete include the chamber walls (labial and buccal movement and sensation, palatal anatomy, and sensation), condition of the mucosal covering and, of course, the tongue (size relative to its chamber, symmetry, range of motion, agility, or shaping, strength, and coordination).

*Interpretation:* Determination of the meaning and implications of fluoroscopic observations of oral clearing is dependent on correlation with detailed patient complaint, clinical oral motor and speech evaluations, and the various histories (feeding/dietary, dental, developmental, neurological, surgical, medical, etc.) of the individual patient. Poor clearing can be due to xerostomia postradiation therapy, to structure deficits associated with oral cancer surgery, and to movement deficits either due to restriction because of scarring or sensation and movement deficits associated with neurologic diagnoses.

### Posterior Linguapalatal Valving

*Analysis:* Posterior linguapalatal or "retro-oral portal" (Bosma, 1957a, p. 901) valving is central to DSS analysis because, in this scheme, timing of all subsequent evens is compared to the beginning of bolus entry into the oropharynx. Timing of linguapalatal valving is the only oral chamber event that is measured.

Normally, if the patient is instructed properly, once the linguapalatal valve is opened, all remaining events will proceed apace. Confidence that the instruction is understood and that the patient is doing his or her best to comply are essential, since there are normal variations in bolus transfer to the pharynx during eating and drinking. For example, it is not abnormal to let some part of the bolus fall into the oro- or hypopharynx prior to initiation of swallow gestures when eating, espe-

cially during chewing, unless one has been instructed to prevent it. Inability to attend to or understand the instruction complicates interpretation of linguapalatal valving.

Assessment of linguapalatal valving competence requires that, at least at the beginning of the fluoroscopic study, the position of the head/neck should be neutral (not flexed or extended). Even small changes in head/neck position can alter the valving task. A dysphagic patient may spontaneously flex his neck prior to swallow. Because this would compensate for incompetent valving it should not allowed during the DSS until it has been demonstrated to be necessary for swallow safety.

Standardized control of valving initiation and head/neck position facilitates determination of linguapalatal valve competence or incompetence in its major functions:

1. Closure achievement and maintenance
2. Opening range adequate for the task (bolus size)
3. Coordination of opening with onset of pharyngeal swallow gestures.

*Interpretation:* If linguapalatal valving fails in the above functions even though the patient is able to follow the instruction, components of the valve to be inspected include palatal anatomy and sensation, lingual anatomy (especially relative to posterior oral space), movement range, strength, and control, and sensation. Suspected impairment of any component should correlate with detailed patient complaint, clinical oral motor and speech evaluation, and the multiple relevant histories of the particular patient (see previous discussions).

Complaints associated with impaired linguapalatal valving can be nonspecific (potentially due to several kinds of failure), for example, coughing on liquids and mixed consistencies. Findings on oral sensory motor and, especially, speech evaluations can be very specific (e.g., poor posterior tongue elevation strength or distortion, absence of, or compensatory articulation of back stops [k/g]).

If fluoroscopic and clinical findings are consistent with each other, they should in turn be consistent with history, depending on the impairment identified. For example, poor linguapalatal valving would be consistent with neurologic diagnoses that affect movement and/or sensation, or with surgical therapies that might affect the size or movement of the posterior tongue or palatal anatomy. If no consistencies in the constellation of histories of a given individual patient can be found, referral to a physician should be considered.

### Oropharynx: Oropharyngeal Chamber, Nasopharyngeal Valve, Epiglottis

#### Timing

*Transit Time:* Oropharyngeal transit begins when the linguapalatal valve begins to open, that is, when the soft palate and tongue separate, giving up control of the bolus to the oropharynx. Oropharyngeal transit ends when the head of the bolus passes the base of the valleculae.

*Analysis:* Pharyngeal gestures that contribute to timing of bolus transit include linguapalatal valving behaviors (see previous discussion), lingual retraction

capability, posterior and lateral wall anatomy and medialization capability, and the influence of these on the epiglottis and on the lateral gutters between the sides of the epiglottis and the lateral pharyngeal walls.

When oropharyngeal transit time is prolonged, the following components should be inspected:

- Competence of linguapalatal valving: failure, either of bolus control or of coordination of onset with onset of other gestures
- Anatomic abnormalities of the pharyngeal tongue, lateral and posterior pharyngeal walls, and epiglottis affecting chamber shape and impeding bolus flow
- Mucosal dryness may slow movement of the bolus, especially when combined with other abnormalities
- Changes in head/neck and body position that alter the effects of gravity

Prolonged oropharyngeal transit associated with complete bolus control and evidence of precautionary closure can also be a voluntary caution strategy in some patients.

*Interpretation:* The presence and relative contribution of abnormalities identified in the components above, as well as plans for intervention and/or counseling, are developed by correlation with what is known about the patient from clinical evaluations and historical reviews. Because of the potential for behavioral interference (such as fearfulness), prolonged oropharyngeal transit that is not explained by impairments identified as above, and/or consistent with clinical or historical findings might be judged as precautionary.

**Oropharyngeal Clearing.** Because of the effect of gravity on whatever residue might remain, incomplete oropharyngeal clearing of liquids is often characterized by residue in the valleculae after or between swallows. The actual site of failure is best identified and measured at the time of maximum chamber space obliteration.

*Analysis:* Because incomplete clearing can fall within the normal range for age, determination of clearing abnormality requires measurement (see Chapter 17). When clearing is abnormally incomplete, the range of movement and coordination of movement of chamber structures should be inspected, including:

- Retraction of the pharyngeal tongue. Incomplete lingual retraction can be bilateral or unilateral, and consistent with neurological conditions, surgical and trauma histories that change lingual or mandibular anatomy and development of scarring, and radiation therapies for head/neck cancer.
- Lateral and posterior pharyngeal wall medialization. Lingual retraction alone is unlikely to be sufficient if the pharyngeal chamber walls do not medialize or lack tone. Normally, a descending wave of medialization is identifiable in the posterior and lateral walls. A prominent (perhaps compensatory) posterior wall wave may be associated with inadequate lingual retraction.

- Size of the oropharyngeal chamber or space in baseline position. Chamber space, when a component of dysphagia, is generally larger than normal, but occasionally is abnormally small. Measurement of lateral area at baseline is necessary to determine whether size is abnormal. Changes in chamber size can be seen in neurological conditions where pharyngeal constrictor and/or suspensory muscles are weakened, and in head/neck cancer patients where structures have been removed or irradiated. Abnormally small chamber size, when present, is generally post head/neck or spinal surgeries, frequently when observed acutely.
- Complete obliteration of the oropharyngeal space is the goal, but is insufficient if lingual and pharyngeal wall gestures are not appropriately sequenced. When oropharyngeal obliteration is complete but not sequenced, some or all of the bolus may be forced back into the mouth or into the nasopharynx. Inability to sequence constriction for swallow is seen most often in patients whose anatomy is distorted by surgical intervention or trauma. It can be distinguished from voluntary pharyngeal constriction during nonswallow tasks (i.e., hawking) if it occurs during attempts to swallow and is coupled in a timely fashion to gestures essential to swallow, namely, hyoid and laryngeal displacement and PES opening.

- Mucosal dryness can result in diffuse pharyngeal wall residue. Xerostomia is not uncommon in patients post radiation therapy for head/neck cancer. Many medications can cause some dryness and some medical diagnoses are associated with changes in the mucosa.
- Competent velopharyngeal or epiglottic valving (see next section)

*Interpretation:* It should be obvious from the examples above that the meaning and implications of pharyngeal events observed fluoroscopically really cannot be determined without correlation with history. In addition, as noted earlier, swallow events affect each other and the primary event may not be obvious on fluoroscopy. Knowledge of relationships between events, as well as knowledge of patient histories that might bear on pharyngeal structure and function are necessary before fluoroscopic observations can be interpreted. For example, when incomplete clearing is due to incomplete posterior tongue-posterior pharyngeal wall contact, determining whether lingual retraction or pharyngeal wall medialization (or both) are impaired can be difficult. Clarification that will guide prognosis and intervention is often dependent on correlation with what is known about the patient. In this case, patient complaint and speech and dietary histories may be nonspecific but neurological and head/neck surgical histories may reveal consistencies. Similarly, prior knowledge of relevant diagnoses and details of interventions may guide more careful inspection and diagnostic probing of specific gestures during fluoroscopy.

**Oropharyngeal Valving.** The linguapalatal, velopharyngeal, and epiglottic valves divert the bolus to and out of the oropharynx, enable development of descending pharyngeal pressures driving the bolus, and prevent "leaks" into adjacent chambers (oral cavity, nasopharynx, and hypopharynx.)

*Analysis:* The role of these valves is to switch, completely and at just the right times, from respiratory to deglutative positions and back again. Valve opening extent must be adequate for the task and closure must be firm enough to resist pressure on the bolus during swallow. This is even true of the epiglottis which is only arguably a pharyngeal valve: The pharyngeal walls at the level of the epiglottis must provide adequate opening around it for respiration and bolus transfer, but can close against it to prevent bolus entry into the hypopharynx.

The linguapalatal valve (discussed in the oral chamber section):

- opens in a manner adequate for bolus size to begin oropharyngeal transit
- prevents backflow of the bolus into the mouth
- prevents oral contrast residue (after or between swallows) from falling into the pharynx uncontrolled (without initiation of a second swallow) where it would increase potential for aspiration

The velopharyngeal valve closes during swallow and opens during respiration.

- During the swallow, when the bolus in the oropharynx is

under pressure, this valve prevents backflow or reflux of contrast into the nasopharynx. If contrast is extruded into the nasopharynx, some or all of it is likely to fall back into the oro- or hypopharyngeal after or between swallows, increasing aspiration risk. Backflow during the period of maximum velopharyngeal closure is due to bi- or unilateral weakness or anatomic insufficiency of the palate or excessive lateral or A/P dimension of the velopharyngeal space. Cephalometric norms for these structures have long been available.

■ After or between swallows, but also important for eating and drinking, the velopharyngeal valve opens adequately to support nasal respiration. When opening is inadequate, nutrition/hydration and respiration compete for the oral chamber, and both activities require more time and work.

■ When backflow of contrast is seen as the velopharynx begins to reopen post swallow, it is more likely due to a more distal event, such as obstruction, than to valve dysfunction.

The epiglottis, whether it retroverts or not, is an important obstruction to bolus flow, that is, it diverts the bolus to the lateral pharyngeal gutters, away from the larynx. When the epiglottis fails to retrovert, more or less obstruction results. Absence of epiglottic retroversion for swallow of a very small bolus may not be abnormal. When failure to retrovert combines with changes in the lateral and/or posterior walls that reduce the space around the epiglottis, however, obstruction of bolus flow can be excessive, resulting in dysphagia. The epiglottis may retrovert incompletely or not at all due to:

■ inadequate or ill-timed (relative to bolus position) lingual retraction
■ inadequate extent of posterior and lateral pharyngeal wall medialization or lack of descending sequencing of medialization
■ inadequate hyoid and laryngeal displacement (Fink & Demarest, 1978)
■ inadequate space between the epiglottis and posterior pharyngeal wall due to anatomic changes in the pharyngeal wall or the spine (or to cervical appliances). Because head/neck position affects chamber size and shape, neck extension may decrease this distance as well.
■ inadequate flexibility of the epiglottis.

*Interpretation:* Clearly, judgment about which of the many potential causes for inadequate valving is dependent on a detailed description of the abnormality and identification of historical consistencies that explain the particular fluoroscopic observation. Speech and feeding or dietary histories, as noted previously, should be consistent with linguapalatal and velopharyngeal findings. Developmental and/or neurological diagnoses and histories of head/neck (including spinal) abnormalities, surgical intervention, or trauma should reveal consistencies with fluoroscopic observations that will, again, guide decisions regarding prognosis and intervention. If consistencies are not identified, further investigation, including more thorough speech and swallow evaluation and referral to a physician should be considered.

### Hypopharynx: Hyopharyngeal Chamber, Laryngeal Valves, and Pharyngoesophageal Valve

The presence of the bolus in the hypopharynx is associated with increased aspiration risk.

### Hypopharynx: Timing

*Transit Duration*

> *Analysis:* Transit time must be measured to identify abnormality. Hypopharyngeal transit time begins when the bolus head (or some part of it) exits the valleculae and ends with the clearing of its tail from the PES into the esophagus. As in the oropharynx, hypopharyngeal time can be prolonged by failure of gestures that propel the bolus and anatomic or movement abnormalities that impede bolus flow.

> *Interpretation:* Prolonged hypopharyngeal transit may be due to:

> ■ failure to coordinate position of the bolus with onset of hypopharyngeal elevating and medializing (engulfing) gestures. When bolus entry to the hypopharynx is uncontrolled, the bolus may enter the hypopharynx prior to initiation of hypopharyngeal swallow gestures. Such a lag between gestures

and bolus position is likely if the epiglottis is all or partially absent but is also the result of poor bolus containment in the oropharynx.

> ■ incomplete obliteration of the hypopharyngeal space due to inadequate medialization of the posterior and lateral walls and/or inadequate foreshortening, or to excessive hypopharyngeal space. Poor obliteration of the hypopharyngeal space is associated with reduced ability to propel the bolus so that bolus flow is dependent on gravity, increasing time for transfer. Unilaterally or bilaterally, poor or absent pharyngeal wall movement might be consistent with neurological diagnoses, and immobility of the wall is consistent with a history of treatment for head/neck cancer.

> ■ obstruction due to changes in anatomy of the wall, the larynx, the pharyngoesophageal (PES) valve or the spine (including large osteophytes and cervical appliances). More time is required for transit if space at any level is inadequate for bolus size, and the bolus must flow around an obstruction (e.g., impingement on the space by a cervical appliance or associated thickened posterior wall). Obstruction at the PES, discussed later in this section, may prolong hypopharyngeal transit by slowing bolus transfer to the esophagus. The condition of Zenker's diverticulum is an extreme example. In this case,

hypopharyngeal transit is prolonged due to 2 factors: PES obstruction and poor space obliteration because of the diverticulum proximal to the PES.

*Interpretation:* Interpretation of timing abnormalities in the hypopharynx is dependent on recognizing the consequences of abnormalities in the oral and oropharyngeal chambers for swallow demands on the hypopharynx. For example, poor control of oral residue requires that the hypopharynx and larynx adopt defensive postures and be habitually wary of bolus material even after or between swallows. During fluoroscopic observation of swallow, timing relationships between events can be insightful and predictive. For example, closure of the laryngeal valve normally occurs within 0.10 sec of bolus entry into the PES (Kendall, Leonard, & McKenzie, 2004). In stroke patients, failure to achieve this degree of coordination between laryngeal closure and bolus position in the PES has been demonstrated to increase the likelihood of aspiration during fluoroscopy (Leonard, unpublished data).

**Hypopharynx: Clearing.** Because of its proximity to the airway hypopharyngeal clearing failures, like timing failures, can be associated with greater risk than in the oral and oropharyngeal chambers. As noted, voluntary and passive (suctioning) expulsion of residue is easier when residue is in the latter. Hypopharyngeal residue can be diffi-

cult to remove if it can't be swallowed. Fortunately, the lateral gutters (around the epiglottis) and the pyriform sinuses divert and store residue if they are intact. When these spaces are missing because of changes in the pharyngeal walls or due to impingement, their value for laryngeal protection is obvious. When the pyriform sinus spaces are filled due to changes in the hypopharyngeal wall, the bolus may be funneled directly into the larynx.

*Analysis:* Because some residue is normal, especially in elderly patients, determination of abnormally incomplete clearing is dependent on measurement. Because of gravity effects, site of incomplete clearing may be best identified at the point of maximum pharyngeal constriction. A/P observation is especially helpful in specifying asymmetry. Additionally, overlap between the pyriform sinuses and the larynx in the lateral view, occasionally a source of confusion, can be more clearly understood by comparison to the A/P view. Hypopharyngeal clearing abnormalities can be due to:

- inadequate bilateral or unilateral pharyngeal wall tone or descending sequential medialzation. Pulsion diverticulae may contribute to residue, but their contribution to dysphagia may or may not be significant.
- inadequate pharyngeal foreshortening associated with incomplete anterior-superior hyoid and laryngeal displacement. Reliable determination of abnormality requires measurement. If hyoid and laryngeal displacement is not correctly

judged, incomplete clearing may be incorrectly attributed to obstruction at the PES.

- insufficient mucosal lubrication
- obstruction at any level, due to thickening of structures (laryngeal cartilages, pharyngeal walls, impingement by spinal abnormalities or appliances on the spine). Obstruction can be acute or chronic, depending on the etiology. Secondary effects such as proximal dilation and backflow into the oro- or naso-pharynx or mouth will suggest the degree of obstruction. Although safety may preclude it, obstruction can only be completely assessed by swallow of a large bolus.
- laryngeal and pharyngoesoph-ageal valve failures (see next section)

*Interpretation:* Suspected abnormalities leading to incomplete hypopharyngeal clearing must be correlated with neurological, surgical (including head/neck and spine), and trauma histories. Because of the health risks and implications of abnormalities in the hypopharynx, referral to an ENT physician is indicated.

**Hypopharynx: Valving.** The epiglottic, laryngeal, and pharyngoesophageal valves divert the bolus away from the airway and draw it into the esophagus. Failure of adequate opening of the pharynx at the epiglottis and PES will slow bolus flow and may prevent complete bolus clearing. Inadequate PES closure increases potential for backflow of material in the esophagus (either a just-swallowed bolus or material re-fluxed from the stomach). Inadequate supraglottic closure is associated with supraglottic residue. Of course, inadequate glottic valving increases the likelihood of aspiration.

As discussed previously, the epiglottis with its surrounding pharyngeal walls diverts, controls, and at times prevents transfer of the bolus into the hypopharynx. Please see that discussion.

*Laryngeal Valve:* Supraglottic and glottic laryngeal valving provides primary defense for the trachea and lungs. Compared to other valves involved in swallow, this valve differs markedly in complexity and behavioral capabilities. Competence of the laryngeal valve for swallow requires, in addition to range, agility, and coordination of movement, intact sensation and ability to respond to stimulation protectively, even to anticipate a threatening situation. Laryngeal closure adequate to withstand bolus pressures during swallow depends on sensory as well as motor competence. Laryngeal reopening and maintenance of a sufficient laryngeal airway is required for oral nutrition/hydration.

*Analysis:* Supraglottic penetration (contrast material that stays above the glottis) is judged to be abnormal when it is frequent and/or is not extruded during the swallow.

Aspiration during fluoroscopy is defined as contrast material that passes into and through the glottis. By far the most helpful construct for describing aspiration timing is that developed by Logemann (1983, p. 65). In our experience, however, rather than referencing aspiration timing relative to "the swallow" or triggering of the swallow reflex, we have found it more useful to specify aspiration timing relative to achievement of laryngeal closure, once the bolus has entered the pharynx (regardless of other swallow gestures). Logemann's description, with this modification, is as follows:

- Aspiration before laryngeal closure for swallow, after the bolus has entered the pharynx.
- Aspiration during maximum laryngeal closure for swallow, as the bolus passes the laryngeal aditus
- Aspiration after or between swallows, following reopening for respiration

*Interpretation:* Aspiration *prior* to laryngeal closure for swallow is considered a failure of timing due to inadequate bolus control, inability to coordinate initiation of swallow gestures or altered structural (such as epiglottic) protection. The longer the bolus takes to transit the pharynx, the more likely it will be aspirated. In patients post CVA, prolonged pharyngeal transit has been shown to increase the risk of developing aspiration pneumonia, even if aspiration is not detected during the fluoroscopy (Johnson, McKenzie, & Sievers, 1993). Risk of aspiration during the DSS also increases when closure is not coordinated with bolus arrival in the PES (Leonard, unpublished data). Aspiration prior to laryngeal closure for swallow is almost always associated with abnormalities of other swallow events: among them, inadequate control of the bolus, inability to coordinate onset of pharyngeal gestures with onset of pharyngeal transit due to movement or sensory deficits, structural deficits that direct bolus flow toward instead of away from the lar-

ynx. Cognitive deficits (poor attention, distractibility, difficulty suppressing other behaviors) and unstable head/neck posture make aspiration prior to laryngeal closure more likely as well.

Aspiration *during* laryngeal closure for swallow is due to incompetent laryngeal valving and may only become apparent when the maximally closed valve is exposed to pressure from the bolus as it passes the aditus. Thus, if it is judged unsafe to swallow a large liquid contrast bolus during fluoroscopy, this valve cannot be completely tested. Aspiration during laryngeal closure is, of course, more likely when both supraglottic and glottic closure is incompetent. The observation of aspiration during the swallow should be consistent with the findings of voice evaluation, patient complaint, and feeding, especially drinking history. Management of patients with laryngeal dysfunction is directed by the ENT physician. If incompetent laryngeal valving is suspected, referral should be made immediately.

Aspiration *after* the swallow is always of oropharyngeal or hypopharyngeal residue so is a consequence of inadequate pharyngeal clearing (discussed in previous sections).

*Hypopharynx: PES Valve:* The pharyngoesophageal segment (PES) valve opens to draw the bolus into the esophagus, expands depending on bolus size and closes, preventing backflow of bolus material into the pharynx from the esophagus. Between swallows the PES remains closed to prevent any gastroesophageal reflux from reaching the airway. During DSS, questions most often arise regarding timing and extent PES opening. Occasionally, PES closure is inadequate.

*Analysis:* Determination of PES opening abnormality is not always clear. Prominence of the PES on fluoroscopy (cricopharyngeal bar) does not necessarily mean opening is restricted. Atrophy of the pharyngeal wall just above the PES complicates interpretation by making the PES appear more prominent. If swallow safety does not permit swallow of a large liquid bolus, the PES cannot be completely tested. In addition, the standard deviation for normal opening extent is large. Thus, measurement of the PES in both A/P and lateral views increases confidence in identifying restriction. Consequences of obstruction (proximal dilation and backflow) may help to confirm poor PES opening in the absence of other obstruction. Abnormal timing of PES opening cannot be determined without measurement and comparison to other timing measures. For example, PES opening that appears delayed relative to bolus arrival in the hypopharynx may be normally timed relative to other swallow gestures. In this case, then, arrival of the bolus may be early (due, perhaps to poor control) rather than PES opening being late.

Determination of PES closure abnormality is fairly clear: contrast should be entirely cleared from the walls of the PES once the swallow is complete.

*Interpretation:* Abnormal PES opening extent may not be due to failure to relax or structural abnormalities of the PES but to inadequate movement of structures that pull the relaxed PES open (hyoid and laryngeal displacements) and structures that propel the bolus through the PES (tongue and pharyngeal walls). (Please see previous discussions of these components.) If these components are normal, structural, or neuromuscular aspects of PES function are implicated. If the PES is indeed obstructive, consistencies should be found in detailed patient complaint and dietary history. PES obstruction in patients without histories of surgical intervention, radiation therapy, and so forth is often attributed to chronic GER.

The finding of abnormal PES closure should correlate with neurological, surgical, or radiation therapy history.

## REPRISE

Accurate analysis of swallow during fluoroscopic studies like DSS is dependent on detailed knowledge of the biomechanical relationships between normal swallow events, and the ability to distinguish normal from abnormal behaviors despite the variability associated with different swallow tasks and multiple additional influences on swallow performance. Accurate assessment is also best guided by prior knowledge of performance on speech, feeding, and voice evaluations; detailed patient complaint; and a complex array of histories (neurological, developmental, dietary, medical, and surgical among them) that are particular to an individual patient. This means having a working knowledge of what the potential impacts of various diagnoses and conditions might be on swallow and on the direction of the fluoroscopic study.

Interpretation, or derivation of meaning and implications from analysis, is the process of correlating fluoroscopic observations with what is known about the individual patient from historical review, interview, and clinical performances and ferreting out consistencies and inconsistencies, both of which will guide recommendations and interventions. If consistencies are not identified, analysis may suggest additional investigation. Accurate interpretation of fluoroscopic swallow studies like DSS cannot be achieved in isolation, but leans heavily on awareness of the roles and interests of a variety of medical specialties and interaction with those professionals.

Most important for the patient, accurate analysis and interpretation of fluoroscopic swallow studies improves efficacy of dysphagia management by improving specificity of intervention.

## REFERENCES

Bosma, J. (1957a). Studies of the pharynx. I. Poliomyelitic disabilities of the upper pharynx. *Pediatrics, 19*, 881–907.

Bosma, J. (1957b). Deglutition: Pharyngeal stage. *Physiological Reviews, 37*, 276–299.

Fant, G. (1970). *Acoustic theory of speech production*. The Hague, Mouton.

Fant, G. (1980). The relations between area functions and the acoustic signal. *Phonetica, 37*, 55–86.

Fink B. R., & Demarest, R. J. (1978). *Laryngeal biomechanics*. Boston: Harvard University Press.

Flanagan, J. (1972). *Speech analysis, synthesis, and perception*. Berlin, Springer-Verlag.

Johnson, E. R., McKenzie, S. W., & Sievers, A. (1994). Aspiration pneumonia in stroke. *Archives of Physical Medicine and Rehabilitation, 74*, 665.

Kendall, K. A., & Leonard, R. J. (2002). Videofluoroscopic upper esophageal sphincter function in elderly dysphagic patients. *Laryngoscope, 112*, 332–337.

Kendall, K. A., Leonard, R. J., & McKenzie, S. (2004). Airway protection: Evaluation with videofluoroscopy. *Dysphagia, 19*, 65–70.

Kennedy, J. G., & Kent, R. D. (1985). Anatomy and physiology of deglutition and related functions. *Seminars in Speech and Language, 6*, 257–272.

Leonard, R., Belafsky, P. C., & Rees, C. J. (2006) Relationship between fluoroscopic and manometric measures of pharyngeal constriction: The pharyngeal constriction ratio. *Annals of Otology, Rhinology and Laryngology, 115*, 897-901.

Leonard, R., Kendall, K., & McKenzie, S. (2004a). Structural displacements affecting pharyngeal constriction in nondysphagic elderly and nonelderly adults. *Dysphagia, 19*, 133-141.

Leonard, R., Kendall, K., & McKenzie, S. (2004b). UES opening and cricopharyngeal bar in nondysphagic elderly and nonelderly adults. *Dysphagia, 19*, 182–191.

Logemann, J. (1983). *The evaluation and treatment of swallowing disorders*. San Diego, CA: College-Hill Press.

Maeda, K., Ono, T., Otsuka, R., Ishiwata, Y., Kuroda, T., & Ohyama, K. (2006). Modulation of voluntary swallowing by visual inputs in humans. *Dysphagia, 19*, 1–6.

Martin-Harris, B., Michel, Y., & Castell, D. O. (2005). Physiologic model of oropharyngeal swallowing revisited. *Otolaryngology-Head and Neck Surgery, 133*, 234–240.

McConnel, F. M. (1988). Analysis of pressure generation and bolus transit during pharyngeal swallowing. *Laryngoscope, 98*, 71–78.

# 16

# *Dynamic Swallow Study*

## *Objective Measures and Normative Data in Adults*

### Katherine Kendall
### Susan McKenzie
### Rebecca Leonard

## INTRODUCTION

This chapter is divided into two main sections. First, a brief history of our team's use of objective measures obtained from dynamic swallow studies (DSS) will be presented. Though we have subsequently used these measures for research purposes, our initial interest in them arose primarily from a shared dissatisfaction with the credibility of our fluoroscopy (DSS) interpretation and recommendations for treatment, based as they were on subjective observations. Even though our team included very experienced medical, surgical, and radiology professionals, as well as speech pathologists and

nurses, no one at that time had broad experience in observing and interpreting these types of evaluations. As soon as objective measures appeared in the literature, we incorporated them in our patient studies. As more information was published on swallow and as our experience grew, we adjusted and developed new measures to reflect new developments in the literature, our understanding of swallow and the particular problems presented by the head and neck cancer population. Our experience in this pursuit may be of interest to other clinicians, and is included here for this reason.

In the second portion of the chapter, the specific measures we collect, and the rationale for each, will be discussed. Normative values and reliability data for each measure will also be provided, as will differences according to age, gender, and bolus size or consistency. Our own experience with the clinical utility of particular measures will also be discussed.

## BACKGROUND AND RATIONALE

### The Path to Objective Measures

Our interest in making objective measures started at about the same time our team began meeting weekly to discuss patients. In reviewing their dynamic swallow studies, it became apparent that we sometimes disagreed about what we were seeing, even when we watched a recording repeatedly, and in slow motion. In general, and consistent with many subsequent literature reports (Ekberg et al., 1988; Gibson & Phyland, 1995; Karnell & Rogus, 2005; Kuhlemeier, Yates, & Palmer, 1998; McCullough et al., 2001; Perlman, Booth, & Grayhack, 1994; Scott, Perry, & Bench, 1998), we were usually in agreement for binary observations, for example, whether or not there was aspiration, penetration, velopharyngeal reflux, or significant post-swallow residue. Swallows that appeared greatly prolonged typically produced consensus, as well. Times that were possibly prolonged, on the other hand, were problematic. For other observations—how normally did the hyoid move, the pharynx constrict, or the pharyngoesophageal segment (PES) open—our judgments frequently differed. Beyond our problems with

subjective reliability, and in fact even when we did agree, there was a strong feeling within our team that, without objective information, our impressions and recommendations lacked credibility.

In the interest of harmony, improved objectivity, and enhanced credibility, we searched available resources for information that would lead to improved assessments. We had been performing fluoroscopy studies in our craniofacial anomaly patients, and referred frequently to the cephalometric literature for help in evaluating velopharyngeal function in a quantitative manner. When the fluoroscopic evaluation of swallow was introduced by Logemann and her colleagues (Blonsky, Logemann, Boshes, & Fisher, 1975; Logemann, 1983; Logemann, Boshes, Blonsky, & Fisher, 1977), we recognized that it also lent itself to quantitative analysis. We adopted Logemann's recommended protocol with its emphasis on standardization, and have been employing it with little change ever since. With the exception of some work on timing, however, which began to emerge in the 1980s, quantitative guidelines pertinent to swallowing were slow to emerge. Though limited, the data available were quite useful; very quickly, we added timing information to our studies.

Initially, we used conventions described by Logemann (1983) for measuring transit times, but the parameters she was using were not always present or identifiable in our studies. For example, the faucial pillars were not easily visualized, and neither the angle of the mandible nor the faucial pillars were always present in patients who had undergone head and neck resections. In time, we modified our scheme to facilitate measurement, in particular, in our head and neck population. Our first effort to collect normative timing data was in a group of 16 adults who were undergoing upper gastrointestinal (GI) studies for distal esophageal GI complaints (unpublished data, 1988; Johnson, McKenzie, Rosenquist, Liberman, & Sievers, 1993). The resulting data were consistent with those reported by other investigators (Cook et al., 1989; Curtis, Cruess, Dachman, & Maso, 1984; McConnel, 1988a, 1988b), and our standard deviations were small, which encouraged us to move forward.

Soon after adding timing information to our studies, we explored possibilities for displacement measures. Our explorations led us to strategies for getting video images into a computer (or "digitizing" them). Fortunately, the technology for doing this easily, relatively inexpensively, and effectively improved just as our interest piqued. Once the digitization problems were solved, we worked on techniques for measuring hyoid displacement and PES opening. When several members of our own team, as well as outsiders recruited for the task, made measurements that demonstrated good inter- and intrajudge reliability, we again felt we were moving in the right direction. As always, we incorporated measurements into routine patient assessments and our measurement techniques reflect this perspective. When our data appeared comparable to values reported by other investigators using different techniques (Cook, 1993; Dantas et al., 1990; Dodds, Man, Cook, Kahrilas, Stewart, & Kern,1988; Dejaeger, Pelemans, Ponette, & Joosten, 1997; Ekberg, 1986; Jacob, Kahrilas, Logemann, Shah, & Ha,

1989; Kahrilas, Dodds, Dent, Logemann, & Shaker, 1988; Perlman, VanDaele & Otterbacher, 1995), our confidence improved further.

## Normative Data

Ultimately, we collected additional normative data, using the same equipment and measurement strategies we used for patients. In time, we performed fluoroscopy studies on large groups of younger and more elderly normal subjects, respectively (Kendall, 2002; Kendall & Leonard, 2002; Kendall, Leonard, & McKenzie, 2001; Kendall, Leonard, & McKenzie, 2003; Kendall, Leonard, & McKenzie, 2004a, 2004b; Kendall, McKenzie, Leonard, Gonsalves, & Walker, 2000; Kendall, Leonard, & McKenzie, 2004a, 2004b; Leonard, Kendall, McKenzie, Gonzales, & Walker, 2000). As a team, we were now able to use our particular measurement scheme to compare patient data to nondysphagic subjects according to age and gender. Observations from these studies also provided us with a much better idea about normal variability, and of the range of behaviors, both times and displacements, that characterize normal swallow. Normative data for the measures we obtain, for adults younger than 65 years of age, and for a more elderly population of adults over 65 years, are presented in Table 16–1.

## Data Display

Having now worked out strategies for both timing and displacement measures, and having collected these measures

**Table 16–1.** Normative values for timing, duration and displacement measures, for subjects under and over age 65 years.

| NORMAL DISPLACEMENT *mean with 2 SD* | | | | | | | |
| MEASURE (cm) | < AGE 65 yrs | | | MEASURE (cm) | > AGE 65 yrs | | |
| | 1 CC | 3 CC | 20 CC | | 1 CC | 3 CC | 20 CC |
|---|---|---|---|---|---|---|---|
| Hmax (M) | 2.00 1.42 | 2.12 1.38 | 2.4 1.36 | Hmax (M) | 1.98 1.41 | 2.08 1.62 | 2.48 2.04 |
| Hmax (F) | 1.39 1.0 | 1.62 1.12 | 1.81 1.46 | Hmax (F) | 1.63 1.06 | 1.79 1.54 | 2.07 .45 |
| HL (M) | 1.33 .92 | 1.30 1.08 | 1.25 .83 | HL (M) | 1.50 .68 | 1.71 1.43 | 1.58 1.35 |
| HL (F) | 1.10 1.48 | 1.08 1.17 | 1.07 1.10 | HL (F) | 1.27 .87 | 1.24 1.2 | 1.23 1.30 |
| PESmax | .39 .38 | .51 .30 | .90 .55 | PESmax | .37 .34 | .50 .37 | .80 .40 |
| Pamax (M) | .13 .22 | .24 .36 | .28 .38 | Pamax (M) | .24 .49 | .35 .46 | .90 1.06 |
| Pamax (F) | .10 .18 | .12 .23 | .17 .33 | Pamax (F) | .25 .46 | .52 1.04 | 1.38 3.33 |
| Pam/Pah (M) | .02 .04 | .04 .05 | .06 .12 | Pam/Pah (M) | .02 .04 | .03 .04 | .13 .28 |
| Pam/Pah (F) | .02 .03 | .02 .04 | .03 .06 | Pam/Pah (F) | .02 .06 | .07 .15 | .14 .28 |
| Hmax+HL (M) | 3.33 1.86 | | 3.72 1.82 | Hmax+HL (M) | | | 4.06 .98 |
| Hmax+HL (F) | 2.49 1.7 | | 2.88 .86 | Hmax+HL (F) | | | 3.30 .55 |
| PA HOLD (M) 7.9 (4.2) (F) 6.5 (3.4) | | | | PA HOLD (M) 11.4 (6.0) (F) 8.09 (4.0) | | | |

**Morphometry of the Cartilaginous Larynx (mm)**

| | (M) | (F) |
|---|---|---|
| Cric | 24.6±1.9 | 21.6±1.5 |
| Aryt | 16.6±1.9 | 12.6±2.1 |
| | Total = 41.2 mm ±15.1 mm | 34.2 mm ±13.6 mm |

Sprinzl GM, et al. Head & Neck, December (1999).

**Increased aspiration pneumonia risk post CVA**

2–3 sec = 33%
3–5 sec = 48%
>5 sec = 90%

**Hyoid to mandible @ baseline (cm)**

| | <65 | >65 | >65+bar |
|---|---|---|---|
| (M) | 2.67 (.8) | 2.68 (.62) | 2.63 (.84) |
| (F) | 1.86 (.53) | 2.02 (.68) | 2.08 (.53) |

**Hyoid to larynx @ baseline (cm)**

| | <65 | >65 |
|---|---|---|
| (M) | 3.79 (.54) | 4.20 (.74) |
| (F) | 2.95 (.59) | 3.36 (.55) |

## NORMAL DURATION mean with 2 SD

| MEASURE (cm) | < AGE 65 yrs | | | MEASURE (cm) | > AGE 65 yrs | | |
| --- | --- | --- | --- | --- | --- | --- | --- |
| | 1 CC | 3 CC | 20 CC | | 1 CC | 3 CC | 20 CC |
| H max | .22 .20 | .21 .20 | .24 | H max | .13 .12 | .12 .14 | .20 |
| PES max | .34 .16 | .41 .14 | .50 .21 | PES max | .47 .20 | .62 .50 | .64 .21 |
| AE closed | .53 .28 | .60 .30 | .72 .50 | AE closed | .66 .28 | .84 .62 | .85 .93 |
| OP transit | .50 .33 | .41 .34 | .23 .26 | OP transit | .50 .64 | .49 .46 | .42 .36 |
| HP transit | .41 .46 | .43 .34 | .64 .24 | HP transit | .65 .37 | .76 .62 | .77 .26 |
| AEcl-Aest. | .27 .18 | .27 .29 | .25 .31 | Aecl-Aest | .48 .65 | .50 .66 | .54 .69 |
| Em | 1.07 .59 | 1.01 | 1.0 .36 | Em | 1.30 .88 | 1.30 .95 | 1.30 .57 |

## Maximum phx expansion, a-p (cm)

| | <65 | >65 |
| --- | --- | --- |
| (M) | 3.60 (.44) | 3.99 (.59) |
| (F) | 3.07 (.43) | 3.41 (.50) |

**Invariant Sequence Pairs**

AEs before Pop
  AEc no more than .1 sec after Pop, BP1
  HL after Pop
PAmax after PESmax
Pop before/same time as BP1
Pcl after/same time as BP2

**UES Max Openings, a-p (cm)**

| | <65 | >65 | >65+bar |
| --- | --- | --- | --- |
| (M) | 1.69 (.18) | 1.54 (.32) | .65 (.17) |
| (F) | 1.35 (.25) | 1.40 (.32) | 1.21 (.21) |

for normal subjects, we needed to display the information in a clinically useful way. After several attempts, we arrived at the method currently used and illustrated in Figure 16–1. In the Swallow Time/Duration/Displacement plot (STDD), *bolus transit* times are tracked separately from *swallow gesture* times. Bolus movement through the pharynx for a 20-cc swallow is represented along the lower portion of the plot by hatched lines and small circles. The "*B*" values on this axis (*B1, BV1*, etc.) represent bolus arrival or departure from certain anatomical sites.

The timing of various swallow gestures is also indicated along the horizontal axis by a solid line and small boxes. These points represent structural movements critical to swallow, for example, onset of hyoid elevation (H1), point of maximum pharyngoesophageal opening (PESmax), and closure of the supraglottic airway (AEclose). For both *bolus transit* and *swallow gestures*, an individual patient's values, in red, are plotted against our normative mean values (± 2 SD), in blue. This presentation allows us to consider both the coordination between bolus transit and the timing of various swallow gestures, and also how our individual patient compares to normal.

Displacement and duration data, respectively, appear in boxes inserted at the top of the plot (Figure 16–1). As before, an individual patient's values, in red, are plotted on vertical lines representing the normative mean (± 2 SD) for each measure, in blue. Patients' data are graphed separately for ages under and above 65 years, respectively, and for gender, when appropriate. Again, the plot permits ready comparison of the patient's performance to a group of comparable normal subjects.

Our team discussions now included presentation of the objective measures we had obtained from the DSS, and the advantages of this were several. We had anticipated that improved objectivity would reduce our disagreements and enhance our credibility, and this proved true. The ability to compare our patients to normal subjects was, of course, a significant development as well. Other benefits became apparent over time.

## Data Storage

Once we had a large amount of patient data (a few hundred patients per year), we wanted to be able to store the information, preferably in a database. This option allows the user to retrieve results quickly, and even link them to a report generator—a definite timesaver in clinical situations (Figure 16–2A–C). But perhaps the real power of a database is that, once patient information is added to it, the program can be "queried" to organize and summarize the data in a particular manner. If it is of interest to review transit times in all patients with cerebrovascular accident (CVA), or all patients with reduced PES opening size, or even all the patients seen in a certain time interval who are of a certain age or gender, the information can be produced in minutes (Figure 16–3). If we are discussing a particular patient, and want to know how other patients with similar pathologies or impairments compare to this individual, we simply query the database (Figure 16–3).

**Figure 16-1.** Plot (in Graphpad Prizm) displays objective data from fluoroscopic study.

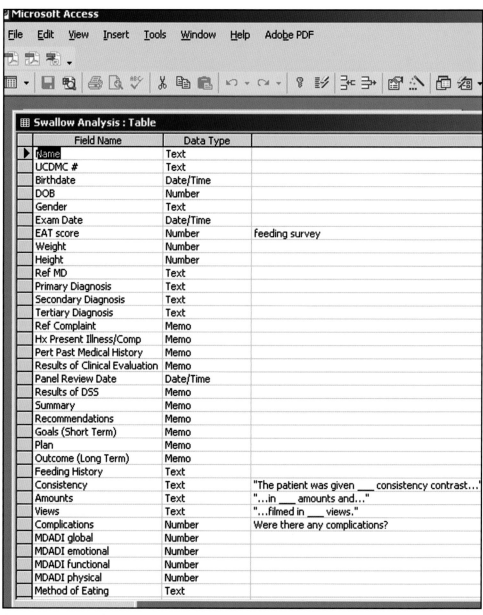

**Figure 16–2. A.** Database fields for which information will be obtained. *(continues)*

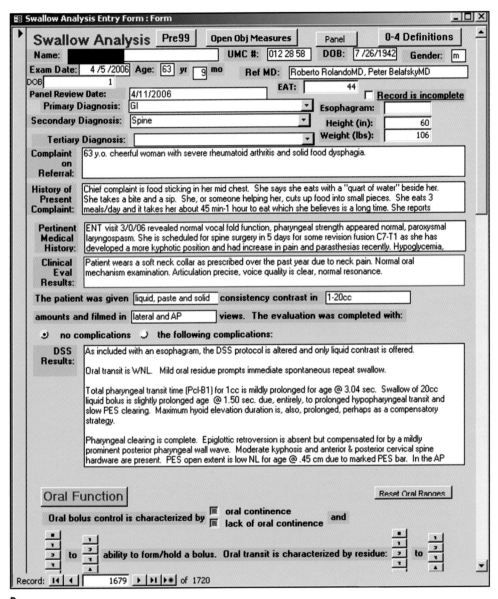

**B.**

**Figure 16-2.** *(continued)* **B.** Form created in Access database is used to enter pertinent patient information, including objective measures. *(continues)*

*DYNAMIC VIDEOFLUOROSCOPIC SWALLOW STUDY*
*Speech Pathology Report*

Name:                                  Referral:
UCDMC #:                               Birth Date:
Exam Date:                             Panel Review Date:


**ASSESSMENT:**                 **EAT:** 44        **WT(lbs):** 106        **HT(in):** 60

*Complaint on Referral:*

   63 y.o. cheerful woman with severe rheumatoid arthritis and solid food dysphagia.

*History of Present Illness/Complaint:*

   Chief complaint is food sticking in her mid chest. She says she eats with a "quart of water"
   beside her. She takes a bite and a sip. She, or someone helping her, cuts up food into small
   pieces. She eats 3 meals/day and it takes her about 45 min-1 hour to eat which she believes is
   a long time. She reports things like salad as easy, and sandwiches as hard to get down. She
   complains of extremely dry mouth. Eating is described as effortful and painful. Pain is
   described in throat, esophagus, chest and stomach (rated as 3 on the EAT). She also reports
   choking on pills, when this happens she can become unable to breathe. She also reports
   occasional difficulty with feeling of water sticking (does not go down). She reports an
   approximate weight loss of 10 lbs over the past 2 years but does not believe this is related to
   swallowing problems. Her BMI is in the "normal" range. She reports coughing at times other
   than meals. She wakes up at night choking, and this is reported as better since her visit
   with and Lisinopril was changed. She has a 7-8 year history of reflux and
   bleeding ulcers. She sleeps with her head elevated on pillows and avoids spicy foods and takes
   Prilosec daily. She is on oxygen at night (2.5 L) and has CPAP for sleep apnea, but hasn't
   been using it.

*Pertinent Past Medical History:*

   ENT visit 3/0/06 revealed normal vocal fold function, pharyngeal strength appeared normal,
   paroxysmal laryngospasm. She is scheduled for spine surgery in 5 days for some revision fusion
   C7-T1 as she has developed a more kyphotic position and had increase in pain and
   parasthesias recently. Hypoglycemia, reactive airway disease, hypertension, tachycardia,
   rheumatoid arthritis. Multiple orthopedic surgeries (knees, elbow, hands). History of uterine
   cancer with hysterectomy, history of thyroid cancer (unknown type) with thyroidectomy,
   meningitis, cataract surgery. Meds: Actonel, Accolate, Synthroid, Prilosec, Celebrex,
   Varapamil, Zyrtec, Ditropan, Arava, iron, acidophilus, calcium citrate, Centrum silver.

*Results of Clinical Evaluation:*

   Patient wears a soft neck collar as prescribed over the past year due to neck pain. Normal oral
   mechanism examination. Articulation precise, voice quality is clear, normal resonance.

*Description of Dynamic Swallow Evaluation  (see Radiology Report)*
*Results of Dynamic Swallow*

C.

**Figure 16–2.** *(continued)* **C.** Report is generated from information included in Form.
Information here does not have to be re-entered. *(continues)*

As included with an esophagram, the DSS protocol is altered and only liquid contrast is offered. She has other medications as needed.

Oral transit is WNL. Mild oral residue prompts immediate spontaneous repeat swallow.

Total pharyngeal transit time (Pcl-B1) for 1cc is mildly prolonged for age @ 3.04 sec. Swallow of 20cc liquid bolus is slightly prolonged age @ 1.50 sec. due, entirely, to prolonged hypopharyngeal transit and slow PES clearing. Maximum hyoid elevation duration is, also, prolonged, perhaps as a compensatory strategy.

Pharyngeal clearing is complete. Epiglottic retroversion is absent but compensated for by a

**SUMMARY:**

DSS findings indicate subjective (timing) and objective (PES bar) observations that could be considered consistent with uncontrolled GER. Prolonged hypopharyngeal transit could be in response to impaired esophageal function. Delay in airway closure may increase aspiration risk, particularly of thin liquids, before maximum glottic closure is achieved although no aspiration is detected. Findings are consistent with history and complaint.

**RECOMMENDATIONS:**

Consider return to review videotaped exam, analysis and Panel discussion and recommendations, including early airway closure to minimize aspiration risk.

Return to Dr. _____ for follow-up and monitoring.

Oral hygiene.

Careful behavioral GER precautions.

**SIGNATURE:**

Rebecca Leonard, Ph.D.
Susan McKenzie, M.S.
Alice Walker, M.S.
Cheryl White, M.S.

Jan Pryor, M.A.
Ann Sievers, R.N.
Susan Goodrich, M.S., Pediatrics

C.

**Figure 16–2.** *(continued)*

**Figure 16–3.** Once information is in the database, it can be queried to answer specific questions. Here, for example, the database is queried for patients with cricopharyngeal bar.

Generalizations about given populations, or insights into the unique characteristics of certain types of patients, are possible. This capability adds insights into individual patients, but also allows us to consider groups of patients, and to investigate them in ways that allow us to predict their impairments, or their responses to certain interventions. Many of our resulting efforts are reviewed in this text.

## PROS AND CONS OF OBJECTIVE MEASURES

In discussions with our peers, we sometimes hear that what we are doing is too time consuming, comprehensive,

cost-prohibitive, and/or too technically difficult to be replicated in most clinical settings. This is somewhat surprising to us because our fluoroscopy evaluation, including performance of the procedure, its analysis, and report preparation, takes no more time than other comparably billed procedures, such as a language or voice evaluation. It is perhaps the case that many clinicians consider the DSS to be primarily a screening exam with limited goals, that is, to determine if a patient aspirates, and if so, to identify strategies that prevent aspiration. The DSS is also used by many clinicians to make recommendations about diet, and dietary advancement. These are worthwhile objectives, and are routine components of our study, as well.

But our goal has always been to make the DSS study the most powerful diagnostic and treatment tool we can. The adherence to a uniform protocol for administration and the availability of normative data allow our approach to meet at least some of the criteria for a standardized test. This improves the power and credibility of interpretation and treatment recommendations in our own eyes, and in those of other medical professionals. For example, from the DSS we can identify and describe aspiration during fluoroscopic observations. But we can also also extract information predictive of aspiration risk, even if no aspiration is observed during the study. Similarly, dietary recommendations based on a standardized approach to the DSS permit generalizations beyond the conditions of the fluoro suite.

We would argue, further, that there is value in elaborating swallowing impairment in a manner that permits an explanation of the mechanics of dysphagia in individual patients, allows for generalizations between and among patient groups, as well as comparisons to normal and, eventually, predicts impairment in a wide variety of pathologies. The fluoroscopy study, at best, is still a sample of a patient's swallowing capability at one point in time, and is only one piece of the information that must be considered in the management of that individual. But if certain findings can be reliably related to other variables associated with swallowing health, and if these can be used to improve treatment or minimize consequences of swallow impairment, in future patients as well as current, then they are of value. It is this kind of information that may help us not only get patients out of hospitals more quickly,

but also keep them from returning with pulmonary or other complications. In our experience, it is the objective measures we collect that are most helpful to these purposes.

Once we understand patient groups well enough, we are also likely to find that some measures are of particular value for one group of patients, and others are more critical in other populations. In fact, one of our ongoing long-term objectives is to identify selected measures—even one or two—that may be of great value in individual patients. Transit times, for example, have been shown to predict aspiration pneumonia requiring repeated hospitalization in CVA patients (Johnson, McKenzie, & Sievers, 1993), whereas a measure of pharyngeal constriction predicts aspiration in other types of patients (Yip, Leonard, & Belafsky, 2006), and possibly, outcomes on other instrumental studies, such as manometry (Leonard, Belafsky, & Rees, 2006). When this kind of information is available, we can begin to apply measures selectively in individual patients, or patient populations. The task of measurement may then be expedited without loss of significant information.

To conclude this section, we return to the beginning. That is, we first became interested in acquiring objective measures from our fluoroscopy studies because of our concerns about the reliability of subjective impressions, and about the credibility of studies based solely on nonstandardized assessments. These concerns arose quickly in our setting because we were meeting as a team, and trying as a group to extract both useful and accurate information from our evaluations.

In today's health care settings, it is not uncommon for clinicians to summarize studies immediately upon their completion, possibly with only brief review. A usual rationale offered for this practice (in inpatient settings) is that demand for patient turnover is high, and that time constraints permit nothing further. But the decisions made from the study have important, perhaps huge, consequences for individuals. Of course it is important to determine the competence of a patient's swallow in terms of safety and effectiveness, and it is a decision that should be made with deliberation. Presumably, we would not be subjecting patients to an invasive procedure if we did not feel the potential for valuable information was good. We would suggest again, however, that our success should be measured not simply by how many patients we discharge from hospitals, but by how many patients we discharge who are not readmitted and who are eating in a way that truly befits their capabilities, because we have made the soundest decisions possible about their care.

## OBJECTIVE MEASURES

In this section of the chapter, the actual measures obtained from the dynamic study will be discussed, and the rationale for their selection will be presented. When available, reliability data for each measure will be included in the discussion, as will gender and age differences identified in our normal populations. Reliability has been determined for most of our measures across four individuals who made measures (using measurement criteria presented here) on a subset of swallows from 15 normal subjects. As new clinicians and interested individuals have become available, reliability checks have been continued. Reliability on many of our measures has by now been established across 8 to 10 raters. Instructions for actually making the measures will be the focus of Chapter 17. The DVD accompanying this text also includes an animated tutorial (DSS TUTOR) that should be helpful in making the measures.

## Timing Measures

In our clinical studies, we typically obtain timing measures from the 1-cc bolus swallow, and from the largest bolus swallowed. As noted, five of these measures represent points in *bolus transit*, which define the rate at which the bolus travels through the pharynx. Seven additional measures represent the timing of *gestures*, or structural movements, during the swallow. By tracking the bolus separately from the gestures responsible for transporting the bolus, it is possible to assess the coordination between various swallow events. In this scheme, "delay" is characterized as an increased latency between two events, as between a swallow gesture and a point of bolus transit. Swallows that require a greater than usual amount of time are then characterized as "prolonged," not delayed. A video clip labeled "DSSnormswall" will be found in the materials folder for Chapter 16. The reader is encouraged to play through this clip while reading the section on timing measures. All of the *bolus transit* and *swallow gesture* times described here are identified on the clip. *Bolus transit* measures include:

## B1

*B1* is defined as the time of the first movement of the head of the bolus past the posterior nasal spine. This measure is used to establish a zero point marking the beginning of the entry of the bolus into the pharynx. All other timing measures are compared to *B1* to determine the relative time of their occurrence during the swallow. This definition of the onset of pharyngeal transit time, *B1* in our scheme, differs from author to author (Bisch, Logemann, Rademaker, Kahrilas, & Lazarus, 1994; Curtis, Kruess, Dachman, & Maso, 1984; McConnell, 1988a).

It is important to recognize that these differences in definition will likely affect comparisons across investigators. McConnel (1988a; 1988b) defines the beginning of pharyngeal transit time as the moment the hyoid begins its anterior and superior movement. This is a swallow *gesture*, rather than a measure of bolus position, and thus does not describe transit. Other authors (Logemann, 1983) define the onset of pharyngeal transit relative to the mandible, for example, the time when the bolus crosses the lower or anterior rim of the mandibular ramus. In oropharyngeal cancer patients, however, the mandibular ramus may be absent. And if a patient's head is rotated during the x-ray study, the position of the mandible will be changed relative to the midline of the pharynx, with a subsequent effect on the measured value of *B1*. The alternative we have chosen,

that is, the first movement of the bolus past the posterior nasal spine, is more constantly available and readily identified in most cases. The posterior nasal spine is also a midline structure and therefore its position is less likely to be affected by rotation of the patient. If the palate is absent, the anterior border of the ramus can be used if care is taken not to allow rotation of the patient's head. The interrater reliability of our clinicians in identifying *B1* on normative studies is 99%.

## BV1 and BV2

*BV1* and *BV2* describe transfer of the bolus from the oropharynx to the hypopharynx. The division of pharyngeal transit into multiple components is consistent with, for example, the concept of "pharyngeal transit time" as comprised of "pharyngeal delay" time and "pharyngeal response" time, as defined by Logemann (1987).

## BV1

*BV1* is defined as the moment that the bolus reaches the base of the vallecula. *BV1* is measured because it demarcates the boundary of the oro- and hypopharynx and, as such, marks the end of oropharyngeal transit and the beginning of hypopharyngeal transit. In patients with reasonably normal anatomy, it is easily found. This is reflected in an *r* value of 0.99 for *BV1* in our normative data. Patients post head and neck cancer may present with absent valleculae or valleculae severely altered in position and anatomy, however, making it impossible to measure *BV1*. *BV1* is another option to use as a reference point in the calculation of transit measures, in particular, in cases where *B1* for some reason cannot be identified.

### BV2

*BV2* represents the first exit of the head of the bolus from the valleculae and the beginning of hypopharyngeal transit. In larger bolus sizes, *BV1* and *BV2* are essentially indistinguishable in normal subjects, that is, the bolus does not rest in the valleculae but simply passes by it. But for a 3-cc bolus, for example, there is a significant difference between these two bolus transit points in normal subjects. By the time the bolus reaches this point, there is an increased urgency of swallow success.

### BP1 and BP2

*BP1* and *BP2* describe bolus movement through the PES and can be used to examine the coordination of PES opening and closing with other events.

### BP1

*BP1* is defined as the first entrance of the head of the bolus into the upper esophageal sphincter as the sphincter begins to open. Typically, this occurs immediately upon the opening of the pharyngoesophageal sphincter (PES) in normal subjects. The sphincter can occasionally be seen to open before the arrival of the bolus in patients who are not able to move the bolus effectively through the pharynx, however. Opening of the sphincter following its relaxation is considered to be the result of the anterior and superior movement of the hyoid bone and laryngeal structures.

### BP2

*BP2* is defined as the moment that the tail of the bolus clears the PES and is fully within the esophagus. This timing measurement marks both the end of pharyngeal bolus transport and, in normal subjects, the end of PES opening.

### Pharyngeal Transit Times

Once bolus transit times have been identified, it is a straightforward matter to calculate pharyngeal transit times. In our scheme, three such measures are determined, including: *Total pharyngeal transit time*, which is defined as the difference between *BP2* and *B1* and represents the total time of bolus passage through the pharynx. This can be further divided into *oropharyngeal transit time* (*BV1-B1*) and *hypopharyngeal transit time* (*BP2-BV2*). Interjudge reliability for *total pharyngeal transit time* in our normative data was 98%.

### Age, Gender, and Bolus Size/Consistency Differences in Transit Times

The analysis of our 60 younger normal swallow subjects (age 18–65) revealed no change in pharyngeal transit time across bolus size or consistency. This finding has implications for cases in which very small or very large boluses are unmanageable. That is, if a patient is unable to propel a very small liquid bolus into the oropharynx secondary to anterior tongue and mouth abnormalities, a larger liquid bolus can be substituted for this measure and the expected time for a normal response will not be affected. In the same fashion, if a patient cannot control a large liquid bolus, or transfers the bolus to the pharynx in a piecemeal manner, timing measures made on the smaller bolus size will still accurately reflect the patient's pharyngeal transit time. In addition, if thin consistencies are difficult for the patient, then paste can be substituted and the evaluation of pharyngeal transit time should remain accurate. Our results contradict previous studies in which the subject numbers were smaller (Dodds, Stewart, & Logemann, 1990; Johnson et al., 1992).

Pharyngeal transit time did not increase significantly with increasing age in our first group of normal subjects, who ranged in age from 18 years to 65 years (Kendall, McKenzie, Leonard, Goncalves, & Walker, 2001). This finding differs from that reported by other investigators (Cook et al., 1994; Curtis et al., 1984; Logemann, 1987; Robbins, Hamilton, Lof, & Kempster, 1992; Shaw et al., 1995). Subjects in our first group of normal subjects were chosen without regard to age, and the age distribution of the subjects is weighted more heavily toward the middle of the age range. Our findings did not change, however, when subjects were grouped by age and the means for specific age categories compared using linear regression analysis.

However, in a comparison of 62 normal subjects under 65 years to a group of 83 normal, nondysphagic subjects over 65 years, transit times were significantly different for 1-cc, 3-cc, and 20-cc bolus sizes. In general, transit times were prolonged in the elderly group. The elderly group was then further subdivided into those with no medical problems typical of an aging population (hypertension, diabetes, and osteoarthritis), and those who had one or more of these conditions. When the younger normal subjects were compared to 23 normal elderly subjects with no medical conditions, all transit times for the elderly were still significantly prolonged. We typically use the values from this subgroup for comparison to our elderly patients with dysphagia (see Table 16–1).

## Clinical Implications of Prolonged Bolus Transit Times

Prolonged bolus transit times have frequently been implicated in swallowing difficulty (Bisch et al., 1994; Johnson et al., 1992; Johnson & McKenzie, 1993). The longer bolus material remains in the airway, the greater the challenge to airway protective mechanisms. Previous studies in stroke victims have shown an increased risk of aspiration pneumonia in patients with prolonged pharyngeal transits as measured from a dynamic swallow study, even when no aspiration was identified on the examination (Johnson et al., 1993). In a study of elderly individuals with dysphagia with no obvious medical or surgical causes of their impairment, prolonged bolus transit times were identified in 61% of the patients (Kendall & Leonard, 2001). Delayed or prolonged pharyngeal transit time has also been shown to be associated with an increased incidence of aspiration pneumonia in several populations (Johnson et al., 1992; Johnson et al., 1993; Rademaker, Pauloski, Logemann, & Shanahan, 1994). As such, its clinical significance is well-established. We interpret prolonged pharyngeal transit times as an indication of increased risk for aspiration and make recommendations accordingly.

## Swallow Gesture Times

In addition to bolus transit times, we identify times when critical swallow gestures occur. Typically, these involve the onset of a structure's movement, and when it achieves maximum displacement during the swallow. In the case of the PES, we also note when it closes. The reader is encouraged to continue to move through the video clip, "DSSnormswall" to identify swallow gesture points described here. The swallow gesture times are as follows:

### AEstart and AEclose
### (Airway Closure)

The aryepiglottic folds and the outline of the arytenoid cartilages are visible against the relative hypodensity of the pharyngeal space in the lateral projection on the x-ray. During swallowing the arytenoid cartilages are seen to elevate and approximate the down-folding epiglottis, effectively closing the supraglottic larynx and protecting the airway. During frame by frame analysis, it is possible to identify movement of these structures, in particular, when the most superior part of the arytenoid cartilages begins to elevate, and again when it makes contact with the down-folding epiglottis (Logemann, 1987). The points of onset (AEstart) and completion (AEclose) of supraglottic closure can therefore be measured. The timing of these events can then be compared to other events that occur during the swallow. In particular, it may be impor-

tant to determine the relative timing of aryepiglottic fold closure relative to bolus transit through the pharynx in patients observed to aspirate. Normally during a swallow, the arytenoid cartilages begin to move towards the epiglottis as the bolus enters the pharynx. By the time the bolus arrives at the upper esophageal sphincter (designated as **BP1**), the down-folding epiglottis is seen to approximate the arytenoid cartilages, effectively obliterating the supraglottic passage.

### H1, H2, and H3 (Hyoid Displacement)

In our measurement scheme, **H1** is defined as the first superior–anterior displacement of the hyoid that results in a swallow. **H2** is marked by the first frame in which the hyoid bone has reached its maximum superior–anterior excursion during the swallow, and typically occurs in close relationship to PES opening (Cook et al., 1989; Jacob, Kahrilas, Logemann, Shah, & Ha, 1989). In our normative data, comparison of the values of **H2-B1** and **Pop-B1** (**Pop** represents the first opening of the PES during swallow) were found to be identical. **H3** indicates the first retreat of the hyoid from its maximum displacement.

The frame chosen to represent **H2** is also used when measuring the distance of maximum hyoid excursion. Reliability in defining **H1** and **H2** in normal subjects was 99% and 98%, respectively. A number of authors have described the first movement of the hyoid (**H1** in our scheme) as the onset of the swallow reflex. We recently described the relationship of **H1** in our normal nonelderly and elderly subjects to a number of bolus transit points, including **B1**, **BV1**, **BV2**, **BP1**, and passing the angle of the mandible (Leonard & McKenzie, 2006).These data provide a number of options for considering the relationship between first movement of the hyoid and bolus transit and can be used to relate specific latencies to various concepts of pharyngeal swallow delay.

The onset of hyoid elevation is one of the first visible gestures in the swallow sequence and, as such, signals the onset of hypopharyngeal elevation and preparation to receive the bolus. Information about timing of the onset and maximum swallow movement of the hyoid can be especially helpful in patients whose coordination of swallowing gestures with bolus transit is in question, for example, in conditions affecting neural transmission, that is, amyotrophic lateral sclerosis, multiple sclerosis.

Although our $r$ values for **H1** and **H2** are quite good, it is nevertheless true that neither of these points may be obvious, even in normal swallowers. "Preparatory" hyoid movements are common and can complicate identification, in particular, of **H1**. It is helpful that hyoid movement for swallow is more vigorous and stereotypic than other hyoid movements (sometimes characterized as a blur on the fluoro study), and is often preceded by a few frames of stability. In both normal and dysphagic individuals, identification of **H2** also may be problematic because the hyoid does not always move at the same rate or in a straight line to its maximum excursion. Rather, it may follow a graceful clockwise or counterclockwise curve or figure eight, slowing significantly as it curves. The measurer must review the study carefully

and fix one point in the patterned movement that best represents maximum hyoid anterior and superior displacement as **H2**. If necessary, several displacement measures can be made to determine which frame represents maximum displacement.

The point at which the hyoid returns to rest following the swallow has sometimes been used to indicate the end of the swallow. However, large variability in the measured values from our normative data for this event suggests significant behavioral overlay affecting its timing. We recommend that the return of the hyoid to a rest position be used to define the end of pharyngeal transit as a last resort, and only then with caution (McConnell, 1988a, 1988b). It is not routinely assessed in our dynamic swallow studies.

### Pop, PESmax, and Pcl (PES Opening and Closing)

**Pop** is the time of the first frame on which the PES is open. **PESmax** represents the first time at which the PES achieves its maximum opening size. **Pcl** is the time of the first frame on which the PES closes (usually on the tail of the bolus), marking the end of pharyngeal transit.

PES timing is of obvious importance as the culminating gesture of the swallow and the literal and figurative "bottom line" of pharyngeal transit. If the concept is not debatable, the definition of the measurement can be. Selection of a single point in time when the PES opens or closes requires selection of a precise point that can be called the PES. The location (and therefore the best place to make measures) of the PES as seen on a dynamic videofluoroscopic swallow study is unclear. It has previously been defined as a point 1.5 cm below the beginning of the tracheal air column (Kahrilas, Dodds, Dent, Logemann, & Shaker, 1988).It seems likely, however, that the position of the upper esophageal sphincter varies from subject to subject, depending on size of the individual and possibly other variables. In addition, the location of the top of the air column is often difficult to identify with precision. In our setting, acceptable reliability for precise designation of this site has not been achieved, even with quite experienced evaluators (though this has improved with improved fluoroscopy units). We have therefore chosen to define the upper esophageal sphincter as the narrowest part of the opening from the level of C3 (superior), above, to the level of C6 (inferior), below. The decision to use this definition was based on the idea, supported by experience, that the narrowest site is always the most clinically significant, that is, what limits rate of bolus passage.

Closure of the PES (**Pcl**) is almost universally used to define the end of the swallow. If hypopharyngeal transit is even partially successful, **Pcl** will coincide with all or part of the bolus entering the cervical esophagus.

### Em (Epiglottic Displacement)

This measure is the time of the first frame on which the epiglottis has returned to its preswallow position, marking the reopening of the supraglottic airway or return to respiratory posture following the swallow. Typically, it occurs after the closure of the PES. **Em** has been used to mark the end of pharyngeal transit (Johnson et al., 1992; Johnson & McKenzie, 1993); not surprisingly, transit times reported using this marker are longer than others reported. The measure has been particularly useful in identifying segments of the CVA population at risk for development of aspiration pneumonia (Johnson & McKenzie, 1993). Nevertheless, application of **Em** in this manner can be debated. Epiglottic return is not a critical gesture for accomplishment of pharyngeal transit and it also appears subject to behavioral interference. However, it does signal re-establishment of the pharyngeal airway, that is, a return to respiratory mode. As the calculation of **H1-Em** may reflect respiration interruption time, **Em** can be a useful measure for patients with respiratory compromise. It is included for these reasons. Reliability for this parameter on normative data was 99.9%.

### Swallow Gesture Durations

Once the times of various structural events have been calculated, it is possible to determine the durations between the events. The durations we obtain include the duration of maximum hyoid displacement (**H3-H2**), PES opening duration (**Pcl-Pop**), and duration of airway closure (**Em-AEc**). Our intermeasurer reliability for the value of **Pcl-Pop** was 92%.

### Age, Gender, and Bolus Size/ Consistency Differences in Swallow Gesture Times

In contrast to *bolus transit* times, certain *swallow gesture* times in our two groups of normal subjects did vary with bolus size and consistency. PES opening time (**Pcl-Pop**) increased with increasing size of the bolus (see Table 16–1). Jacob et al., (1989) also found that the duration of PES opening increased with increasing bolus size, whereas the overall duration of the swallow remained constant. These authors interpreted this finding as indicating that the *speed* of bolus transport through the PES is increased with larger boluses. As noted previously, we did not find (in our younger normal subjects) differences in bolus transit times between the 3-cc liquid bolus and a comparably sized paste bolus (Kendall, Leonard, & McKenzie, 2001). However, we did find that, for the 3-cc liquid bolus, the hyoid remained maximally elevated longer, as compared to the paste bolus. PES opening, on the other hand, was significantly longer for the paste bolus, as compared to the liquid bolus. Our data indicated further that **EM-AEclose** also increased with bolus size, suggesting that the airway is protected longer depending on bolus size.

It is of further interest that the duration of maximum hyoid displacement (**H3-H2**) was significantly reduced in our elderly normal subjects as compared to the younger normal subjects, for the 1-cc, 3-cc, and 20-cc bolus sizes. In contrast, there was a tendency for PES opening (**Pcl-Pop**) and airway closure (**Em-AEclose**) to be longer in the elderly normal subjects as compared to the younger subjects, but these differences were not significant. No gender differences were identified for swallow gesture times.

## Clinical Implications of Swallow Gesture Times

Of these measures, duration of PES opening (**Pcl-Pop**) is perhaps of particular interest. The capability of the upper esophageal sphincter to open in a timely manner is critical to a normal swallow. An inability to do so results in incomplete or absent transit of the bolus into the esophagus. When the PES fails to open, decreased hyoid or larynx elevation or failure of cricopharyngeal relaxation may be the etiology. In addition, poor pharyngeal constriction, secondary to pharyngeal constrictor weakness or lack of tongue mobility, can impact PES opening. Whether it is a problem with timing, extent of opening, or the duration of opening, the spatial measures discussed further in this chapter can provide insight to the etiology of the dysfunction.

## Coordination Between *Bolus Transit* and *Swallow Gesture* Events

Coordination of events during the pharyngeal phase of swallowing has been considered to be reflexive, involuntary, and automatic in nature. Central mechanisms are thought to be primarily responsible for the pattern of events that propel a bolus from the oral cavity into the esophagus. Sensory feedback information and voluntary behaviors are believed secondarily to influence the sequence. Tracking of *bolus transit* separately from *swallow gesture* times permits evaluation of the coordination between and among these events. To determine normal variability in the sequencing and coordination of the swallowing gestures and points of bolus transit, we analyzed the sequence of events during swallowing of a 1-cc, a 3-cc, and a 20-cc liquid bolus in our 60 normal younger adult volunteers (Kendall, 2002). Of 180 swallows evaluated, no two swallows matched in the sequence of all the events, indicating sequence variability between subjects and within individuals depending on changes in bolus size. Predominant patterns could be identified but no sequence could be ruled out as abnormal based on the findings from these 60 individuals. Variability was less during deglutition of larger bolus volumes, perhaps as a result of faster bolus transit times and less opportunity for behavioral overlay. Certain bolus and gesture timing relationships were found to exist during hypopharyngeal bolus transit that did not vary between subjects or across bolus categories. These included the following:

- The elevation of the aryepiglottic folds (**AEstart**) always began *before* opening of the pharyngeal esophageal sphincter (**Pop**).
- The sphincter always opened (**Pop**) *before* the arrival of the bolus at the sphincter (**BP1**); similarly, the sphincter closed simultaneously with or just after the tail of the bolus cleared the sphincter (**BP2**);
- Maximum hyoid to larynx approximation (**HLx**) always occurred *after* the onset of upper esophageal sphincter opening (**Pop**);
- Maximum pharyngeal constriction (**PAmax**) always occurred *after* maximal distension of the upper esophageal sphincter (**PESmax**). Some variability in the relative timing of all other event sets analyzed by this study was found. The lack of variability in the relationships noted, however, make these useful in considerations of coordination between and among swallowing events.

For example, one timing relationship that we have investigated (Kendall, Leonard, & McKenzie, 2004) and found to be of particular clinical relevance is the timing of supraglottic closure (**AEclose**) relative to the arrival of the bolus at the upper esophageal sphincter (**BP1**). As noted, the arytenoid cartilages elevate and approximate the downfolding epiglottis (**AEclose**) during swallow, effectively closing the supraglottic larynx and protecting the airway. This mechanism may be incomplete or delayed in patients complaining of dysphagia and may lead to "penetration" of bolus material into the airway. Aspiration that occurs *during* passage of the bolus into the upper esophageal sphincter is usually the result of incomplete upper airway closure.

To evaluate the relationship of supraglottic airway closure and bolus arrival further, we analyzed the timing of these two events in our group of 60 young control subjects and also in 23 elderly control subjects (65–88 years old) without dysphagia, and without medical conditions typical of an elderly population (diabetes, hypertension, and osteoarthritis). Event timing was measured in 0.01 second intervals from videofluoroscopic studies for two liquid bolus size categories. Results of the analysis revealed that in most individuals, the arytenoid cartilages approximate the epiglottis, closing off the airway, *before* the arrival of the bolus at the pharyngoesophageal sphincter. However, in both bolus size categories, there were individuals who achieved complete supraglottic closure after the bolus had arrived at the sphincter, but *never greater than 0.1 seconds later*. No difference in the timing of supraglottic closure relative to bolus arrival at the sphincter was found between the young and the elderly subject groups. The information from this study has allowed us to objectively determine if supraglottic closure timing is delayed in patients with dysphagia and to address any delay with strategies and exercises designed specifically to correct the delay.

## Spatial Measures

The acquisition of spatial (distance and area) measurements is somewhat more complicated than obtaining timing information. It requires that images of interest be digitized and subjected to computer analysis, adding both hardware and software to the instrumentation setup (described in Chapter 17). Extracting valid estimates of distance and area requires particular attention during the dynamic swallow study so that measures, and comparisons among measures, can be made for the calibration frame, the referent frame, and the frame on which the target movement is seen. Critical aspects of technique include a true lateral patient upper body position and uniform patient-to-fluoroscope arm distance, not to mention good visibility of target anatomy over the course of the exam.

Spatial measures routinely made at our facility include the following:

- **Maximum hyoid displacement**—change in hyoid position from a referent frame, **Hold**, to maximum anterior–superior displacement, **H2** (**Hold** is defined as the relationship between structures with a 1 cc bolus held in the oral cavity);
- **Pharyngeal constriction ratio**—a ratio of pharyngeal area measured in lateral view at its point of maximum constriction during a swallow, to pharyngeal area measured in the **Hold** posture. The ratio is referred to as the pharyngeal constriction ratio (**PCR**);
- **Maximum opening of the PES**—maximum distention of the site designated PES during swallow; and
- **Maximum approximation of the larynx and hyoid**—difference in distance between hyoid and larynx at **Hold**, and at their point of maximum approximation during the swallow.

Normative data for each of these measures, respectively, are presented in Table 16–1. The reader is again encouraged to move through the "DSSnormswallow" clip (in materials folder for Chapter 16) while reading this section to identify frames used in making displacement measures.

### Reference Position

To measure how much a pharyngeal structure or complex of structures is displaced during swallowing, the identification of the "nondisplaced" or a reference position is obviously critical for comparison. Selecting such a position for structures of the oral cavity and pharynx has proved particularly challenging. The difficulty is related to both behavioral and conceptual issues, that is, what constitutes a "rest" position for the larynx? Conceptually, options for "rest" might include a position assumed by the patient when asked not to move, or a position at the end of a vegetative gesture, such as a sigh. In our experience, however, huge variability has been observed in these behaviors both within and between subjects. We have forgone the idea of a "rest" position, and are using a referent preparatory measure identified as "hold." In doing so, we have knowingly sacrificed the idea of measuring total range of movement because there is often displacement *to* the preparatory position. We have essentially focused on what we believe to be more meaningful and useful concepts: Range of movement related to swallow, and the identification of a reliable position to which maximum displacements can be compared. Still, behavioral interference is not eliminated, because movement for preparation for swallow varies greatly in normal and dysphagic swallowers. Nevertheless, use of the "hold" referent has enabled us to make reliable spatial measurements.

### Hold—The "Reference" Position

The **Hold** position is defined by giving the subject of the study a 1-cc bolus of contrast with the instruction to hold it in the mouth before swallowing. For the purposes of the videotaped swallow analysis, the frame just before any posterior movement of the bolus that results in a swallow from the hold position is defined as **Hold**. When a patient is unable to "hold" the bolus, the measure is made on the frame before onset of efforts toward oral transit.

### Hyoid Displacement

**Hmaxd.** Hmaxd is defined as the distance traveled by the hyoid to the point of maximal elevation during a swallow from its position during **Hold**.

PES opening depends primarily on the elevation of the hyoid and larynx (Cook et al., 1989; Jacob et al., 1989). The anterior movement of these structures pulls open the relaxed PES, thereby creating a vacuum, or area of low pressure, at the PES site. This action, combined with gravity and pressure applied by the base of tongue and pharynx, will propel the bolus into the upper esophagus (Dodds et al., 1990; Jacob et al., 1989; McConnel, 1988b). Measurement of maximum displacement of the hyoid during swallow provides valuable insight into the forces contributing to PES opening in a given patient. Diminished hyoid elevation is seen in conditions that affect muscles that attach the hyoid to the mandible, for example, surgical resection of the floor of the mouth, with tissue fibrosis after radiation therapy, and neuromuscular diseases. Inability to elevate the hyoid/larynx is often accompanied by difficulties with PES opening. In fact, identification of diminished hyoid bone elevation can help distinguish failure of PES opening because of failure of cricopharyngeal relaxation from failure of PES opening because of a loss of anterior traction on the sphincter. Given the relationship between hyoid and PES, and the relative ease of identifying the hyoid on the fluoroscopic study, we feel that measurement of hyoid displacement is an important part of the dynamic swallow study interpretation.

Because **Hmaxd** is measured at **H2**, difficulty in identification of the precise frame of maximum displacement may lead to an inaccurate measurement of **Hmaxd**, as discussed earlier. Our inter-measurer reliability for **Hmaxd** was 95%, however, suggesting that with experience it is possible to accurately estimate this point.

### Pharyngeal Area

**Pahold.** The area of the pharynx, that is, the two-dimensional space of the pharynx apparent in lateral view, is calculated on the **Hold** frame and is designated as **Pahold**. Our intermeasurer reliability for **Pahold** was found to be 92%. Linear regression analysis of the effects of subject height and weight on pharyngeal area at the hold position in our younger group of normal subjects failed to reveal any significant differences in pharyngeal area related to these variables.

**PAmaxd.** A second measure of pharyngeal area is made when the pharynx is maximally constricted during the largest bolus swallow, and is designated as **Pamaxd**. As with **Pahold**, for normal subjects this measure was found to differ significantly depending on the gender of the subject (see Table 16–1). Our normative data for this parameter were collected during a 20-cc bolus swallow. Intermeasurer reliability for **Pamaxd** was 96.6%.

*Pamaxd/Pahold: Pharyngeal Constriction Ratio.* A ratio of the pharyngeal area at maximum constriction to the pharyngeal area during hold is calculated. The use of a ratio minimizes gender differences noted for each of the area measurements. Although larger in the elderly normal group as compared to younger subjects, the ratio of pharyngeal area at maximum constriction and pharyngeal area at rest, referred to as the pharyngeal constriction ratio (PCR), is quite low, between 0 and 0.14 cm$^2$. Intermeasurer reliability for *PCR* was 95.6%.

The posterior and downward driving force of the tongue base within the contractile chamber of the pharyngeal walls acts in concert with upper esophageal sphincter opening to ensure successful transfer of the bolus through the pharynx (Cook et al., 1989; Dodds et al., 1990; Jacob et al., 1989; McConnel, 1988a, 1988b). On the dynamic swallow study, the tongue base is seen to move posteriorly toward the posterior pharyngeal wall and combined with pharyngeal shortening (as the hypopharynx elevates) results in the obliteration or narrowing of the pharynx during the swallow. The critical role of the contractile chamber walls against which the piston must work should not escape appreciation. When the role of lingual retraction is limited because of anatomic or neurologic impairment, the compensation provided by the pharyngeal constrictors can still result in complete pharyngeal constriction. From the fluoroscopic study, some evidence pertinent to both pharyngeal constriction and tongue movement is available. Measurement of pharyngeal area represents a possibility for objectively assessing this information, in a manner that takes into account all forces accomplishing pharyngeal transit, not just the tongue.

The lateral view of the pharynx on the swallow study is a two-dimensional representation of a three-dimensional space, and we often rely on the amount of residual barium seen in the hypopharynx to define the size of the space at maximum constriction. These limitations notwithstanding, we feel that the measures provide a useful way to evaluate the "piston" action of the tongue working against the descending constriction of the pharyngeal walls. Pharyngeal area measures have the additional advantage of being relatively easy to obtain in most subjects.

When poor pharyngeal constriction is identified on the swallow study by measurement and calculation of an increased PCR, a loss of tongue mobility or bulk may be the primary etiology. If the tongue activity is relatively normal, weakness of the pharyngeal constrictors (as is often seen in stroke victims) may be the reason. The result is usually persistent pharyngeal residue. Patients will be at an increased risk for aspiration of the residue when the glottis reopens for respiration. Strategies such as the "double swallow" or "effortful swallow," directed at clearing the residue before resuming respiration, may be recommended.

### PES Distension

**PESmaxd.** The maximum opening of the PES during a swallow, **PESmaxd**, is measured. As discussed earlier for **Pop-Pcl**, PES is defined as the narrowest point in the opening between C3 and C6 during the swallow. Because efficient transfer of the bolus into the esophagus is dependent on adequate PES opening, some measure of PES opening is an obvious choice for inclusion in any measurement battery. As discussed previously, however, the actual location of the point designated PES is arguable. By defining the PES as the narrowest point between C3 and C6, we were able to achieve an $r$ of 0.95 on this measure for normal subjects.

### Age, Gender, and Bolus Size/ Consistency Differences for Spatial Measures

Several differences in these variables were identified for spatial measures. Age differences were identified for **PESmaxd** and **PCR**; **PESmaxd** is reduced

in the elderly, and **PCR** is increased, as compared to younger subjects (see Table 16–1). **Hmaxd** was reduced in elderly females, as compared to younger females, but this difference was not identified for younger and elderly males (see Table 16–1). Gender differences were also identified as significant for all displacement measures, on all bolus sizes and consistencies investigated, with the exception of **PESmaxd**, which did not differ significantly according to gender on any bolus considered (see Table 16–1).

Bolus size differences were noted for all displacement measures except maximum approximation of the larynx and hyoid during swallow (true for all bolus sizes). Our interpretation of this finding is that larynx to hyoid approximation (**HLx**) may have more to do with airway protection, and maintaining a constant level of such during swallow, as opposed to making adjustments in size of the PES. **PESmaxd** did increase with increasing bolus size, presumably to accommodate the larger bolus size or in response to changes in intrabolus pressures. Increased PES opening with increasing bolus size corresponds to an increase in **Hmaxd** with increasing bolus sizes (in both age groups and for both males and females), and may reflect the anterior traction on the PES by the forward movement of the hyoid, as well as increased intrabolus pressures (see Table 16–1).

## Clinical Implications of Impaired Spatial Displacements

Impairments in spatial displacements are an important reason for aspiration and dysphagia in many patient populations. Their calculation can provide excellent insights into causes of impairment, as well as therapeutic objectives that might be considered. Our own research, for example, has demonstrated the following:

- Increases in **PCR** appear to be a near-hallmark feature of swallowing in patients with myotonic muscular dystrophy (Leonard, Kendall, Johnson, & McKenzie, 2001). In some patients investigated, in fact, the pharyngeal area when maximally constricted (for a 20-cc bolus) was actually *larger* than in the **Hold** position. This suggests that pharyngeal weakness associated with this disease may become so pronounced that the presence of a large bolus causes the pharynx to distend or expand, rather than constricting to propel the bolus into the esophagus. In monitoring our myotonic muscular dystrophy patients (and others who demonstrate similar weakness), we pay particular attention to this measure in counseling patients regarding a possible transition from oral to non- or partial-oral feeding.

- **PCR** has been further shown to be associated with aspiration in a variety of patient populations (Yip, Leonard, & Belafsky, 2006). Data from 260 sequential patients undergoing dynamic swallow studies were examined for those who aspirated, and those who did not aspirate. Those patients who did aspirate (on the largest bolus swallowed) demonstrated a mean **PCR** of 0.32 cm$^2$, whereas those who didn't had a mean **PCR** of 0.20 cm$^2$ (both values were elevated, as compared to normal). Further, individuals with a **PCR** greater than 0.25 cm$^2$ were three times more likely to aspirate, as compared to other patients. In evaluating patients, we are seriously concerned about safe swallowing in patients with **PCRs** of this value, even when we do not observe aspiration on the dynamic swallow study.

- In a subsequent study, stroke patients (CVA) who did and did not aspirate on the largest bolus swallowed on the DSS were considered (Leonard, unpublished data). The group consisted of 300 patients. Patients with a **PCR** of 0.25 cm$^2$ were six times more likely to aspirate than those with values below 0.25 cm$^2$.

- **PCR** may be a useful surrogate measure of pharyngeal strength. In a comparison of maximum pharyngeal pressures obtained on manometry, and **PCR** from a separate dynamic swallow study in the same patients, a negative correlation of −.7 was found for the two measures (Leonard, Belafsky, & Rees, 2006). Further, only two patients with a **PCR** significantly elevated from normal (for age and gender) were found to have maximum pharyngeal pressures within the normal range on manometry, and pressures for these two patients were very low, 60 and 61 mm Hg, respectively. We are currently investigating these two parameters on simultaneous manofluoroscopy studies, and hope to elaborate our earlier findings soon. If current findings hold, the dynamic swallow study may provide useful inferential information regarding pharyngeal pressures when manometry is not available or possible.

- In an investigation of elderly patients with no obvious medical or surgical cause of their dysphagia (Kendall & Leonard, 2001), 74% of patients demonstrated an elevated **PCR**. Elevated **PCR** was also found to be a factor in 75% of cases of aspiration identified in this population. Interestingly, the timing of maximum pharyngeal constriction remained appropriately coordinated with the position of the bolus in the pharynx in these same patients.
- Our comparison of younger and more elderly nondysphagic individuals revealed a large percentage of the elderly subjects with cricopharyngeal bars (31%) (Leonard, Kendall, & McKenzie, 2002). Interestingly, no bars were identified in our younger group of subjects. Not surprisingly, **PESmaxd** was also reduced in the elderly group, as compared to the younger group. Evaluation of elderly individuals should consider the increased likelihood of apparently asymptomatic cricopharyngeal bars.
- In an investigation of factors affecting pharyngeal constriction in nonelderly and elderly

normal subjects, several findings were of interest (Leonard, Kendall, & McKenzie, 2004). As described, **PCR** was elevated in the elderly, as compared to younger subjects, suggesting a reduced ability to constrict and possibly clear the pharynx during swallow. In addition, the two-dimensional pharyngeal area measured in the **Hold** position was larger in the elderly subjects, as was the distance between the larynx and the hyoid at **Hold**. The distance from the hyoid to the mandible did not differ between groups; however, the distance between the hyoid and larynx at **Hold** was significantly greater in the elderly subjects. A measure of the anterior–posterior view of the pharynx at **Hold** was also wider in the elderly subjects. These data, as well as additional information we have obtained, suggest that the pharynx in elderly subjects may be larger, or longer, as compared to younger individuals. In addition, the pharynx did not constrict as completely, and the larynx did not elevate to the same extent, in elderly subjects. These data comprise an important reference in assessing swallow in elderly dysphagic patients, in particular, in differentiating normal from abnormal in this group.

- In an investigation of normal subjects and elderly dysphagic patients (Kendall & Leonard, 2001), it was found that maximum hyoid displacement was actually greater on smaller bolus sizes in the elderly group, as compared to individuals without dysphagia. This was interpreted as a possible compensation for the decreased duration of the hyoid at maximum displacement, and may represent a strategy that can be used with other patients.

The kinds of observations reviewed here represent just a few that can be made when large amounts of objective data become available for patients representing different disorders. In short, the use of a standardized DSS and objective measures have, in our opinion, allowed us to use the fluoroscopy study as a powerful diagnostic tool. It

- permits us to compare our patients to normal subjects according to age and gender;
- provides an objective means of tracking changes in patients across time and treatments;
- supplies us with a basis for characterizing dysphagia in unique patient populations;
- allows us to go beyond the determination of aspiration versus no aspiration, or appropriate dietary recommendations, to understand the biomechanical deviations from normal deglutition that contribute to the dysphagia, and how these present a risk to patients *outside* the environment of the DSS evaluation;
- reveals information that, increasingly, we are finding can be related to other instrumental measures of swallow function; and

- is now, in our practice, a part of the repertoire of diagnostic tests routinely ordered by many physician specialists charged with evaluating and treating dysphagic patients.

## STUDY QUESTIONS

1. Which structural displacements during swallowing differ in younger and older individuals? According to gender?
2. Do pharyngeal transit times differ according to age and/or gender?
3. What subjective impressions from fluoroscopy studies have demonstrated reasonable interjudge reliability?
4. Define bolus transit at "B1," "BV1," "BV2," "BP1," and "BP2."
5. Why was the "Hold" position selected as a referent for measures of structural displacements? (as compared to a "Rest" position).
6. What are some problems in using the angle of the mandible as a marker for the onset of bolus transit?
7. What is the advantage of tracking *bolus transit* times separately from *swallow gesture* times?
8. What relationships between swallow gestures, or between swallow gestures and bolus transit, appear to be invariant in both younger and older normal individuals?
9. The measure of pharyngeal constriction, "PCR," may be a reasonable surrogate for what other instrumental measure?
10. What was unique about PES opening in the normal elderly population described?

## REFERENCES

Bisch, E. M., Logemann, J. A., Rademaker, A. W., Kahrilas, P. J., & Lazarus, C. L. (1994). Pharyngeal effects of bolus volume viscosity, and temperature in patients with dysphagia resulting from neurologic impairment and in normal subjects. *Journal of Speech and Hearing Research, 37,* 1041–1059.

Blonsky, E. R., Logemann, J. A., Boshes, B., & Fisher, H. B. (1975). Comparison of speech and swallowing function in patients with tremor disorders and in normal geriatric patients: A cinefluorographic study. *Journal of Gerontology, 30,* 299–303.

Cook, I. J., Dodds, W. J., Dantas, R. O., Massey, B., Kern, M. K., Lang, I. M., et al. (1989). Opening mechanisms of the human upper esophageal sphincter. *American Journal of Physiology, 257,* G748–G759.

Cook, I. J., Weltman, M. D., Wallace, K., Shaw, D. W., McKay, E., Smart, R. C., et al. (1994). Influence of aging on oral-pharyngeal bolus transit and clearance during swallowing: Scintigraphic study. *American Journal of Physiology, 266,* G972–G977.

Dantas, R. O., Kern, M. K., Massey, B. T., Dodds, W. J., Kahrilas, P. J., Brasseur, J. G., et al. (1990). Effect of swallowed bolus variables on oral and pharyngeal phases of swallowing. *American Journal of Physiology, 258,* G675–G681.

Dejaeger, E., Pelemans, W., Ponette, E., & Joosten, E. (1997). Mechanisms involved in postdeglutition retention in the elderly. *Dysphagia, 17,* 63–67.

Dodds, W. J., Man, K. M., Cook, I. J., Kahrilas, P. J., Stewart, E. T., Kern, M. K. (1988). Influence of bolus volume on swallow-induced hyoid movement in normal subjects. *American Journal of Roentgenology, 150,* 1307–1309.

Ekberg, O., Nylander, G., Fork, F. T., Sjoberg, S., Birch-Jensen, M., & Hillarp, B. (1988). Interobserver variability in cineradiographic assessment of pharyngeal function during swallow. *Dysphagia, 3,* 46–48.

Gibson, E., & Phyland, D. (1995). Rater reliability of the modified barium swallow. *Australian Journal of Communication Disorders, 23,* 54–60.

Jacob, P., Kahrilas, P. J., Logemann, J. A., Shah, V., & Ha. T. (1989). Upper esophageal sphincter opening and modulation during swallowing, *Gastroenterology, 97,* 1469–1478.

Johnson, E. R., & McKenzie S. W. (1993). Kinematic pharyngeal transit times in myopathy: Evaluation for dysphagia. *Dysphagia, 8,* 35–40.

Johnson, E. R., McKenzie, S. W., Rosenquist, C. J., Liberman, J. S., & Sievers, A. (1992). Dysphagia following stroke: quantitative evaluation of pharyngeal transit times. *Archives of Physical Medicine and Rehabilitation, 73,* 419–423.

Johnson, E. R., McKenzie, S. W., & Sievers, A. (1994). Aspiration pneumonia in stroke. *Archives of Physical Medicine and Rehabilitation, 74,* 665.

Kahrilas, P. J., Dodds, W. J., Dent, J., Logemann, J. A., & Shaker, R. (1988). Upper esophageal sphincter function during deglutition. *Gastroenterology, 95,* 52–62.

Karnell, M. P. & Rogus, N. M. (2005). Comparison of clinician judgments and measurements of swallow response time: A preliminary report. *Journal of Speech Language and Hearing Research, 48,* 1769–1779.

Kendall, K. A. (2002). Oropharyngeal swallowing variability. *Laryngoscope, 117,* 547–551.

Kendall, K., & Leonard, R. (2001). Bolus transit and airway protection coordination in older dysphagic patients. *Laryngoscope, 111*(11 Pt. 1): 2017-2021.

Kendall, K. A., Leonard, R. J., & McKenzie S. W. (2001). Accommodation to changes in bolus viscosity in normal deglutition: A videofluoroscopic study. *Annals of*

*Otology, Rhinology and Laryngology, 110,* 1059–1065.

Kendall, K. A., Leonard, R. J., & McKenzie S. W. (2003). Sequence variability during hypopharyngeal transit. *Dysphagia, 18,* 85–91.

Kendall, K. A., Leonard, R. J., & McKenzie S. (2004a). Airway protection: Evaluation with videofluoroscopy. *Dysphagia, 19,* 65–70.

Kendall, K. A., Leonard, R. J., & McKenzie S. (2004b). Common medical conditions in the elderly: Impact on pharyngeal bolus transit. *Dysphagia, 19,* 71–77.

Kendall, K. A., McKenzie, S., Leonard, R. J., Goncalves, M. I., & Walker, A. (2000). Timing of events in normal swallow. *Dysphagia, 15,* 74–83.

Kuhlemeier, K. V., Yates, P., & Palmer, J. B. (1998). Intra- and interrater variation in the evaluation of videofluorographic swallowing studies. *Dysphagia, 13,* 142–147.

Leonard, R., Belafsky, P. C., & Rees, C. J. (2006). Relationship between fluoroscopic and manometric measures of pharyngeal constriction: The pharyngeal constriction ratio. *Annals of Otology, Rhinology and Laryngology, 115,* 897-901.

Leonard, R. J., Kendall, K. A., Johnson, R., & McKenzie, S. (2001). Swallowing in myotonic muscular dystrophy: A videofluoroscopic study. *Archives of Physical Medicine and Rehabilitation, 82,* 979–985.

Leonard, R., Kendall, K., & McKenzie, S. (2004a). Structural displacements affecting pharyngeal constriction in nondysphagic elderly and nonelderly adults. *Dysphagia, 19,* 133–141.

Leonard, R., Kendall, K., & McKenzie S. (2004b). UES opening and cricopharyngeal bar in nondysphagic elderly and nonelderly adults. *Dysphagia, 19,* 182–191.

Leonard, R. J., Kendall, K. A., McKenzie, S., Goncalves, M. I., & Walker, A. (2000). Structural displacement in normal swallowing: A videofluoroscopic study. *Dysphagia, 15,* 146–152.

Logemann, J. (1983). *Evaluation and treatment of swallowing disorders.* San Diego, CA: College-Hill Press.

Logemann, J. A., Boshes, B., Blonsky, E. R., & Fisher, H. B. (1977). Speech and swallowing evaluation in the differential diagnosis of neurologic disease. *Neurologia, Neurocirugia, and Psiquiatria, 18*(2–3 Suppl.), 71–78.

McConnel, F. M. S. (1988a). Analysis of pressure generation and bolus transit during pharyngeal swallowing. *Laryngoscope, 98,* 71–78.

McConnel, F. M. S. (1988b). Timing of major events of pharyngeal swallowing. *Archives of Otolaryngology-Head and Neck Surgery, 114,* 1413–1418.

McCullough, G., Wertz, R. T., Rosenbek, J. C., Mills, R. H., Webb, W. G., & Ross, K. B. (2001). Inter-and intrajudge reliability for videofluoroscopic swallowing evaluation measures. *Dysphagia, 16,* 110–118.

Perlman, A. L., Booth, B. M., & Grayhack, J. P. (1994). A study of interrater reliability when using videofluoroscopy as an assessment of swallowing. *Dysphagia, 13,* 223–227.

Rademaker, A. W., Pauloski, B. R., Logemann, J. A., & Shanahan, T. K. (1994). Oropharyngeal swallow efficiency as a representative measure of swallowing function. *Journal of Speech and Hearing Research, 37,* 314–325.

Robbins, J., Hamilton, J. W., Lof, G. L., & Kempster G. B. (1992). Oropharyngeal swallowing in normal adults of different ages. *Gastroenterology, 103,* 823–829.

Scott, A., Perry, A., & Bench, J. (1998). A study of interrater reliability when using videofluoroscopy as an assessment of swallowing. *Dysphagia, 13,* 223–227.

Shaw, D. W., Cook, I. J., Gabb, M., Holloway, R. H., Simula, M. E., Panagopoulos, V., et al. (1995). Influence of normal aging on oral-pharyngeal and upper esophageal sphincter function during swallowing. *American Journal of Physiology, 268*(3 Pt 1), G389–G396.

Yip, H., Leonard, R., & Belafsky, P. Can a fluoroscopic estimation of pharyngeal constriction predict aspiration? *Otolaryngology-Head and Neck Surgery, 135*(2), 215–217.

# 17

# *Dynamic Swallow Studies: Measurement Techniques*

## Rebecca Leonard
## Susan McKenzie

## TIMING AND DISPLACEMENT MEASURES

The measures described in this chapter represent our current best thoughts about what types of data are usefully obtained from the dynamic swallow study (DSS). They reflect our "borrowings" from other clinicians and investigators, as well as many of our own conventions, and over time have proven useful to us in assessing our patients (Crary, Butler, & Baldwin, 1994; Dejaeger, Pelemans, Ponette, & Joosten, 1997; Dengel, Robbins, & Rosenbek, 1991; Logemann, Kahrilas, Begelman, Dodds, & Pauloski, 1989; Perlman, VanDaele, & Otterbacher, 1995) But we also believe strongly that a great way to study swallowing, normal and disordered, is to try to "measure" it. The dynamic swallow study affords a unique opportunity to do this, to sample and quantify at least some events that are critical to the complex swallow sequence. It is in the interest of the study not only as an excellent diagnostic and treatment planning tool, but also as a tool for learning, that this chapter is included.

Once familiar with the strategies used, readers will be able to make their own measurements from the sample swallow studies included in the Chapter 17 materials folder, and to compare their results with ours. Shareware programs used in analysis, for both PC and Mac computers, are also included in this folder. In addition, an animated tutorial, "DSSTUTOR" is included on disk to facilitate the mechanics of measurement. Once you have gone through the tutorial, and read this chapter, it will be relatively simple to have both "DSSTUTOR" and the program for making measures open at the same time on the monitor. You can watch us make a measurement and then try it, yourself. For readers who are currently involved in performing and analyzing studies, comparisons to the scheme used in our setting may be of interest. For readers who have not had extensive experience with the dynamic swallowing study, the materials provided should represent an in-depth introduction to the value and potential of this assessment tool, as well as to a number of issues that befuddle both clinicians and investigators working in this area.

## HARDWARE AND SOFTWARE

### Timing Measures

A good quality videocassette recorder (VCR) with stop frame and slow motion reverse and forward capabilities has for many years been the basic component for review and analysis of dynamic swallow studies, and still works well. With an accurate frame advance feature, the time between two events can be calculated simply (if tediously) by determining the number of frames between them, recognizing that each frame is equal to 1/30th of a second. Rapidly, however, VCR technology is being replaced by digital recording systems. Consequently, the methods discussed here, and materials provided for readers, will be primarily directed to digital media.

Our DSS studies are currently recorded on a Sony DVO-1000MD (Sony Corporation of America, New York City, NY) digital video recorder (DVR) using DVD+RW disks. Timing information in hundredths of a second is recorded on the disk from a timing generator interfaced between the x-ray camera and the DVR during filming of the study. Several timing generators will serve this purpose. One used at our Center is the Horita Video Stopwatch VS-50 (Horita, Mission Vijeo, CA). The cable coming from the x-ray camera (same one usually attached to the VCR or DVR) is attached to the "video in" port of the Stopwatch. A second cable is then attached to the "video out" port on the back of the timing device. The other end of this cable is connected to the "video in" port of the DVR. By interfacing the timer between the fluoro and the recorder in this manner, timing information can be superimposed on the recording. The user has the option of where to position the timing information on the monitor, and of adjusting the size and color of the numeric display. The ability to place the time signal in different positions, that is, all four corners, on the disk is a desirable feature in whatever generator is used. If timing information can only be positioned in one location on the screen, it may occasionally cover up events or landmarks in the x-ray study that are critical to visualize.

With the timing generator activated, timing information will appear on the monitor. Because timing information will appear on every frame recorded, it is not necessary to start every swallow attempted by a patient at time "0." Our typical practice is to just turn on the timer when we begin recording, and to leave it on throughout the study. All timing measures are then calculated from whatever time marks the beginning of an event, to the time that marks the end of the event.

Once the study is recorded, there are several options for playback of the DVD disk. A stand-alone DVD player (or player-recorder) may be used. Alternatively, any computer with a DVD drive is sufficient for this purpose. In either case, the particular disks used for recording must be in a format the drive or player can read, for example, DVD+RW, DVD-R (disk included with this text is DVD+RW). Most computers are also equipped with software programs that permit playback of the DVD ("Windows Media Player" for PC, "DVD Player" for Mac). A PC program that we use is "WinDVD" (Intervideo, Fremont, CA). The particular value of "WinDVD" is the great flexibility it permits the user in manipulating the recorded study, including variable playback speeds in forward and reverse, frame advance, and options for adjustment of the video image (contrast, brightness, etc.). Viewing the study in this manner, we attempt to identify and note the times described in Table 17–1, all of which are made from the lateral view x-ray. Typically, we acquire these times for a 1-cc bolus, and for the largest bolus swallowed. As previously described, both *bolus transit* and *swallow gesture* times are noted.

Once the timing events have been determined, it is also possible to calculate durations of critical events during the swallow. In our scheme, the following durations are considered of interest:

> **Oropharyngeal transit time**— duration of bolus transit through the oropharynx, from the posterior nasal spine (**B1**) to the time of bolus exit from the valleculae (**BV2**).
>
> **Hypopharyngeal transit time**— duration of bolus transit through the hypopharynx, from the time the bolus head exits the valleculae

(**BV2**) to the time of bolus tail clearance of the PES (**BP2**).

> **Total transit time**—sum of oropharyngeal and hypopharyngeal transit times (**BP2-B1**).
>
> **PES opening time**—time from PES opening to PES closing (**Pcl-Pop**).
>
> **Airway closure time**—time supraglottic airway remains closed during the swallow (**Em-AEc**).
>
> **Hyoid maximum duration time** —duration of maximum hyoid displacement (**H3-H2**).

## Displacement Measures

Displacement measures are obtained in one of two ways, depending on whether a VCR or DVR is used. If recordings are on videotape, then the images of interest, that is, selected frames from the study, are first digitized so that they can be manipulated by a computerized image analysis program. In our setting, videotaped images are input to either a Macintosh (any one from a Mac 11 to current generation) or PC/Pentium or newer style computer using digitizing boards from Data Translation, Inc. (Marlboro, Massachusetts) or Scion Corporation (Frederick, Maryland).

A cable from the VCR attaches to the digitizing board in the computer so that, when you open the software program and set it to "Capture," images from the VCR monitor also appear on the computer screen. The software program used for capturing images obtained in this manner is "IMAGEJ." It was developed by Wayne Rasband and his

**Table 17-1.** Timing Measures

| | |
|---|---|
| *B1* | Onset of bolus transit through the pharynx. In our studies, this time represents the "zero" point to which all later events during the swallow are compared. It is defined as the first movement of the bolus past the posterior nasal spine that leads to a swallow. If the bolus is large, its head may extend beyond the posterior nasal spine at "Hold." If a portion of bolus material falls in or towards the valleculae early, this is regarded as valving failure or inadequate instruction/attention and is considered a part of oropharyngeal transit, that is, B1 would start with the early bolus loss. OPT would likely be prolonged in this case, and the explanation for it (inability to contain the bolus orally, inattention, etc.) would be included in the narrative. |
| **AEs** | Start of arytenoid-epiglottis approximation to close the supraglottic airway. |
| **H1** | First onset of hyoid displacement that leads to a swallow. The hyoid sometimes moves around prior to the swallow. Try to be certain you identify H1 as the *first movement that leads to the swallow*. The nature of this movement is typically quite distinctive, so rapid and abrupt that it is blurred/hard to recognize in the fluoro study. In some patients, the hyoid is elevated at "Hold," possibly in response to expected difficulty. This can be noted in the narrative and may explain hyoid displacement that appears reduced during the swallow. |
| *BV1* | Bolus head arrival at the base of the valleculae. |
| *BV2* | Exit of bolus head from the valleculae (apparent with small bolus sizes; with larger sizes, BV1 and BV2 are typically the same because the bolus does not stay in the valleculae or is flowing laterally.) |
| **AEc** | Arytenoid-epiglottis approximation indicating supraglottic airway closure is maximally achieved. |
| **H2** | Hyoid arrival at maximum displacement (typically, anterior and superior). In some cases, the hyoid may pause at this point; if not, it may take checking several spots to know which represents the maximum displacement from Hold. |
| **Pop** | First opening of the lumen at the PES during swallow (defined as the narrowest point between C3 and C6). |
| *BP1* | Head of bolus enters PES. If it doesn't, this is noted in the narrative. |
| **PES max** | PES achieves maximum opening during the swallow. |
| **H3** | Hyoid begins to retract from maximum displacement. |
| **HL max** | Hyoid and larynx achieve maximum approximation during the swallow. |
| **PA max** | Pharyngeal chamber is maximally obliterated/constricted during the swallow. |
| *BP2* | Tail of bolus clears PES. If it doesn't, this is noted in the narrative. |
| **Pcl** | PES closes. If it doesn't, no time is recorded for this event. In normal swallowers, Pcl and BP2 are typically the same. |
| **Em** | Epiglottis returns to its upright position; supraglottic airway opens. |

*Note.* Timing measures are presented for both *bolus transit* and *swallow gesture* events during swallow. Exact order may vary depending on characteristics of bolus and on individual impairment to normal swallow.

colleagues at the National Institutes of Mental Health and is available free as shareware (http://rsb.info.nih.gov/nih-image). The precursor to this program was "NIH IMAGE," which can also be used. There are versions of "IMAGEJ" for both Macintosh and PC computers and both are frequently updated (both versions are provided in the Chapter 17 materials folder accompanying this text). "IMAGEJ" is also the program used in our setting for image analysis.

If recordings are made directly on to a DVD, and hence already digitized, then the disk can simply be placed in the DVD-drive of a PC or Macintosh computer for playback. Again, in our setting "WinDVD" for the PC is used for this purpose (Figure 17–1), but other programs, including "IMAGEJ" in some cases, can be used. The displacement measures that we routinely obtain, all from the lateral view x-ray, include (1) maximum displacement

**Figure 17-1.** Intervideo's WinDVD 7 is used to playback DVDs. Multiple playback speeds are possible, and frame advance/step reverse feature (*arrow on left*) allows precise control over the clip. When images of interest are identified in the study, the user can (1) click on the camera icon at the top (*top arrow*); (2) then click the "+" sign; (3) now view the picture when it appears in an inset on the right (*lower arrow*). Pictures are then labeled and can be opened in "IMAGE J" to be used in measurements. On Apple computers, "DVD Player" and the utility program "Snag and Drag," which can be downloaded from the Internet, will perform similar functions.

of the hyoid during swallow (**Hmaxd**); (2) maximum opening of the PES during swallow (**PESmaxd**); (3) maximum approximation of the hyoid and larynx during the swallow (**HLmaxd**); and (4) a measure of pharyngeal constriction (**PCR**). In patients who demonstrate reduced PES opening in lateral view, we also obtain a measure of maximum PES opening in the anterior–posterior view (**PESmaxap**).

With the exception of maximum PES opening, the displacement measures are made from two images, one representing the structure at rest, or in a stable position that can be reliably achieved on a repeat study, and another representing the structure at its point of maximum displacement during the swallow. The pseudo rest position we use is obtained with a 1-cc bolus held in the oral cavity, a position we refer to as "**Hold**." To measure maximum hyoid displacement, we determine the difference between the location of the hyoid in the "**Hold**" position, and its location when maximally displaced during the swallow (**Hmaxd**). With either of the software programs noted ("IMAGEJ" when studies are videotaped, "WinDVD-7" when they are digitally recorded), it is a straightforward matter to first identify these frames, and to then save them for later analysis. Once all of the appropriate frames required for displacement measures have been obtained in this manner, we are ready to make the measures.

## HANDS-ON EXPERIENCE

Materials for this section of the chapter are included here in the materials folder for Chapter 17. They include several dynamic swallow studies, of patients and normal subjects, and both PC and Macintosh versions of "IMAGEJ." The swallow studies included have already been digitized and are in a video file format that can be used on both PC and Mac computers (.avi) using software available for PC or Macintosh computers. Clips of normal subjects can also be opened using the appropriate version of "IMAGEJ." As noted, "DSS-TUTOR," an animated tutorial of all the mesurements, is also available.

## PLAYBACK AND IMAGE MANIPULATION

You will first need to copy the appropriate "IMAGEJ" program (Mac or PC) from the materials folder to your own computer. Open the folder labeled "Chapter 17 materials" under Chapter 17 (on the DVD accompanying the text). The "IMAGEJ" programs are labeled for PC or Mac, respectively, and can be copied on to your own hard disk ("C" drive, desktop). Also copy the .avi files labeled "DSS1ccdemo," "DSS20ccdemo" and "DSSdisplframes" onto your desktop. This will ensure that you keep the originals intact, and the clips will play best from a hard drive, as opposed to playing them from the DVD. When you have copied the program and demo clips onto your computer, open the "IMAGEJ" folder and click on the microscope icon. You may also want to open the text of Chapter 17 on the disk, so that this information is on your screen while you are making measurements. If you adjust the size of both "IMAGEJ" and the text, they should fit nicely on your monitor. Otherwise, you can just refer to this hard copy text while making the measures, or to the examples provided in "DSSTUTOR."

With "IMAGEJ" open, you should see a toolbar at the top of your monitor, and the IMAGEJ menu just above this (Figure 17–2). Tools used for analysis of the x-ray images include the polygon, pencil, heart, line (ruler), and angle. Also note the MENU BAR just above the toolbar, that is, FILE, EDIT, etc. Clicking on any one of these (keep the mouse button depressed) will open a submenu of functions that can be selected. Clicking the mouse on any one of the options will open or activate the function.

Go to "PLUGINS" on the toolbar and click on it. Move the cursor to "AVI Reader" and click on it (Figure 17–3). In "Look in: _____" at the top of the "Select AVI File" dialogue box that opens, you can search for the "DSS20ccdemo" video clip, which you copied to your desktop or hard disk.

When the "Select AVI File" box appears, find the video clip you need and double-click on it. You will see a rectangular box under the toolbar filling as the clip is "loaded" into the program.

The clip will open in a few seconds and you should see the first frame on your monitor (Figure 17–4). You can play the clip by clicking on the arrow keys at the bottom of the clip, sliding the bar between the two arrows, or by using the "<" and ">" buttons on your keyboard. The latter is a good choice for frame advance and reverse. You can also modify the image quality, for example, brightness and contrast, by entering the Menu under IMAGEJ. Click on "Image" and then "Adjust." Under "Brightness/Contrast," experiment with the adjustments for "Minimum" before you apply settings to the whole clip (called "Stack" in "IMAGEJ").

## CALCULATING TIMES AND DURATIONS

Play around with the clip until you are comfortable manipulating it. It is the 20-cc swallow of a 53-year-old male with a primary complaint of solid food dysphagia. When you are comfortable with the controls, go through the clip and decide which times correspond to the *bolus transit* and *swallow gesture* times previously described. *Be sure to play back and forth through the clip several times when you are trying to identify precise times.* It can be difficult trying to do this frame by frame until you have watched the action a few times. The timing events, and the times we decided on, are presented here, in the order of their occurrence on the clip (go down first column, then second, then third).

**Figure 17–2.** When the IMAGEJ program is opened, this is what is seen on the monitor. Menu bar is at top, and tools used for analysis are just below the menu.

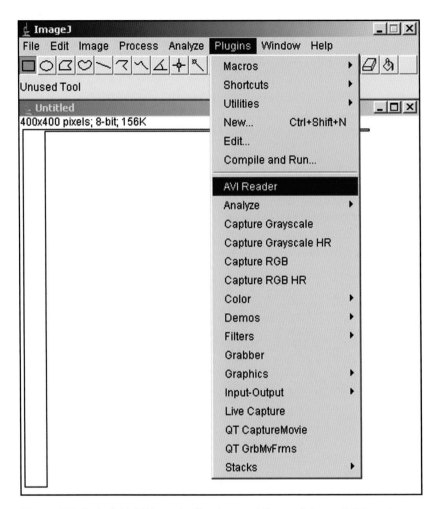

**Figure 17–3.** In IMAGEJ, go to Plugins and then click on AVI Reader.

Incidentally, the average measurement error across 5 to 7 judges approximated 0.06 seconds (about 2 frames) for timing measures. Further, reliability across judges for all timing measures was at least 0.90, and often greater than 0.95. This means that, if you are within a frame or two (each frame = 0.03 sec) of our values, you are making judgments quite similar to ours.

| | |
|---|---|
| H1 —53.19.33 | HLm —53.19.73 |
| BV1—53.19.33 | H3 —53.19.79 |
| BV2—53.19.33 | PAm —53.19.88 |
| AEc—53.19.39 | BP2 —53.20.03 |
| Pop—53.19.43 | Pcl —53.20.03 |
| H2 —53.19.64 | Em —53.20.18 |
| Pop—53.19.43 | |

| | |
|---|---|
| B1 —53.18.79 | BP1 —53.19.43 |
| AEs— 53.18.79 | PESm—53.19.68 |

Once you decide on the times, you can also calculate durations between events

**Figure 17–4.** With "DSS20ccdemo" open in IMAGEJ, your monitor should look like the above.

(in seconds). Here are some examples, including our calculations:

Oropharyngeal transit time, (*BV2-B1*) 0.54 secs

Hypopharyngeal transit time, (*BP2-BV2*) 0.70 secs

Total transit time, (*BP2-B1*) 1.24 secs

PES opening duration, (Pcl-Pop) 0.66 secs

If you compare the values obtained to the normative data (under 65 yrs) presented in Chapter 16, you will be able to determine how this patient compares. In general, his times and durations are prolonged as compared to the normal population, although they are within 2 SD of the means for these values. Transit time is prolonged primarily due to prolonged oropharyngeal transit. The patient does have a PES bar with slight jet (reflecting increased flow rate through the PES).

For all transit times currently in use, our reliability across several judges is greater than 0.90. The average deviation from the mean across judges is on the order of 0.06 seconds for all timing measures, which is about two frames (each time you advance one frame on tape or disk, you are advancing 0.03 seconds). As noted, if your measures are within a click or two of ours (within 0.06 seconds), your values added to ours would likely produce comparable reliability results.

## Measuring Displacements

As noted, images used to make displacement measures from the study of interest are first "saved" and then reopened in "IMAGEJ" for measurement. Images you will need are listed in Table 17–2. For convenience, we have saved the images needed in the .avi file (video clip) called "DSSdisplframes" in the Materials folder. Close the "DSS20ccdemo" clip and open "DSSdisplframes" (open with "AVI Reader" under "Plugins.") Each of the eight frames is labeled, as "1cc Hold," "20ccHmaxd," "20ccPESmaxd," "20cc-HLmaxd" and "20ccPAmaxd." The "1cc Hold" will be used several times in

**Table 17–2.** Images Required for Displacement Measures.

| | |
|---|---|
| **1cc Hold** | Identifies a pre-swallow frame "referent" to which movement of structures during the swallow can be compared. In our scheme, "**Hold**" is defined as the position of structures with a 1-cc bolus held in the oral cavity. A frame from the imaging study representing **Hold** is identified and saved. This will serve as the **Hold** referent for the 1cc swallow, and for all subsequent swallows, i.e., 3 cc, 20 cc. |
| **Hold: Hyoid** | Hyoid position relative to the third and fourth vertebrae is marked in the **Hold** frame and saved. This position of the hyoid will be compared to its maximally elevated position during the swallow. |
| **Hmaxd** | Hyoid position maximally elevated (at time H2) relative to the third and fourth cervical vertebrae is identified and saved. The difference between the hyoid in this position and in the **Hold:Hyoid** position defines maximum hyoid displacement during the swallow. |
| **PESmaxd** | The greatest expansion during swallow of the site designated PES (narrowest opening in lateral view of upper esophagus at maximum distension). |
| **Hold: HL** | The distance between the hyoid and larynx at **Hold** is measured. |
| **HLmaxd** | The distance between the hyoid and larynx at the point of their maximum approximation during the swallow is measured. The difference in this distance and the distance between the two structures at **Hold** defines maximum approximation of the hyoid and larynx during the swallow |
| **Hold: PA** | The boundaries of the pharynx before swallow are outlined in the **Hold** frame and this area is calculated for later comparison to the pharynx maximally constricted. |
| **PAmaxd** | The boundaries of the pharynx when it is maximally constricted are outlined, and this area is calculated and noted. The ratio of **PA Maxd** to **Hold: PA** is referred to as the pharyngeal constriction ratio (**PCR**). |

calculating displacements (all of the measures in Table 17–2 with **Hold** in their label). Again for convenience, we have included several copies of the "1cc Hold" frame in the clip and labeled them as "Hold:Hyoid," "Hold:HL," and "Hold:PA," respectively. There are two cautions that we would advise the reader to remember in working on the measurements:

- **Do not work from the original studies, that is, be sure to copy them onto your hard disk before doing anything else (possibly 3 to 4 copies of "DSSdisplframes).** In case you make errors, or do something you cannot "Undo," all you have to do is recopy the original study; and
- If you get stuck, or make a mistake that seemingly cannot be undone, just close the study **without saving** anything. That is, when the program asks you if you want to "Save changes . . . ," say **NO**! Then just go back to Plugins, AVI Reader, and open the study again.

If you want to find the frames yourself, open the "DSS1ccdemo" clip and move through it until you find an appropriate **Hold** frame. Go to "IMAGE" on the Menu, click on "Duplicate" and save the frame as **1cchold.** (Save only the one image, not the whole stack, and save it in .tif format.) Leave your saved frame open and close the 1-cc clip. Now open "DSSdemo20cc." Move through the 20-cc bolus swallow until you find the point at which the hyoid is maximally elevated. Go to "IMAGE" on the Menu, click on "Duplicate" and save

the frame as **Hmax**. Continue through the study in this manner, finding and saving images representing the maximum approximation of the hyoid and larynx (**HLmax**), maximum opening of the PES (**PESmax**) and maximum constriction of the pharynx (**PAmax**), respectively. Once you have saved all of the images listed in Table 17–2, (1) close the "DSS20ccdemo" clip; (2) click on "IMAGE" in the menu; (3) go to "Stacks"; and then (4) highlight and click "Convert Images to Stack." Now your saved images will be converted into a small video clip, and you can begin to make the measurements in Table 17–2. As you play through the images, you will see your name for them at the top left of each.

### Calibration

The first step in actually calculating displacements is "calibration." In short, the computer monitor is divided into "pixels," not linear measurement units like inches (in.) or centimeters (cm). We must input to the computer how many pixels equal how many (cm) or (in.), so that meaningful distances can be calculated. Because the image size on the recorded fluoroscopy exam varies depending on the patient's distance from the fluoroscope, the image must be calibrated with each change in distance so that the actual size of structures can be determined. To solve this problem, a radiopaque object, usually a metal ring, is affixed to the midline of the patient's chin (Figure 17–5) at the beginning of a study. The dimensions of the device are known (1.9 cm in diameter, in our case) so that distance and area measurements can be made. If the distance between the patient and the fluoroscope changes,

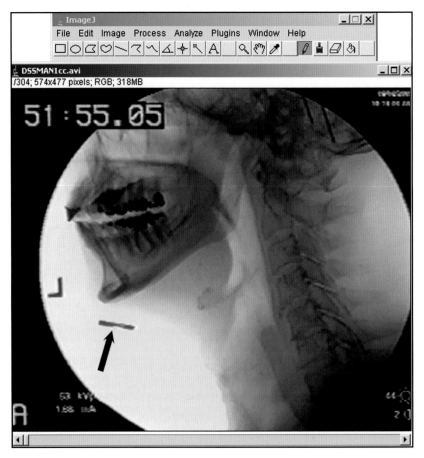

**Figure 17–5.** A radiopaque ring of known diameter is attached to the patient's chin. The diameter of the ring is used to convert "pixels" into centimeters.

or if the position of the patient changes, as in moving from a lateral to an anterior–posterior view, the ring will need to be repositioned, remeasured, and calibration repeated. For each such change, it is necessary to set the calibration referent in "IMAGEJ." Typically, calibration must be done once for the lateral view, and again for the anterior–posterior views.

A.  To establish the calibration referent for this exercise, go to the first image/frame in the "DSSdispl-

frames" clip (the frame is labeled "1cc Hold"). The bolus is held in the mouth and you can clearly see the referent ring on the subject's chin.

B.  Click on the line tool and draw a preliminary line along the referent ring (Figure 17–6). The thickness of the line can be changed by double-clicking on the tool and changing the thickness setting. If you want to change both the color and thickness of this line, you can do so by going under "EDIT" in the menu

**Figure 17–6.** "Line tool" is selected and options for thickness and color determined. Line tool is used to project a line along the diameter of the reference ring (*at arrow*) on patient's chin.

and highlighting "Options." The "Line Width" option is immediately visible. Click on it and enter a number to increase its thickness. To change the line's color, go under "Options" again, click on "Colors" and use the pull-down menu for "Selection." Choose a color ("Selection:" for line).

C. When you have a line of desired color and thickness selected, re-draw the line along the ring under the subject's chin so that it exactly equals its length/diameter (see Figure 17–6).

D. **Keeping the mouse button depressed**, look immediately under the toolbar. To the right of **Length** you will see the number of pixels (units that the monitor screen is divided into) the line you have drawn equals (Figure 17–7). If you

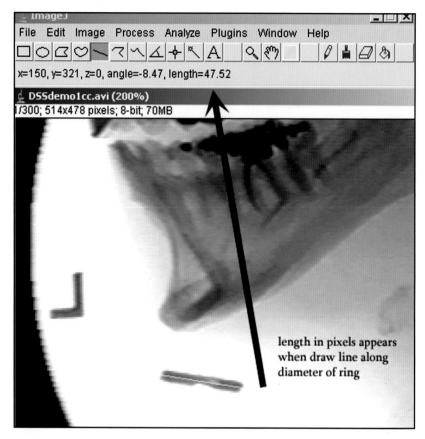

**Figure 17–7.** Using the line tool, extend a line the exact diameter of the ring. Number of pixels is presented as "length = _____" at top.

release the mouse button early, you will have to repeat this step. You may want to project the line two or three times, just to see how uniform your measurements are across trials. (Actual value may vary depending on resolution of monitor).

E. Under ANALYZE, select "Set Scale." (Figure 17–8).

F. In the "Set Scale" dialog box, select "cm" from the choices to the right of "Unit of Length:" (Figure 17–9)

G. Now type in the known length of the ring in centimeters (cm)— in the examples provided, 1.9 cm.

The program will calculate how many pixels equals a cm, as shown in the last line in Figure 17–10, "Scale: _____." This conversion factor will be retained until it is changed.

H. Click OK.

I. If you now draw a line along the ring, keep the mouse button depressed and observe the information box, you will note that the information beside "length" is in cm, hopefully consistent with the calibration you have just completed. Periodically remeasuring

**Figure 17–8.** Under "ANALYZE," "Set Scale" is selected. Click this to open the "Set Scale" box.

the ring in this manner will assure that no changes requiring recalibration have been made.

### Referent Positions

As noted, the 1-cc **Hold** frame is used several times in the calculation of displacements. Hyoid and larynx positions, and pharyngeal area, are first established on the **Hold** frame. Remember that **Hold** is defined as the point where the bolus is held (in as stable manner as possible) in the oral cavity, prior to any posterior movement. Often, the bolus is on the anterior tongue in this position (Figure 17–11). Maximum changes in position of the hyoid, larynx, and pharynx area are compared to the positions and area of these structures, respectively, on the 1-cc **Hold** frame. The **Hold** frame is the frame just prior to bolus movement that results in *B1*, that is, the beginning of pharyngeal transit. The palate is typically resting on the base of the tongue. Check your

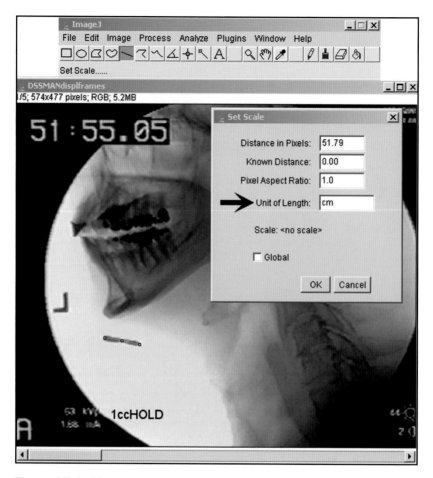

**Figure 17–9.** "Set Scale" box is open and ready for entries. Enter "cm" by Unit of Length.

selected **Hold** frame to see if it meets these criteria.

### Hyoid Displacement

Maximum hyoid displacement is determined by comparing its position on the **Hold:Hyoid** frame to its position on the **20-ccHmax** frame (Figure 17–12). Comparison is made by establishing hyoid position relative to the third and fourth cervical vertebrae in the following manner:

A. Go to **Hold:Hyoid** (Figure 17–13).

B. Highlight/select the angle tool in the Menu.

C. On this image, you will use the angle tool to draw the first limb of a right angle from the anterior corner of C3 to the inferior-anterior border of C4.

D. First find the anterior portion of C3 and click the mouse at that spot. (Just click once, let go and then start moving the mouse down to C4; you will see the angle line

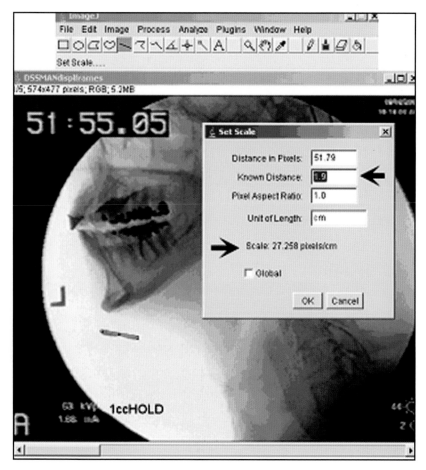

**Figure 17–10.** "Scale: _____." This conversion factor will be retained until it is changed.

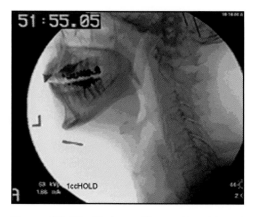

**Figure 17-11.** Note positions of hyoid and larynx, pharyngeal area and bolus at "**Hold**."

appear when you start moving the mouse.)

*E.* Click the mouse button again at the inferior–anterior border of C4.

*F.* From this second point, move the mouse to the right, perpendicular to the first line.

*G.* As you move the mouse, watch the angle size change under the toolbar (Figure 17–14).

*H.* Release the mouse when the angle is 90° (as close as possible to 90°, 89.9°, 90.1°) and the second limb is approximately the length of the first.

**Figure 17-12.** Hyoid position at **Hold** (1 cc) (*left*) and maximally displaced (**Hmax**) during a 20-cc bolus swallow (*right*).

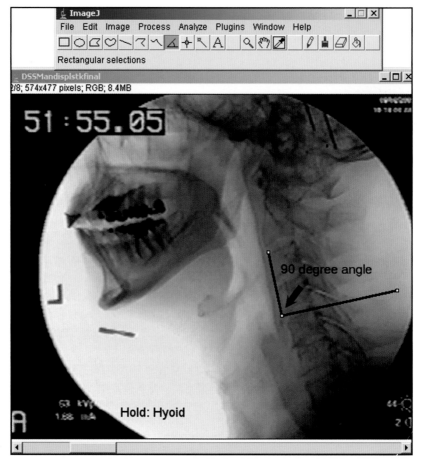

**Figure 17-13. Hold:Hyoid** frame. Using the angle tool, a 90° angle is extended along cervical vertebrae C3–C4.

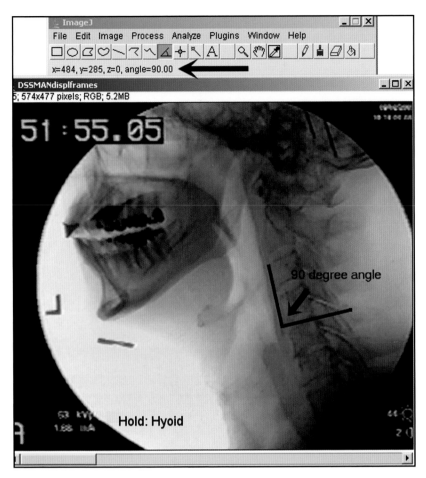

**Figure 17-14.** Note change in angle size under the tool bar as you attempt to create a right angle at C4.

*I.* Click on "Draw" under the EDIT menu. This will fix solid lines on the angle limbs. (If you do not like the angle you have drawn, you can go into EDIT and click on "Undo" and it will disappear).

*J.* When the solid lines are fixed on the vertebrae, outline the anterior-inferior border of the hyoid with the pencil or one of the line tools. (Double-click on the pencil tool to change its thickness.) Now both the vertebrae and hyoid should be outlined (Figure 17–15). Once the hyoid and vertebrae have been outlined, the task is to create a segment that contains both landmarks, and that can be used to compare **Hold:Hyoid** position of the hyoid with the **20-ccHmax** position, that is, its maximally elevated position.

*K.* To obtain the segment, use the Heart tool to encircle a portion of the anterior hyoid, and portions of both limbs of the perpendicular lines on the vertebrae (Figure 17–16).

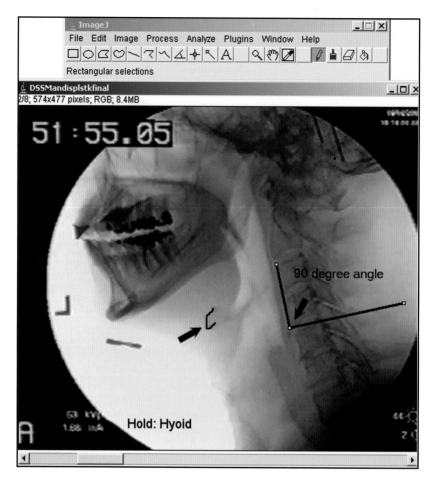

**Figure 17–15.** Vertebrae and hyoid outlined.

**Figure 17–16.** Make selection containing portion of hyoid and portion of 90° angle on vertebrae.

If you do not like your segment, move the mouse cursor anywhere outside of the segment and click. The segment will disappear and you can try it again.

L. When you are satisfied with the selection, go to the Menu and open EDIT. Click on "Copy." The segment can now be pasted on the image representing **20-ccHmax**.

M. Now advance through the clip to the image labeled **20-ccHmax**. Again, draw a 90° angle along C3-C4; then outline the anterior hyoid again using the pencil or line tool.

N. Go to EDIT and click on "Paste." You will see the selection from **Hold:Hyoid** appear on the **20-ccHmax** image (Figure 17–17).

O. Highlight the heart tool. Using the arrow keys on the keyboard, superimpose the right angles outlining the vertebrae by lining up the limbs and vertex of the angles.

P. If the patient has moved and the right angle on the **20-ccHmax** frame does not line up with the right angle on the **Hold:Hyoid** segment, as illustrated in Figure 17–17, the **Hold** frame will need to be rotated.

Q. Estimate how much the **20-ccHmax** frame needs to be rotated in order for the right angles on **Hold:Hyoid** and **20-ccHmax** to line up (on the order of 10° in this case).

R. Go to "EDIT" on the Menu and click on "Undo." Then, being sure the heart tool is still highlighted,

click on the image outside the outline of the pasted segment—this should completely remove the pasted segment.

S. Open "Rotate" under IMAGE on the Menu and click on "Arbitrarily" (Figure 17–18).

T. Enter the amount you want to rotate the **Hold:Hyoid** frame to the right of "Angle" (–90° to 90°). A positive value will rotate the image clockwise; a negative image will rotate the image counterclockwise. In this case, something between 6–10° should be about right (Figure 17–19). Click OK when you have entered the angle value.

U. Just rotate one frame, not the entire stack (Figure 17–20).

V. With the **20-ccHmax** frame rotated to the desired degree, repaste the **Hold:Hyoid** segment on the rotated **20-ccHmax** frame, and align the limbs using the arrow keys on the keyboard (Figure 17–21).

W. Measure the distance between two comparable points on each hyoid using the line tool (Figure 17–22). Our value for Hmaxd was a little over 3 cm. The average measurement error across judges for this measure was 0.18 cm (reliability was 0.95), so if you are within this range, that is good!

### Pharyngeal Constriction

Open the **Hold** image again, this time representing **PAhold**, or the two-dimensional area of the pharynx at **Hold**. Our estimate of pharyngeal constriction is defined as the ratio of **PAmaxd:PAhold**, and is referred to as the **pharyngeal constriction ratio (PCR)** (Figure 17–23). Use the polygon or

**Figure 17–17.** Hyoid is outlined and 90° angle formed again on **20-ccHmax** frame. Segment from **Hold:Hyoid** frame is pasted onto **20-ccHmax** frame. Note if right angles from both frames can be aligned. If not, **20-ccHmax** frame needs to be rotated.

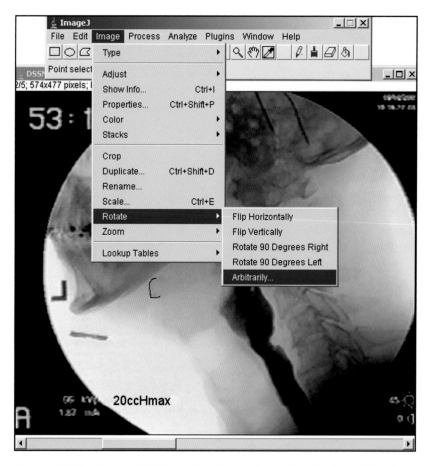

**Figure 17–18.** Go to IMAGE on the Menu, then "Rotate," and "Arbitrarily." When the information box opens, indicate how much you want the image to be rotated (about 10°, in this case).

heart tool to outline the air-filled pharynx (left) in the lateral view (Figure 17–24) as follows:

A. Start on the posterior pharyngeal wall just anterior to the tubercle of the atlas.
B. Trace the posterior pharyngeal wall to the floor of the hypopharynx, and up the posterior arytenoids.
C. Trace over the tops of the arytenoid cartilages and directly anteriorly to the laryngeal surface of the epi-

glottis (do not include laryngeal vestibule).
D. Continue up the laryngeal surface of the epiglottis, over the lip of the epiglottis and down into the curve of the valleculae.
E. Continue along the pharyngeal tongue to a point where the soft palate contacts or is closest to the tongue.
F. Draw a straight line to the soft palate (if necessary), outline the velum and continue up its nasal

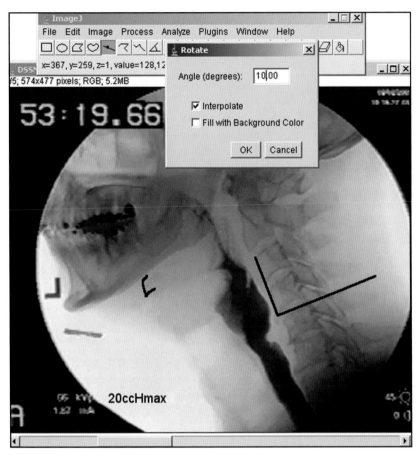

**Figure 17–19.** Enter number of degrees image needs to be rotated (estimate).

surface to the posterior nasal spine. (If the mouse button is released at this point, the tracing will close itself with a straight line.)

G. Under the ANALYZE menu, click on "Measure," then "Show Results" for the calculation. Record the calculation for use as a referent. Our value for **PAhold** in this example was 15.63 cm$^2$.

Now move to the **20-ccPAmax** image, representing the pharynx when maximally constricted during swallow (Figure 17–25). Little air space or residue is observed, so that this value is quite small. In normal swallows it often approximates "0."

A. Using the polygon or heart tool, outline the walls of the pharynx (often marked only by a small patch of contrast) when it is most constricted. **20-ccPAmax** often occurs at about the time the posterior pharyngeal wave is in the hypopharynx.

B. Once the area is outlined (assuming an area greater than "0"), go to

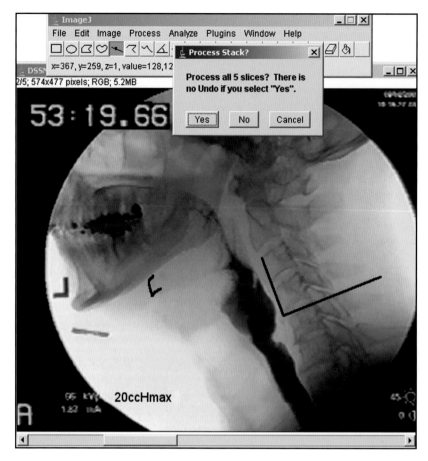

**Figure 17–20.** Only one frame needs to be rotated; click on "No."

"Measure," then "Analyze," then "Measure," and "Show Results." The calculated area is shown. Our calculation was 0.31 cm$^2$.

C. To calculate **PCR**, divide **20ccPAmaxd** by **PAhold**. Using our data, the value is 0.02 cm$^2$, which again, is typical of a normal swallow for age/gender. Average measurement error for **PCR** across five judges was 0.06 cm$^2$.

### PES Opening

PES opening represents the maximum distention of the PES during the swallow. In most cases, it falls between C4 and C6; occasionally, it may be closer to C3.

Open the saved image labeled **20-ccPESmax** (Figure 17–26). Then, using the line tool, measure the distance between the anterior and posterior PES walls at the narrowest point between C3 and C6. In this patient, the location is easy to identify because there is a cricopharyngeal bar present. Note this value. Our calculation was 0.83 cm (average measurement error across 5 judges was 0.09 cm). Even with a PES bar, this opening is within normal limits.

**Figure 17-21. 20-ccHmax** frame is rotated 10°. Segment from **Hold:Hyoid** is repasted and now angle lines are aligned (using arrow keys on keyboard).

**Figure 17-22.** With angles aligned, distance between two comparable points on the hyoid can be calculated using the line tool. Our value for hyoid displacement was slightly over 3 cm.

**Figure 17-23.** Pharyngeal area for **PA Hold** (*left*) and at point of maximum constriction (**PAmax**) (*right*) for a 20-cc bolus.

**Figure 17-24.** Use heart tool to measure area, as illustrated here. Go to "ANALYZE," "Measure" and "Show Results." Area measured will be listed as "_____ cm².''

**Figure 17-25.** Remeasure area at point when pharynx is maximally constricted.

**Figure 17-26.** Line tool is used to measure maximum opening of PES during 20-cc bolus swallow.

### Hyoid to Larynx Approximation

Hyoid to larynx approximation is defined as the difference between these two structures at **Hold**, and at their point of maximum approximation during the swallow (Figure 17–27)

A. Open the **HL:Hold** frame.
B. Using the line tool, measure the distance from the top of the tracheal air column to the hyoid, as shown in Figure 17–28.
C. Open the **20-ccHLmax** frame and repeat this measurement (Figure 17–29).
D. Subtract the difference to determine the approximate degree of change in these two structures during the swallow. Our calculation for this measure was 1.48 cm. Average measurement error across five judges was 0.13 cm for this measure.

### PESa-p

Occasionally, as when patients with cricopharyngeal bars and reduced

**PESmaxd** are identified, it is useful to measure the PES from the anterior–posterior view during the largest bolus swallowed. This measure is illustrated in Figure 17–30. Remember that, with the change in patient position, the ring must be repositioned to be in the same approximate plane as the structures of interest (as on the neck, rather than on the chin). Recalibration, that is, remeasuring the ring and resetting the pixels/cm conversion, is then completed.

## ADDITIONAL PRACTICE EXERCISES

The materials folder for Chapter 17 includes additional swallow studies from both normal subjects and patients. The patient studies represent a variety of pathologies and impairments, which are documented in team reports included in the materials folder. The video clips of these studies are rather large, and are best played using whatever software is available on the

**Figure 17–27.** Position of larynx and hyoid at **Hold** (*left*), and at point of maximum approximation during 20-cc swallow (*right*).

**Figure 17–28.** Using the line tool, draw a line from the inferior portion of the hyoid to the top of the tracheal air column. Note this distance.

reader's computer, that is, Windows Media Player for PC, or DVD Player for Macintosh. They can also be opened in "ImageJ" by going under "File," then "Import" and "Using Quicktime." Additional clips illustrating the use of various strategies to facilitate swallowing are included in the materials folder for Chapter 18. These typically have audio; the others generally do not. The normal studies include clips from six individuals under 65 years of age, and five subjects over 65 years of age. For each normal subject, the 1-cc and 20-cc swallows are included, respectively. These clips can all be opened in IMAGEJ (using AVI Reader under "Plug-ins"). IMAGEJ does not support audio, so there is no sound on these clips. We encourage the reader to make measures from these studies, using the same strategies used on the "DSSDemo" studies. Our values for these subjects are included in the materials folder, as well. The reader can calculate timing and duration measures, first, followed by displacement measures. Alternatively, he can go through the study and note times, save appropriate images, and so on in the same order they occur. The advantage of this sequence is that it permits the viewer to actually play through a recorded study one time, identifying and noting times, and also saving frames that will be required to make displacement measures. The order may differ slightly from study to study; however, a typical order is listed here:

1. **Calibration** Establishes the IMAGEJ-real size relationship, that is, allows conversion of the number of "pix-

**Figure 17–29.** Distance between hyoid and top of tracheal column (inferior boundary of larynx) is calculated.

**Figure 17–30.** Maximum distension of the PES as illustrated in the a-p view.

els" on the computer screen into centimeters so that spatial or displacement measures can be made.

2. **Hold:** Identifies (on a 1-cc bolus) a preswallow frame "referent" to which movement of structures during the swallow can be compared.

3. **Hold: Hyoid** Hyoid position relative to the third and fourth vertebrae is marked in the "**Hold**" frame and saved. This position of the hyoid will be compared to its maximally elevated position.

4. **Hold: PA** The boundaries of the pharynx before swallow are outlined in the "**Hold**" frame and this area is calculated for later comparison to the pharynx maximally constricted.

5. **B1** The time of onset of bolus transit through the pharynx is noted. In our studies, this time represents the "zero" point to which all later events during the swallow are compared.

6. **BV1** The time of bolus arrival at the base of the valleculae is noted.

7. *BV2* The time of the first exit of bolus material from the valleculae.

8. **H1** The time of onset of hyoid displacement for swallow is noted.

9. **H2** The time of hyoid arrival at maximum displacement is noted.

10. **Hmax** Hyoid position maximally elevated (at time H2) relative to the third and fourth cervical vertebrae is marked. A saved segment showing hyoid position on the Hold frame (see #3) is pasted on the H2 image. The difference in position is measured and noted.

11. **Pop** The time of first opening of the lumen at the site PES during swallow is noted.

12. **PES max** The greatest expansion during swallow of the site designated PES is measured.

13. **PA Max** The boundaries of the pharynx when it is maximally constricted are outlined, and this area is calculated and noted.

14. **Pcl** The time of closing of the lumen at the site PES is noted.

15. **Em** The time of epiglottis return to its upright position is noted.

## STUDY QUESTIONS

1. How is "PESmaxd" defined? Where is it measured?

2. What is "PCR?" How is it measured?

3. How is airway closure time defined?

4. Why is a ring of known diameter placed on the patient's chin during the DSS? Does the location of the ring ever need to change? Why?

5. What equipment is required to make timing measurements from a fluoro study?

6. What does "Hold" refer to? How is it used in making displacement measures?

7. When might it be of particular interest to measure PES opening size from the anterior/posterior view?

8. Can you describe how maximum hyoid displacement is measured using IMAGEJ?

9. When are BV1 and BV2 likely to be the same?

10. How is approximation of the larynx to the hyoid measured?

## REFERENCES

Crary, M., Butler, M., & Baldwin, B. (1994). Objective distance measurements from videofluorographic swallow studies using computer interactive analysis: technical note. *Dysphagia, 9*, 116–119.

Dejaeger, E., Pelemans, W., Ponette, E., & Joosten, E. (1997). Mechanisms involved in postdeglutition retention in the elderly. *Dysphagia, 12*, 63–67.

Dengel, G., Robbins, J., & Rosenbek, J. (1991). Image processing in swallowing and speech research. *Dysphagia, 6*, 30–39.

Kay-Pentax, 2 Bridgewater Lane, Lincoln Park, NJ. Swallowing Workstation.

Logemann, J., Kahrilas, P., Begelman, J., Dodds, W., & Pauloski, B. (1989). Interactive computer program for biomechanical analysis of videoradiographic studies of swallowing. *American Journal of Roentgenology, 153*, 277–280.

Perlman, A., VanDaele, D., & Otterbacher, M. (1995). Quantitative assessment of hyoid bone displacement from video images during swallowing. *Journal of Speech and Hearing Research, 38*, 579–585.

# 18

# *The Treatment Plan*

Rebecca Leonard
Katherine Kendall
Susan McKenzie
Susan Goodrich

Patients referred to the dysphagia team are evaluated and then presented at a weekly team meeting. At the team presentation, relevant information from the patient's medical history/chart review, results of current physical examinations or clinical evaluations, findings on bedside or clinical swallow evaluations, and results of videofluoroscopic study are discussed. If related exams have been completed (i.e., esophagram, manometry, endoscopy), these are considered as well. Patients' medical records, pertinent test results, and related information are available for review by team members who were not part of the patient's clinical evaluation. Following the review of each patient, the team determines if there is a problem with the individual's ability to eat safely, efficiently, and/or in a timely manner and identifies specific factors that characterize and account for the dysphagia. The information is assimilated by members of the team, who then summarize and prioritize team recommendations. Typically, the speech pathology members of the team assume responsibility for presenting patients and preparing reports. In this chapter, we will discuss how recommendations are translated into a treatment plan, and review the major categories of therapies that are recommended for individual patients. In addition, record-keeping details that permit the simultaneous generation of a written report and entry of information into a dysphagia data-base will be described.

## PRELIMINARY CONSIDERATIONS

To be most effective, treatment recommendations must take into account *the patient's living situation* and *acuity of care*. For example, one patient may be hospitalized, but nearing release to home or a care facility. Another may be seriously impaired at the time of evaluation, but be expected to recover, perhaps fairly rapidly, to a normal or near-normal level of function. The impact of treatment recommendations on human resources (caregivers and their capabilities), as well as on technical resources (obtaining and preparing particular food types) must be considered. The team makes every effort to provide preliminary recommendations and precautions for safe feeding as soon as sufficient information is available. In some instances, however, *additional diagnostic studies* are required before a treatment plan can be finalized. Such studies may be necessary to establish a medical diagnosis, when this is in question, or to further elaborate or treat a problem that has been identified. *In infants and young children, special studies* are frequently required before interpretations of findings, and treatment recommendations, can be completed. Some of these were discussed at greater length in Chapter 9. Commonly requested studies, however, include neurodevelopmental assessment and communication skills evaluation. In infants, pulmonary workup is often needed to determine the adequacy of respiratory support for swallowing.

Initial team recommendations may also include a referral of the patient to other medical specialists for further evaluation. For example, if there are concerns about esophageal function in swallowing that have not been addressed, or about the possibility of serious gastroesophageal reflux disease, referral to gastroenterology is indicated. Questions about neuromotor integrity or sensation that have not been previously raised warrant referral to neurology. Issues regarding laryngeal function are most often considered

prior to the team evaluation; if not, an otolaryngology referral is generated. Similarly, concerns about dentition or oral hygiene may warrant a dental evaluation. Very often, the team finds it advisable to secure a dietary consult. This recommendation is so often critical, that, in fact, an entire chapter in this manual has been devoted to nutritional evaluation of patients with dysphagia. In our experience, the advantage of having a network of specialists who act as an extended part of the dysphagia team is extremely useful. These specialists are familiar with team functions and objectives, have had experience with patients with similar problems, and are typically willing to see patients as expediently as possible.

## TREATMENT PLAN

Dysphagia team recommendations directly related to the management and treatment of dysphagia fall into several categories. For our purposes, treatments can be classified as behavioral, medical, or surgical. Examples of these treatments, and the indications for prescribing them in individual patients, or particular groups of patients, are discussed next.

### BEHAVIORAL THERAPIES

A therapist specializing in oropharyngeal swallowing disorders, most often a speech-language pathologist, provides behavioral therapy to patients suffering from dysphagia. Physical therapists and occupational therapists may also provide swallowing therapy, and/or other therapies of value. For example, a physical therapist may be consulted when there are concerns about a patient's head/neck or body posture in support of respiration and swallowing, or about appropriate seating during eating. Occupational therapists may become involved in rehabilitation of motor skills required for a particular function related to eating, as in the use of feeding utensils or adaptive devices used for this purpose. In some instances, nursing professionals also participate in swallowing therapy. In hospitals and other care facilities, the combined efforts of the swallowing-disorder therapist and nurses charged with a patient's care may be used to "mass" patient trials with various therapeutic strategies, and to monitor a patient's response to these strategies.

In general, behavioral therapies are recommended when the strength, endurance, and/or mobility of structures involved in swallowing are diminished, and when diagnostic probes have indicated that swallowing may be facilitated, or made safer, by bolus manipulation, postural compensations, facilitative maneuvers, or adaptive devices. Behavioral therapies are also recommended when it is believed that a more appropriate initiation or timing of certain swallowing events may be induced by selective stimulation of particular structures or systems. Summaries of the rationale and objectives for each of these interventions, and examples of each, are presented here.

## Improving Strength/Mobility/ Endurance of Structures

Related to the model of swallowing discussed in earlier chapters, exercise is directed to improving the effectiveness of valves and chambers involved in swallowing (i.e., lip seal, breath holding, pharyngeal constriction). Indications for therapy directed to improving the strength, range of motion, endurance, and agility of the gestures involved include clear evidence of weakness or limited movement of the mandible, lips, tongue, pharynx, larynx, or pharyngoesophageal segment. Specific examples of this type of problem include failure to contain bolus material in the mouth related to an inability to maintain lip closure, or failure to protect the airway related to an inability to elevate the larynx or close laryngeal valves. Such findings are typical of certain patient populations, for example, patients treated with radiation therapy for head and neck cancer, or patients with muscle weakness secondary to neurogenic disease. Poor structural mobility and muscular weakness should be documented by the physical examination and confirmed with diagnostic studies such as the dynamic swallow study (DSS). Specific exercises should be aimed at improving the capabilities of residual swallowing gestures, and/or those with the most compensatory potential.

A number of swallowing exercise programs have shown promise in recent years. One described by Shaker et al. (1997) demonstrated increased pharyngoesophageal (PES) opening in normal elderly adults and in a group of nonoral patients with dysphagia with abnormal PES function (Shaker et al., 2002). The specific exercise involves lying on the back and elevating the head sufficiently to observe the toes without moving the shoulders. Both sustained head elevation and repetitive elevations are used. The authors reported that normal elderly adults who did the exercise three times a day for a period of 6 weeks demonstrated significant increases in PES opening, as well as the anterior excursion of the larynx, as compared to a sham exercise group. The patient group demonstrated similar findings and was also noted to show improvement in self-assessment of function. In our experience, however, not all patients are able to perform the exercise recommended, and Easterling, Grande, Kern, Sears, and Shaker (2005) have reported a fairly high noncompliance in a group of nondysphagic elderly adults. When this type of therapy is indicated, however, we routinely include this exercise in our home protocol for patients who are able to perform it.

Another exercise demonstrating promise is one described by Robbins, Gangnon, Theis, Kays, and Hind (2005). This exercise requires the placement of a pressure sensitive bulb (Iowa Oral Performance Instrument) into the oral cavity between the tongue and palate. The goal is to compress the bulb as completely as possible with the tongue. In the study noted, normal elderly adults completed the resistance training over an 8-week period. Both swallowing pressures and isometric pressures were significantly increased at the end of the exercise period, and the authors recommend the use of lingual resistance exercise in patient populations with lingual weakness and swallowing disability, in particular, in patients whose difficulties are related to age-related conditions. Of particular interest in this study was the finding of increased lingual volume after completion of the training, as documented by magnetic resonance imaging (MRI) before and after therapy. Addition of muscle mass is the goal of many strength training

programs traditionally directed to limb and trunk muscles, but evidence of vascular and tissue changes in swallow structures with exercise is just beginning to emerge. Tongue strengthening exercises have also been used with some success in dysphagic head and neck cancer patients (Lazarus, 2006; Sullivan, Hind, & Roecker, 2001). Another exercise that has been described is referred to as the "Masako" maneuver (Fujiu & Logemann, 1996). The exercise involves swallowing with the tongue held between the teeth; the intent is to strengthen tongue-pharynx contact. To our knowledge, reports on the effectiveness of the strategy in a large number of patients have not been described.

Therapy directed to respiratory muscles should also be considered in treatment planning for patients with dysphagia. Silverman et al. (2006) reported increases in expiratory muscle strength in patients with idiopathic Parkinson's disease following a specific respiratory muscle training program. The authors suggest that such training leads to improved respiratory driving forces necessary not only for cough and speech, but also for swallowing. In patients with tracheostomy, for example, it has been demonstrated that occlusion of the tracheostomy tube results in improved swallow timing, as opposed to swallows with the tube unoccluded (Gross, Mahlmann, & Grayhack, 2003). The inference is that the increased subglottal pressures associated with occlusion of the tube facilitate swallow. Sapienza and Wheeler (2006) note that expiratory muscle strength training potentially benefits both airway protection and swallow-related behaviors such as hyoid and laryngeal elevation. Electromyography has revealed increased activation of anterior suprahyoid muscles during expiratory muscle strengthening training (Wheeler, Chiara, & Sapienza, 2007). Further study is needed to evaluate the effect of expiratory muscle strength training in other muscle groups and the subsequent impact of the training on the coordination and extent of swallowing gestures.

Of additional interest is evidence that exercise directed to one function or system of the upper aerodigestive tract may produce cross-system benefits. For example, patients with Parkinson's disease and dysphagia underwent fluoroscopic studies of swallowing before and after undergoing a program of Lee Silverman Voice Therapy (LSVT/LOUD) (El Sharkawai et al., 2002). Goals of the therapy were to improve vocal loudness, in part by retraining patients' perceptions of their own loudness levels. Although no specific efforts were directed to swallowing, the authors reported a 51% reduction in the number of oropharyngeal swallow abnormalities observed posttreatment, including reductions in oral and pharyngeal transit times, improved ability to form a bolus, and reduced pharyngeal residue postswallow.

These preliminary studies demonstrate the potential of exercise in treating dysphagia, and provide objective evidence substantiating tools used by dysphagia (as well as speech and voice) clinicians for many years. In addition, recent evidence from studies in animals (primarily) and in stroke patients suggest that exercise therapies lead to changes in brain function or cortical reorganization, as well as to changes in blood flow and muscle volume (Barbay et al., 2006; Gobbo & O'Mara, 2005; Kleim, Jones, & Schallert, 2003; Nudo, 2003, 2005, 2007; Nudo & Friel, 1999). These intriguing findings demand additional inquiry, as do questions regarding which therapies may be indicated for which patients, and how best to deliver these therapies. For example:

- Should an exercise simulate the dynamics of the impaired function as closely as possible, that is, be task specific, or is more general, nonspecific, training directed to strengthening involved structures equally useful? Current thinking widely supports the use of the former, that is, exercise that simulates the impaired function as closely as possible (Cerny & Burton, 2001). But a case might be made that any exercise that strengthens pertinent muscle groups is likely to produce some benefits. Sapienza and Wheeler (2006) note, for example, that if a patient is aspirating, effortful swallow training may not be indicated. Rather, a nonswallowing exercise that is safe, and that promotes improved strength, coordination, or endurance of muscles involved in swallowing, is a useful substitute.

- Related to the first question, what is the role of dynamic versus static muscle training, or isometric (muscle length stays the same) versus isotonic (muscle tension is constant)? Again, dynamic exercises are more likely to simulate target functions involved in swallowing.

Stathopoulos and Duchan (2006) suggest, however, that static exercises designed to improve neuromuscular support for the function may be a useful or necessary prelude to dynamic training. And both the Robbins et al. (2005) and Shaker et al. (2002) studies incorporated static training exercises that improved particular aspects of function, tongue pressures, and PES opening, respectively, that are critical to effective swallow.

- What are the best delivery methods for exercise programs? That is, how many repetitions of the exercise, how many times per day, over how many weeks, constitutes the best approach, and should this protocol be tailored with respect to patient group? In general, available evidence supports the use of multiple repetitions of sets of exercises, several times a day, over a period of several weeks. However, precise combinations likely to be more beneficial than others, and under what circumstances, have not been elaborated. Similarly, little information is available regarding the permanence of exercise effects, or the necessary requirements for maintaining any beneficial gains of exercise.

- Finally, what is "fatigue," what role should it play in designing training programs, and is it more or less important in certain types of patients? Are there some types of patients, in fact, for whom exercise is contraindicated? Interestingly, exercises have been shown to be effective even in some populations with degenerative diseases, such as spinal muscle atrophy and Duchenne's muscular dystrophy (Koessler et al., 2001). But exercise that exacerbates fatigue may not be advisable in particular patients. Investigators are beginning to explore these and related questions, and it is likely that significant gains in our understanding of exercise physiology and its applications in dysphagia therapy will be forthcoming in the next few years (see Stathopoulos & Duchan, 2006 for an excellent review).

Obviously, no behavioral therapeusis is appropriate until disease processes resulting in neural, muscular, or connective tissue changes have been ruled out or identified and managed. The etiology of the impairment dictates the principles and goals of therapy. Because etiologies of specific impairments vary widely between and even within patient groups, the dysphagia therapist will need to carefully question the referring physician or dentist for information regarding the basis for the impairment, and the potential for improvement. These specialists should also caution against some exercises, if necessary. In burn patients, for example, therapeutic approaches must consider scar tissue or regenerating superficial tissues, which are quite fragile. In cancer patients, bony structures may have been removed or weakened, muscle tissue may have been removed or altered by radiation, and muscular attachments may be very different from normal. Exercises undertaken without regard to these possibilities may result, for example, in breaking a weakened bone. Understanding the limitations and alterations unique to a particular patient is critical to designing and implementing appropriate therapy. If the dysphagia therapist is to provide optimally safe and effective therapy, familiarity with principles of exercise therapy will also be of value, even required. In some instances, multiple behavioral therapies, that is, strengthening exercises and movement therapy, or behavioral therapy combined and coordinated with surgical or prosthetic treatments, can interact to facilitate the success of all therapies. Again, it will be incumbent on the dysphagia therapist to recognize the need for, understand the advantages of, and work within the framework of multiple treatment modalities when appropriate.

As noted previously, work to improve the strength, mobility, endurance, and agility of the oral, pharyngeal, and laryngeal structures cannot be done without a stable platform (head/neck and upper body postural stability) from or against which the head, jaw, lips, tongue, palate, and larynx can move. If neck or torso stability is questionable or unsupportive, consultation with occupational or physical therapists is indicated. Collaborative efforts will help to develop a strengthening program and/or compensatory postural support strategies that will allow work on mandibular, labial, lingual, palatal, and laryngeal gestures.

### Performance Feedback Tools

If sensory mechanisms have been affected, alternative or improved sources of feedback will need to be identified or established if patients are to receive the fullest benefit of exercise therapies for deglutition. A number of devices that provide feedback regarding various physiologic events may help serve this purpose. As discussed in Chapter 11, visual feedback provided by a flexible fiberoptic nasopharyngoscope attached to a video camera (alternatively, a scope with a camera in its tip) and monitor can provide excellent information to patient and clinician regarding a number of physiologic events or maneuvers which are otherwise difficult to observe (i.e., pharyngeal constriction, laryngeal elevation, and vocal-fold adduction).

Other commercially available systems provide immediate visual feedback regarding muscle function. Computer-assisted EMG biofeedback systems with surface electrodes present visual evidence of the presence and amplitude of the electrical activity of muscle units close to the electrode. As an objective indication of muscle effort in the area of the electrode, such information may be a very useful clinical tool. There are some limitations to use of EMG in the head and neck, however. For example, surface electrodes cannot be targeted at a particular muscle. Wire or needle electrodes must be used if this is desired. In addition, an increase of effort in a muscle, or group of muscles, does not signal a successful movement of a structure(s) directed to swallow. Accomplishment of the goal gesture(s) must be assessed by some other means. This is of particular concern when the gesture in question, for example, PES opening, cannot be easily visualized by the patient or clinician.

Another commercially available feedback device is the Iowa Oral Performance Instrument (IOPI) (Blaise Medical, Inc., Hendersonville, TN). The system, used by Robbins et al. (2005)

in the study cited earlier, consists of a pressure transducer connected to a battery-operated display unit. The IOPI measures pressure produced by squeezing a small bulb placed on the tongue (a small bulb for hand-squeezing strength is included) and can be used to develop strength or endurance of squeezing. Normative data are presented in the manual that accompanies the device. When the IOPI intra-oral bulb is used to develop tongue strength or endurance, it may be helpful to isolate effort to the tongue by supporting or stabilizing the mandible. The IOPI strengthens lingual muscle groups that accomplish elevation against the palate in a gently rounded shape. Thus, it may strengthen the lingual configuration required to hold the bolus on the mid tongue during oral preparation for swallow. The intraoral bulbs are small and require a normal or near-normal lingual bulk, however, limiting its use in glossectomy patients. A dental laboratory may be able to custom make bulbs for patients postoral cancer or with orofacial anomalies whose tongues do not fill the oral cavity. The bulb can be moved around in the mouth and may be used to strengthen specific tongue sites as long as the bulb and the tongue can be seen (to ensure the exercise is being done correctly). Although there are no norms for this kind of task, the patient's performance on successive trials can be compared. Unfortunately, the bulb can be tolerated only in the oral cavity and, in some patients, not at all sites in the oral cavity.

The Therabite (Therabite Corporation, 3415 West Chester Pike, Suite 302, Newtown Square, PA 19073; 1993) is an excellent tool for feedback regarding range of mandibular opening. It can be used to develop masseter strength in different positions, but gives no feedback regarding strength or effort. Our own experience with Therabite in increasing mandibular opening in patients postoral cancer has been very positive.

### External Stimulation

In addition to specific exercise regimens, there are a number of externally implemented techniques to facilitate stretching of muscles, connective tissue, and scars, including the application of temperature, massage, and ultrasound. Recently, transcutaneous electrical stimulation has been used to treat a wide variety of dysphagic impairments. This stimulation can take different forms, for example, be activated continuously (Freed, Freed, Chatburn, & Christian, 2001) or only during swallow attempts (Leelamanit, Limsakul, & Geater, 2002), and vary according to specific frequency-intensity-duration patterns. Electrodes used may be applied to the skin or inserted directly into muscles. One intent of stimulation has been to enhance contraction of muscles involved in swallowing, in particular, by increasing the number of motor action potentials supplied to the muscle or muscles involved. To date, there has been little investigation of these techniques, and those that are available are somewhat contradictory (Blumenfeld, Hahn, Lepage, Leonard, & Belafsky, 2006; Freed, Freed, Chatburn, & Christian, 2001; Humbert et al., 2006; Ludlow, Humbert, Saxon, Poletto, Sonies, & Crujido, 2007).

In an example of the kind of study likely to shed light on the potential benefits of electrical stimulation, Ludlow et al. (2000) reported the use of electrodes implanted in the thyroarytenoid muscle in dogs. Intermittent stimulation was provided to the muscle over periods of up to 8 months, and appeared to produce changes in muscle function consistent with improved airway protection. Burnett, Mann, Cornell, and Ludlow (2003) described the use of electrical stimulation applied via hooked-wire electrodes into the geniohyoid, mylohyoid, and thyrohyoid muscles of nondysphagic subjects. Interestingly, bilateral stimulation of the mylohyoid and/or thyrohyoid with subjects at rest produced approximately half of the laryngeal elevation typically observed during a swallow. More recently, Burnett, Mann, Stocklosa, and Ludlow (2005) reported an electrical stimulation device that can be self-triggered. That is, when a subject initiates a swallow, defined by the authors as the onset of thyrohyoid activity leading to a swallow, a button can be pushed that delivers electrical stimulation to the suprahyoid muscles. To date, this technique has not been shown to alter muscle activation patterns, but it does represent an interesting concept that deserves further inquiry.

No exercises, especially stretches, should cause pain. Patients, especially aggressive patients, should be counseled regarding potential injury when doing stretching exercises. Frequency and intensity of exercise sessions will depend on patient tolerance, and also on the specific goals of treatment. That is, strength exercises may be more taxing than exercises designed to improve endurance, leading to more rapid patient fatigue and, of necessity, briefer sessions. Therapy strategies and exercises that are directed to mobility/strength/endurance impairments are summarized in Table 18–1.

## BOLUS MANIPULATION

Therapeutic probing during bedside/clinical or videofluoroscopic evaluations may suggest that a patient can manage particular types or amounts of food materials safely and efficiently, but have difficulty with others. Therapeutic strategies directed at elaborating the patient's potential for improved swallowing by manipulating bolus materials, and at establishing the patient's facility with these selected materials, are described here. Strategies are tailored to an individual patient, as there are few if any data establishing the value of particular strategies with particular patient groups.

Bolus characteristics can be manipulated to compensate for timing/coordination or constriction/patency impairments of the oral and/or pharyngeal chamber or of the lingual-palatal, velopharyngeal, laryngeal, or PES valve. Characteristics of the bolus that lend themselves to manipulation include: (1) *Properties that maximize sensory feedback about the bolus and its position*, and (2) *Properties that affect bolus deformability and/or bolus flow in response to gravity or compression*. For simplicity, the properties are presented here somewhat separately, but, in fact, bolus properties combine, heightening some properties and minimizing others.

## Properties that Maximize Sensory Feedback About the Bolus and Its Position

Properties that maximize sensory feedback include temperature, taste, size, and texture. Swallow initiation has been reported to be facilitated with cold instrument stimulation of the faucial pillars (Lazzara, Lazarus, & Logemann, 1986).

**Table 18–1.** Exercises for Improving Movement, Strength and Endurance of Swallowing Gestures

| Impairment may include | Indications | Goal | Tasks |
|---|---|---|---|
| Limited control, agility, or ROM of neck rotation, extension and flexion | Neck mobility is important in development of compensatory strategies to facilitate oral transit, airway protection, or PES opening. | Range, control, agility adequate for needed task | Obtain consult from Physical Therapy. Depending on need, tasks may focus on development of agility of movement as well as control and ROM. |
| Trismus | Before trismus can be addressed therapeutically, etiology must be identified by a physician or dentist. When mandibular opening is inadequate for eating or oral hygiene, and a disease process has been ruled out or treated, therapy may be appropriate. | Adequate opening for feeding route (spoon, fork, cup or biting), for denture or palatal prosthesis placement and for oral hygiene. | Maintain mandible-maxilla alignment while increasing passive and active range of mandible opening. Can be done with a variety of props, from simple to sophisticated. For example, stacked tongue blades placed between the molars can facilitate maintenance of maximal opening. During stretch, the patient can relax, bite gently, then attempt further opening and insert another tongue blade in the stack (while it is in place). Movements should be made slowly. Maximum stretch should be maintained ≥15 seconds. The Therabite is a more sophisticated device, especially useful for marked trismus or when alignment of mandible and maxilla is difficult to maintain. The cost, of course, is greater. |
| Weakness or absence of mandibular support/control | Absence of or asymmetry in achievement or maintenance of mandible-maxilla approximation, or inadequate mandibular stability to support lingual work against the palate for bolus control, mastication or speech. | Symmetric mandible-maxilla approximation supportive of potentials for posture, oral nutrition/hydration and speech | Establish optimal alignment passively or actively, and present exercises graded for endurance. Slowly diminish support (if that is necessary) and increase time position is sustained. Increase strength and control using graded resistance and biting/munching tasks to strengthen muscles of mandibular closure and opening. Mandibular lateral and A/P ROM may be addressed depending on potential. |

| Impairment may include | Indications | Goal | Tasks |
|---|---|---|---|
| Weakness or absence of buccal tone | Inability to prevent food from falling into the buccal sulci in a patient with potential for oral preparation and oral transit. | Increased buccal tone. | Isometric tightening of the buccal area or squeezing of soft objects between the cheek and teeth/gums or from the buccal sulcus to the molar surface. Both oral opening and object size can be graded during squeezing tasks. Maintain mandible alignment throughout. |
| Diminished labial opening | Inadequate opening for eating, speech or oral hygiene (also diminishes mandible opening.) | Adequate labial opening size for eating. Adequate change of shape for speech. | Tasks depend on etiology (scarring, resection of muscle, muscle weakness) and may include passive stretching and exercises to increase range and strength of lateral commissure movement. Maintain mandible alignment throughout. |
| Partial or complete absence or weakness of labial strength and/or ability to close | Inability to maintain labial closure in a variety of mandibular positions, including rest, with oral incontinence for saliva, liquid, food or air during labial pressure consonants. | Oral continence for saliva management, eating/drinking and speech. | Establish closure passively or actively, and present exercises graded for maintenance then endurance: Slowly diminish support (if that is necessary) and increase time position is sustained. Increase strength at selected sites using squeezing and holding tasks with and without resistance. Develop agility for desired range using tasks graded for speed and accuracy. Maintain mandible alignment throughout. |
| Unilateral partial or complete lingual weakness or missing lateral lingual tissue | Diminished or absent ability to form, hold or manipulate the bolus with bolus loss into the lingual sulcus of the weak side. Consonant and mild vowel distortions. | Posterior bolus retention-release control for airway protection. Bolus and airflow control (minimize lateral "leaks") and lingual shaping range and agility | Maximize lingual symmetry at rest and in a variety of nonspeech and speech gestures. Maximize posterior lingual-palatal valve strength and agility and lingual lateralization and lateral lingual elevation (for cupping)on the weak side with passive, then active ROM tasks, resistance to lateral and elevation gestures. Squeezing and lingual manipulation tasks may be appropriate. Palatal prosthesis may facilitate therapy. |

*(continues)*

**Table 18–1.** (continued)

| Impairment may include | Indications | Goal | Tasks |
|---|---|---|---|
| Bilateral anterior lingual weakness or missing anterior lingual tissue | Diminished or absent ability to form, hold or manipulate the bolus with bolus loss into the anterior lingual sulcus. Anterior consonant and vowel distortions. | Bolus and airflow control and lingual shaping range and agility. | Establish target lingual non-speech and speech positions passively or actively, and present exercises graded for maintenance then endurance: Slowly diminish support (if that is necessary) and increase time position is sustained. Increase strength at selected sites using squeezing and holding tasks with and without resistance. Develop agility for desired range using tasks graded for speed and accuracy. Maintain mandible alignment throughout. Palatal prosthesis may facilitate therapy. |
| Bilateral posterior lingual weakness or missing posterior lingual tissue | Diminished or absent ability to form, hold or manipulate the bolus with bolus loss into the oropharynx. Posterior consonant and vowel distortions. | Strength and agility of bolus retention-release and transfer to the pharynx. Improved palatal contact for speech sound production. | Establish target lingual-palatal contact passively or actively, and present exercises graded for maintenance and endurance: Slowly diminish support (if that is necessary) and increase time position is sustained. If squeezing tasks are used, object must be anchored. Palatal prosthesis may facilitate therapy. |
| Bilateral lingual weakness | Diminished or absent ability to form, hold, transfer or manipulate the bolus with bolus loss into the oropharynx, and the lingual sulci | Oral transit with minimum loss into the sulci and maximum coordination with initiation of swallow gestures. | Address sectionally as above. |

| Impairment may include | Indications | Goal | Tasks |
|---|---|---|---|
| Absent tongue | Inability to form a bolus. Inability to transfer a bolus without compensatory strategies. Severely distorted speech sounds | Development of compensatory mandibular, labial, and head/neck movement strategies. | Develop ROM and agility of movements needed for compensations that take advantage of gravity. Consider mandibular or maxillary shaping prosthesis. |
| Unilateral or complete weakness or missing tissue of the palate | Velopharyngeal incompetence for speech and oral and/or oropharyngeal transit. Diminished ability to transfer the bolus through the posterior oral cavity or oropharynx. | Adequate velopharyngeal closure if tissue is adequate. Effective obturation if tissue is inadequate. | Feedback for velopharyngeal closure can be elusive. There is some commercially available, inexpensive equipment, e.g. SeeScape. Sustained blowing against resistance may strengthen closure, as long as tongue facilitation is ruled out. Endoscopic feedback may be helpful for some patients. Exercises may be helpful even with obturation. Obturation may actually recruit improved compensatory participation in closure from the lateral and posterior pharyngeal walls. |
| Unilateral, bilateral, or regional failure of pharyngeal constriction | Poor pharyngeal transit in the affected area increasing risk of aspiration of pharyngeal residue after the swallow. | Improved bolus compression | Maximize lingual retraction range and strength, laryngeal elevation and supraglottic closure, and pharyngeal constrictor participation. Provide resistance by holding the tongue forward manually and retract the tongue against this resistance. Maximize extent of externally visible signs of laryngeal elevation. Practice effortful swallow and "hawking" of secretions for expectoration. |

*(continues)*

**Table 18–1.** *(continued)*

| Impairment may include | Indications | Goal | Tasks |
|---|---|---|---|
| Incomplete glottic closure | Increased risk of aspiration during maximum closure for swallow. Inadequate vocal quality and loudness | Improved glottic closure | Attempt to establish conditions resulting in improved vocal fold approximation while avoiding using pitch, positional, compression, and respiratory support strategies. Increase endurance with tasks graded for time, pitch, onset, loudness, position and respiratory support. |
| Incomplete supraglottic closure | Increased risk of supraglottic penetration prior to closure for swallow and aspiration of this residue when respiration is resumed. May contribute to incomplete hypopharyngeal clearing. | Improved supraglottic closure | Habituate early and effortful laryngeal closure and elevation for swallow. Maximize extent and sustained time of externally visible signs of laryngeal elevation. |
| Inadequate PES opening for swallow | Incomplete pharyngeal transit with increased risk of aspiration of pharyngeal residue after the swallow | Maximum PES opening. | Once the muscles of the PES have relaxed, PES opening is influenced by elevation of the laryngeal/hyoid complex and by intrabolus pressures. Therapeutic approaches to optimizing PES opening thus include maximizing extent and timing of hyoid/laryngeal elevation and the effects of pharyngeal compression of the bolus. |

There is some evidence that a cold bolus may stimulate swallow initiation for some populations (Kagel & Leopold, 1992); and some patients report that thermal characteristics of the bolus affect their dysphagia (Martin, 1994). On the other hand, Bisch, Logemann, Rademaker, Kahrilas, and Lazarus (1994), investigating post-CVA and neurologically impaired patients, did not find significant effects on transit times or durations with a chilled bolus. Temperature is known to affect esophageal function (Meyer & Castell, 1983). We routinely include chilled bolus presentation in evaluation of patients with suspected neural or neuromuscular etiologies.

Common potentially irritating taste characteristics of the bolus may facilitate swallow initiation in some populations (Logemann, Pauloski, Colangelo, Lazarus, Fujiu, & Kahrilas, et al., 1995; Palmer, McCulloch, Jaffe, Neel, 2005), Palmer et al., (2005), for example, reported that a sour bolus produced stronger muscle contractions in mylohyoid, geniohyoid, and anterior belly of the digastricus muscles than a water bolus in normal individuals. Pelletier and Lawless (2003) noted that citrus acid and citric acid-sucrose boluses produced more dry swallows and decreased both aspiration and penetration in neurogenic patients as compared to a water bolus, possibly because of increased gustatory and trigeminal stimulation of the brainstem. However, we have been reluctant to apply this strategy in most patient populations, fearing the potentially noxious effects of bolus materials used should they penetrate the laryngeal, tracheal, and nasal airways and the lungs. Irritating tastes may be safer and still useful when introduced in tiny, dilute amounts to the lips or anterior oral cavity where they will stimulate saliva that must be swallowed. Size, viscosity, and texture of the bolus may add to tactile feedback. For patients who are able, mastication may lead more easily to swallow. When patients are not able to masticate, simply manipulating the bolus briefly may facilitate swallow initiation. Carbonation increases the "texture" of liquids and is known to improve esophageal clearing (Wong & Johnson, 1983). Recently, carbonation has also been reported to shorten pharyngeal transit times and reduce both aspiration and amount of residue (Bulow, Olson, & Esberg, 2003). Alternating thermal, taste, and texture characteristics during therapeutic feeding or a meal may keep the interest of the swallower, supporting vigilance regarding swallow.

Finally, manipulation of bolus placement to maximize available sensory capabilities is a valuable compensatory maneuver for patients with sensory impairment. If a sensory deficit is unilateral, for example, bolus material on the more intact side may facilitate swallow.

## Properties that Affect Bolus Deformability and Flow in Response to Gravity or Compression

*Bolus viscosity* is a powerful tool and is probably the most popular compensatory strategy. Viscosity is referred to in common categories: liquid, thick liquid, puree, soft solid, and so on. However, viscosity characteristics exist as a continuum from water (least) to (for example) hard candy (most) so that a wide range of viscosities exists within each category (please see Chapter 10). Even when a patient with dysphagia is able to eat orally, his or her viscosity tolerance range is likely to be compressed, as compared to normal.

Thin liquids are easily deformed and move very readily in response to gravity and compression. Adequate transit relies less on strength of constriction, patency of the chambers, and mucosal/salivary facilitation, and more on agility and coordination to control the bolus, time its transit through the pharynx and protect the airway. Thin liquids, being almost completely deformable, will pass most easily through narrow sites in transit (e.g., a stricture, an incompletely opened PES, or an incompletely closed airway).

As viscosity of the bolus increases, it moves more slowly in response to gravity or compression. A more viscous bolus, thus, requires less agility and control and is more forgiving when timing of swallow/coordination of transit with gestures is impaired. However, with increases in viscosity, adequate transit becomes more reliant on strength of constriction and mucosal/salivary facilitation. As the bolus becomes less deformable, it is less likely to pass through narrow sites in transit, and may lodge above them instead. Thus, a liquid may be aspirated, but a less deformable bolus may obstruct the airway. The most viscous consistencies require adequate mastication and salivary mixing prior to initiating oral or pharyngeal transit.

Patients with dysphagia, as mentioned, are unlikely to tolerate a full range of bolus viscosities, but may be able to eat orally by compressing the range (see Chapter 10 for examples.).

When viscosity is being considered in treatment planning, it is important to keep these principles in mind:

*Bolus size* affects bolus flow in response to gravity or compression. Large liquid bolus sizes may be compensatory for incomplete oral or pharyngeal constriction and decrease work per meal, but may be risky if laryngeal function is compromised. Small bolus sizes increase swallows/work per meal, but are less reliant on competent laryngeal function to protect the airway.

*Placement of the bolus* at a particular site on the tongue or in the oropharynx can take advantage of the swallower's anatomic and motoric strengths while avoiding his weaknesses.

## POSTURAL COMPENSATIONS

Postural manipulation is indicated when it appears that a patient can either redirect bolus material in a manner that improves swallowing efficiency (i.e., amount of bolus attempted that actually makes it to the esophagus), improves protection of the airway, or both. Changes in head/neck and upper body position, first described by Logemann (1983), can have a powerful effect on bolus flow through the oral and pharyngeal chambers. Tilting the upper body or the head changes the impact of gravity on the bolus and, in some cases on poorly supported anatomy. In addition, capital flexion, extension, or rotation change the size and shape of the pharyngeal chamber and may impact PES opening. Positional changes do not necessarily have to be dramatic to be effective. In our practice, positions are frequently combined to facilitate safe oral and pharyngeal transit.

## Position Strategies that Exploit Gravity

### Tilting the Upper Body

Effective use of upper body tilting requires that the cervical spine remain in neutral relation to the thoracic spine and the shoulders. If neutral position is not maintained, the effects of upper body tilting may be lost. If the upper body is tilted laterally or posteriorly, bolus flow will be biased to the "downhill" side, diverting it (to a point) away from the airway. Upper body tilting is useful when bolus transit and the sequence of pharyngeal swallow gestures are discoordinated, when pharyngeal constriction is incomplete, or pharyngeal transit is prolonged. The degree of "tilt" will impact (depending on bolus viscosity) bolus transit time and the size of bolus tolerated without overflow into the airway. When postural support of the anterior pharyngeal wall structures (the tongue and hyoid/laryngeal complex) is poor, as is the case in some anatomic, neurologic, or neuromuscular conditions, the pharyngeal airway may be improved when the upper body is tilted anteriorly.

### Tilting the Head

If the head is tilted laterally, bolus flow through the oral chamber will be biased to the downhill side. If only the head is tilted, the site of bolus entry to the pharynx is affected (it would enter on the "downhill" side), but not the course the bolus takes through the pharynx. Lateral head tilting may be useful when lingual movement, sensation, or anatomy is unilaterally impaired. Tilting the head anteriorly (*capital flexion*) will keep the bolus in the anterior oral cavity unless it is actively transferred by compression. Thus, neck flexion requires purposeful initiation of pharyngeal transit/bolus entry to the pharynx, and may be useful when linguapalatal valving is impaired. Capital flexion also minimizes the likelihood that oral residue will fall into the pharynx after the swallow. On the other hand, tilting the head posteriorly (*capital extension*) facilitates oral transit of consistencies that will flow with gravity. Safe use requires adequate laryngeal airway protection. Because extension can *at times* be an obstacle to pharyngeal transit, it is usually used in sequence with flexion (extend-flex). An example of a patient with partial tongue resection using the extension strategy to bypass the oral cavity is included in the materials folder for Chapter 18 (Pt. Strategy 1 video clip). A variation of position strategies is illustrated in Strategy 5a and 5b in the materials folder. Strategy 5a illustrates an infant having difficulty extracting bolus material through a nipple; in Strategy 5b, the feeder provides jaw support, which helps stabilize the oral cavity and facilitates the baby's management of the nipple.

### Positions that Impact Pharyngeal Chamber Shape and Function

*Capital flexion, extension, and rotation* change the shape of the pharyngeal chamber, thus impacting bolus flow. *Capital flexion* alters the oropharyngeal space such that airway protection is facilitated for some patients (Logemann, 1983). An example of a patient with supracricoid laryngectomy and only the arytenoid-epiglottis valve available for airway protection is seen using this strategy in the Strategy 4 video clip (materials folder for Chapter 18). In our experience, *capital extension* narrows the pharynx, closes the valleculae, and impacts mobility of the hyoid/larynx complex. Some patients with poor oral capabilities but good ability to protect the airway may benefit from this posture. *Capital rotation* diverts the bolus toward the opposite side and can be very useful when pharyngeal constriction is incomplete, sometimes even when the impairment appears symmetric, but certainly when constriction and PES opening are asymmetric (Logemann, Kahrilas, Kobara, & Vakil, 1989). Because it diverts the bolus to one side of the pharynx or the other (around the epiglottis in some patients), capital rotation may also be useful for patients with incomplete vallecular clearing, especially for a more viscous bolus. In our experience, when capital rotation is used to compensate for asymmetric pharyngeal wall function, the direction of most facilitative rotation is not completely predictable. In other words, in some patients, pharyngeal transit is facilitated by rotation away from the affected side.

## FACILITATIVE MANEUVERS

This category of therapeutic strategy refers to physiologic postures or gestures that have been demonstrated to improve swallowing efficiency or safety, and that a patient can learn to use for these purposes. Such maneuvers differ from strategies discussed earlier in this chapter. Other categories of compensatory strategies (bolus manipulation, positional changes) can to some extent be imposed on the swallower by a feeder. Facilitative maneuvers require sophisticated and active participation by the swallower, good muscular kinesthetic and proprioceptive sense, movement control, and ability to understand, learn, and apply the strategy during the swallow. For some patients, considerable time and effort will be required to develop the strategies to the point of habituation. Thus, facilitative maneuvers are appropriate when less labor-intensive maneuvers fail. Some maneuvers are very familiar. Often patients who perceive their dysphagia are seen to apply these strategies spontaneously: generally increased effort (during a single swallow or by repeating swallows) and expectoration of pharyngeal residue. Other maneuvers are likely to be unfamiliar and more difficult to learn. These involve altering the extent and/or timing of laryngeal behaviors for swallow, with the goals of providing improved laryngeal closure for airway protection and/or improved PES opening for pharyngeal clearing.

Maneuvers that attempt to recruit increased effort are probably the simplest to learn and habituate. For these maneuvers, the patient is instructed to "swallow as hard as you can, squeezing all your swallow muscles harder" or "after you swallow, swallow once (or twice or more)." At least one study has reported increased duration of tongue base contact and increased pharyngeal pressures with *effortful swallow* (Lazarus, Logemann, Song, Rademaker, & Kahrilas, 2002). Other authors reported no change in hypopharyngeal intrabolus pressure with increased effort, however (Bulow, Olson, & Ekberg, 2003). Hiss and Huckabee (2005), using manometry, reported a later onset of swallow but increased pharyngeal pressures on effortful swallows. These authors suggest, thus, that effortful swallow may be more appropriate for patients with weak pharyngeal constriction than those with prolonged pharyngeal transit times. Maneuvers with the goal of providing improved airway protection include the frequently described *supraglottic* and *super supraglottic* maneuvers. These maneuvers seek to develop closure of the airway prior to bolus entry into the hypopharynx and to maintain closure throughout hypopharyngeal transit. These strategies are appropriately offered to patients whose airway closure timing is delayed relative to bolus position in the pharynx for neurologic (i.e., CVA) or anatomic (i.e., supraglottic laryngectomy) reasons and to patients whose *supraglottic* and *glottic* closure is incomplete. On lateral videofluoroscopy, delayed glottic closure is identified by aspiration prior to the swallow, as actual glottic closure cannot be seen in this view. Observation requires an anterior–posterior view of the larynx and vocal folds or, preferably, endoscopic examination of the larynx.

For the *supraglottic* maneuver, the patient voluntarily initiates airway closure before oral transit begins and reopens the airway after the swallow, releasing the breath audibly to blow any residual off the folds. The instruction may be: "Put the bolus in your mouth, hold your breath, and keep holding it as you swallow. When the swallow is done, let your breath go in a sudden, audible breath." We typically do not instruct the patient to cough, because, in energetic and diligent patients this instruction has appeared

to contribute to vocal abuse with characteristic vocal fold changes. However, the power of effective "hawk-spit" is illustrated in Strategy 6 (materials folder, Chapter 18) by a patient with a pill stuck in the valleculae.

For the *"super" supraglottic* maneuver, the patient voluntarily and with effort initiates airway closure before oral transit begins. Effortful closure, such as is achieved when "bearing down" or fixing the upper body for heavy lifting, usually elicits supraglottic laryngeal constriction, thus supplementing glottic airway protection. The instructions are as above, with the addition of this significant effort. Both supraglottic and super-supraglottic maneuvers can be extended to include more than one swallow at a time as long as pulmonary function supports holding the breath for longer than one swallow. Instructions would be: "Hold your breath hard, keep holding your breath while you drink as much as you want from this cup, stop drinking, then let your breath go suddenly and audibly."

The final maneuver, the *Mendelsohn maneuver* (Jacob, Kahrilas, Logemann, Shah, & Ha, 1989), is aimed at improving or prolonging PES opening and has also been noted to normalize the timing of swallow events (Lazarus, Logemann, & Gibbons, 1993). Although prolonged laryngeal closure is one result of this maneuver, this is not the goal. Maximal hyoid/larynx elevation is associated with PES opening (Cook et al., 1989). When maximal elevation is prolonged, PES opening is prolonged. This maneuver is appropriately applied when videofluoroscopy reveals: (1) slowed transit of the bolus through the pharynx and PES, so that the PES closes before the bolus has been completely transferred; and (2) incomplete PES opening so that transit through the PES itself is slowed and it closes before the bolus has been completely transferred. The success of this maneuver in increasing or prolonging PES opening *cannot be* assessed clinically, even using techniques such as EMG feedback regarding activity of the hyoid elevators. Teaching involves identification of maximal hyoid/larynx elevation and then prolongation of this position during swallow.

An additional maneuver that has sometimes been effective, in our experience, is *mandibular advancement*. In patients with limited PES opening but good control of oral structures, this maneuver has been observed on fluoroscopy to apparently facilitate increased opening of the PES. The patient is instructed to jut the jaw forward at the same time swallow is initiated. A video clip illustrating this maneuver is included in the materials folder for Chapter 18 (Strategy 3).

## FACILITATIVE DEVICES

Facilitative devices modify the delivery of bolus material into the swallowing tract or change the shape of the tract in a manner that positively impacts swallowing efficiency and/or safety. For example, a syringe and catheter allow placement and delivery of the bolus to particular areas of the oral or pharyngeal cavities (see an example in the materials folder for Chapter 18, Strategy 2). These instruments may be useful in bypassing certain structures incapable of adequately directing or propelling the bolus to the pharynx,

or in facilitating movements conducive to bolus management.

Devices as simple as a modified spoon or a mandibular sling may allow management of food materials previously prohibited. In children, a variety of different nipples may aid and modify the delivery of liquid to the oral cavity. Different sizes and shapes of cups and bowls can also facilitate feeding and swallowing in both children and adults.

A palatal augmentation appliance, or palatal prosthesis, is sometimes useful in reshaping the oral cavity in a manner that facilitates bolus manipulation. For example, lowering of a particular area of the palate, such as the palatal vault, or certain portions of posterior or lateral palate, may improve tongue-to-palate contact for mashing or sealing a bolus, or for propelling the bolus posteriorly (Logemann, 1983). Palatal appliances are indicated in some patients with dysphagia with restricted lingual mass or motility because of either surgical ablation or neuromuscular impairment (Logemann, Kahrilas, Hurst, Davis, & Krugler, 1989; Wheeler, Logemann, & Rosen, 1980). If nasal regurgitation is present because of structural or neuromuscular impairment of the velopharyngeal port, the prosthesis may be extended to become a palatal lift or obturator. In rare instances, as in a patient with total glossectomy, a mandibular prosthesis may be of value in shunting bolus materials safely into the pharynx (Gillis & Leonard, 1983).

There is some evidence in studies of velopharyngeal dysfunction for speech that prosthetic appliances in the oral cavity (i.e., palatal lift appliances), may stimulate muscle activity (Blakely, 1960,

1964, 1969; Blakely & Porter, 1971; Weiss, 1971; Wong & Weiss, 1972). For the most part, the available reports appear largely anecdotal. In fact, in one study (Shelton, Lindquist, Arndt, Elbert, & Youngstrom, 1971), objective measures were acquired before and after prosthesis reduction, with no significant changes noted for oral or nasal sound pressure level, nasal air pressure, articulation proficiency, or in pharyngeal wall movement as seen on cinefluorography.

In our clinical experience, however, it has occasionally been possible to reduce the size of a prosthetic appliance. It has been presumed that the reductions were possible because of improved or increased muscle function in residual tissues, or even because of an increase in the bulk of residual tissues. Somewhat similarly, in the larynx, it has been our impression that Gelfoam injections to augment a fixed vocal fold on a temporary basis may have improved compensatory activity in the intact vocal fold, and perhaps prevented the development of less desirable compensatory behaviors, such as false-fold constriction/medialization. These clinical impressions are intriguing, and suggest a potential for prosthetic appliances (or augmentative substances) that has not been fully elaborated.

## Improved Initiation and Timing of Swallowing Events by Selective Stimulation

Implicit in some stimulation techniques is the belief that certain sensorineural thresholds critical to swallowing have been impaired and that these can be influenced, in particular, heightened, in a manner that impacts positively on the initiation, timing, and/or completeness of swallow and various swallowing events.

Primary to sensory cueing is orientation, that is, alerting the patient to the task. Reduction of noise, light, and other distractions, selective positioning, and verbal cuing may all enhance the patient's level of alertness. Verbal cues are general, such as the patient's name, or instructive, such as "swallow," "close your lips," or "chew," and may be accompanied by visual cues or demonstration. Children may benefit from additional orientation techniques. Rosenthal, Sheppard, and Lotze (1995) suggest prefeeding preparation may include rituals, attendance to state, including fatigue, readiness/playtime activities, and prosthesis placement. Morris and Klein (1987) have noted that a "ready state" may be enhanced by such factors as soothing music. Sensory cues involving taste or smell can also be used to heighten alertness. During the feeding task itself, pacing of bolus delivery is suggested as a technique to help improve breath control and stamina (Rosenthal, Sheppard, & Lotze, 1995). The usefulness of a particular technique or cue will vary depending on each patient's individual needs and abilities, and may require revision during the rehabilitative process, depending on goals and progress.

Direct stimulation of oral-pharyngeal structures prior to introduction of a bolus has also been used in attempts to facilitate swallowing. For example, rubbing or massaging the gums provides sensory input that may serve to "alert" and "orient" oral structures. Alexander (1987) suggests such preliminary preparation of cheek, lip, and tongue musculature using tactile/pressure input and muscular elongation. Graded pressure stimuli, firm to light touch, can also be applied to various muscles and muscle groups in preparation for functional activities. Special brushes used to stroke the lips, tongue, and gums will provide further oral stimulation and, possibly, facilitate function. Use of an exaggerated suck in the oral stage of swallow has also been described as useful for facilitating the initiation of pharyngeal swallow (Logemann, 1997). Other types of mechanical stimulation have been considered, as well.

Fujiu, Toleikis, Logemann, and Larson (1994) experimented with mechanical tapping, Sinclair (1970) with heavy and light stimulation of the posterior faucial pillars, and Kaatzke-McDonald, Post, and Davis (1996) with single and repetitive touch. Power et al. (2004) used a vibratory stimulus at 5 Hz presented to the faucial pillars and described *inhibition* of corticobulbar projections and *lengthened* swallow response times. Conversely, stimulation with a lower frequency stimulus (0.2 Hz) in the same study appeared to increase corticobulbar excitability, with no observed alterations in swallow initiation latency, pointing to the need for understanding specific effects of various stimuli on brain activity and swallow function *prior* to their wide clinical use. Thermal stimulation, or icing, of the anterior faucial pillars by touching or stroking them with a chilled laryngeal (00) mirror has been shown in some studies to increase the speed of initiation of the pharyngeal swallow and improve timing of subsequent swallowing events

(Kaatzke-McDonald, Post, & Davis, 1996; Lazzara, Lazarus, & Logemann, 1986). Other authors have demonstrated no substantial effect with this technique, however (Ali, Laundl, Wallace, deCarle, & Cook, 1996; Rosenbek, Robbins, Fishback, & Levine, 1991). Rosenbek et al. (1991) reported some immediate effects in CVA patients exposed to thermal stimulation, but no residual effects at one month posttreatment. Martin (1994) reported thermal stimulation to be most effective when combined with other input modalities, including cognitive stimulation and the presence of a bolus. Kaatzke-McDonald et al. (1996) reported an increase in swallow latency (rather than the desired decrease) with cold stimulation, and no changes with touch or chemical (glucose, saline) stimulation. Knauer, Castell, Dalton, Nowak, and Castell (1990) reported no changes in resting pressure of the upper esophageal sphincter or swallow coordination using both thermal stimulation and a variety of pharmacological agents.

Of additional interest are recent studies demonstrating changes in cortical behavior with electrical stimulation which has been used either to increase muscular contractions directly by increasing motor input to involved muscles (as described previously), or to influence sensory input to reflex arcs associated with swallowing. Hamdy, Azia, Rothwell, Hobson, and Thompson (1998) reported that electrical stimulation of the pharynx (5 Hz) produced changes in the size of cortical motor representation involved in swallow. Interestingly, the increased size was bilateral but asymmetric, and appeared to be associated with a decrease in the size of esophageal cortical representation. In a subsequent study, Fraser et al. (2002) monitored the effects of pharyngeal stimulation with transcranial magnetic stimulation in acute onset, hemispheric stroke patients. The authors identified increases in cortical pharyngeal representation and excitability, in particular, in the undamaged hemisphere, with 5-Hz stimulation for a period of 10 minutes. The changes were associated with improved swallowing function, as well. On the other hand, stimulation with other frequencies resulted in inhibition of pharyngeal excitability and longer delays in swallow initiation, as defined by the authors. Such studies not only demonstrate both positive and adverse effects of stimulation on cortical and brainstem structures, but help provide a sound basis for rehabilitation efforts incorporating stimulation techniques in selected populations.

## MEDICAL THERAPIES

Medical therapies designed specifically for the treatment of dysphagia of any cause have not been developed. Rather, therapies designed to treat the underlying medical condition resulting in dysphagia are the mainstay of medical therapy. The need to identify the etiology of the dysphagia becomes all the more important so that appropriate treatment can be instituted.

## Neuromuscular Disease

When a neuromuscular disease is the etiology of the dysphagia, whether or not the medical therapy appropriate for treating the condition has been

maximized must be ascertained. For any patient with dysphagia, a review of other medications prescribed for the patient will help determine if any of them may contribute to dysphagia. Many drugs affect the cholinergic nervous system and are known to have an effect on swallowing (Chapter 2). Occasionally, the same drugs prescribed to treat the neuromuscular disease may have a deleterious effect on swallowing. A balance between therapeutic benefit and side effects must be achieved.

## Gastroesophageal Reflux

Gastroesophageal reflux may contribute to the swallowing difficulties of an individual patient, and to certain patient populations (i.e., asthma [Babb, Notarangelo, & Smith, 1970; Duclone, VanDevenne, & Jovin, 1987], scleroderma, gastroparesis). Patients who demonstrate a cricopharyngeal bar on the dynamic swallow study are also at risk for reflux. In all such cases, an antireflux regimen is indicated. Reflux precautions should also apply in any patient who has been identified by the swallow team evaluation to be at risk for aspiration, for example, a patient with glottic incompetence.

In our practice, antireflux recommendations begin with behavior modifications. Patients are advised not to eat before bedtime. The last meal of the day should be at least 3 hours and preferably 4 hours before the patient assumes a supine position. No bedtime snacks are allowed. Digestion and gastric emptying will have adequate time to be completed while the patient is upright and gravity aids in minimizing the increased risk of reflux that exists during this period. Once the patient does go to bed, it is recommended that the head of the bed be elevated by 4 to 6 inches. The effect of gravity is therefore never completely removed. Patients are advised to use blocks under the front feet of the bed. This is more effective than trying to elevate the head with the use of pillows alone, as with this method patients will often assume a more supine position during sleep. Prior to going to bed, it is recommended that the patient take an antacid medication. This will neutralize any residual acid in the stomach and diminish the irritation to the upper aerodigestive tract should the patient experience reflux during the night.

Throughout the day, but especially at the evening meal, it is recommended that certain foods be avoided. These are foods thought to increase gastric acidity or to lower the lower esophageal sphincter resting tone. In addition, foods that result in a diuresis, such as caffeine-containing beverages, are to be avoided to prevent dehydration. Our list includes coffee, tea, peppermint, chocolate, citrus fruits, and alcohol. Meals high in fat content are known to increase the risk of reflux and a low fat diet in general is recommended. Patients are also advised not to use tobacco.

If behavior modification alone is not adequate to control reflux symptoms, specific medications can be added to the regimen. H2-blockers, such as cimetidine and ranitidine, are a standard therapy and can now be purchased over the counter. Our own preference is to have patients take these medications at a dose proven to be effective. Thus, medications are prescribed for them with specific recommendations for the dose and schedule believed to be most appropriate for their condition. When symptoms persist despite the use of H2-blockers, proton pump inhibitors, such as omeprazole and lansoprazole, can be prescribed. These medications are more powerful than the H2-blockers in terms of decreasing gastric acid production and they are extremely well tolerated. Typically, proton pump inhibitors are prescribed for a period of 2 to 3 months. Once the symptoms of gastric reflux have been controlled for this period of time, the proton pump inhibitors will be replaced by H2-blockers. If the patient tolerates this change, they can be maintained long-term on the H2-blockers, if indicated. Occasionally, medications that increase the rate of gastric emptying such as metaclopramide and cisipride are helpful in the control of reflux disease and can be prescribed along with proton pump inhibitors in patients where reflux has been very difficult to control.

## Xerostomia

Xerostomia impedes bolus lubrication and bolus flow and is deleterious to oral mucosal and dental health and esophageal GER defense (Zide, 1990). Poor bolus flow results in bolus residue on the surfaces on the tongue and palate, in the crevices and on the walls of the pharynx, placing the patient at risk for aspiration after the swallow. Predictably, in a swallower with xerostomia, residue is likely to increase with viscosity of the bolus, increasing the risk of aspiration of a potentially obstructive bolus. Treatment of xerostomia includes maximizing hydration, limiting mouth-breathing, minimizing use of products that would contribute to xerostomia (including many medications, mouthwashes, and toothpastes containing alcohol) or favor increased oral bacterial growth. We also recommend maximizing general hydration and oral hygiene, using one or a combination of over-the-counter products or the prescription drug pilocarpine. Patients with xerostomia need to avoid potentially irritating foods (acidic and pepper-hot) because of oral sensitivity or GERD. Strategies to wet the bolus carefully during oral preparation prior to initiation of oral transit can improve completeness of oral and pharyngeal transit. Certain factors (i.e., Sjögren's syndrome and related autoimmune conditions, radiation effects, medications that dry mucosal tissues or decrease salivary flow, iron or vitamin (B12) deficiency), predispose patients to xerostomia and are therefore important to identify during evaluation.

## SURGICAL THERAPIES

Although many forms of dysphagia respond to nonoperative therapy, selected conditions may benefit from surgical therapy. To identify these lesions and conditions, a thorough understanding of the physiology of swallowing is necessary (see Chapters 1 and 2). Successful swallow depends on the normal functioning of a number of structures acting as sphincters or valves that sequentially close and open to permit bolus material into the upper esophagus. Other structures, including the oral cavity, pharynx, and esophagus, must expand and compress to first propel and then clear bolus material as it moves through the aerodigestive tract. Dysphagia secondary to structural

or anatomic abnormalities that result in incompetence should lead the clinician to consider surgical correction. Careful evaluation of individual cases must be performed to ensure that the defect lends itself to surgical correction. In cases where structural integrity of the oral cavity and pharynx have not been compromised, but muscular weakness is the etiology of the dysphagia, surgery can occasionally improve the condition by repositioning structures into an arrangement more favorable for weakened muscle contraction.

The first sphincter function in swallow is comprised of the lips and oral musculature. Oral-labial incompetence results in drooling and poor bolus preparation. Both the clinical and dynamic swallow study may reveal loss of the test bolus onto the chin and difficulty with bolus positioning within the oral cavity. Surgical therapies designed to release contractures that prevent oral closure or are designed to recreate an intact obicularis oris muscle can improve dysphagia caused by this type of defect (Morris, Bardach, Jones, Christiansen, & Gray, 1995).

During oral preparation of the bolus, the soft palate contacts the base of the tongue to create the oral-pharyngeal valve, which prevents the bolus from entering the pharynx prematurely. Defects of the soft palate, as in the case of a cleft palate or an oropharyngeal cancer resection, can prevent closure of the valve and may allow early entry of the bolus into the pharynx. The soft palate elevates during the pharyngeal phase of the swallow to become a key element of the nasopharyngeal sphincter. Nasal regurgitation, therefore, is another consequence of a soft palate defect. Both early pharyngeal penetration and nasal regurgitation can be identified during a dynamic swallow study. Soft palate tissue defects and soft palate muscular weakness may be surgically repaired with local flaps such as a superiorly based pharyngeal flap (Stepnick & Hayden, 1994). Palatal obturators are also an option for correction of palatal soft tissue defects or muscle weakness and should be considered along with surgical therapy.

The tongue plays a major role in bolus preparation and is a key element of the oropharyngeal valving mechanism. It also creates the primary driving forces in oral and pharyngeal bolus propulsion. Adequate tongue mobility is crucial for these functions, especially for pharyngeal bolus propulsion. When the tongue is tethered anteriorly or laterally, such as after a floor of the mouth cancer resection, a dynamic swallow study may suggest poor pharyngeal contraction as the tongue's restricted mobility precludes adequate contact with the posterior pharyngeal wall during the pharyngeal phase of the swallow. In some cases, reconstruction at the time of resection may include procedures designed to minimize tethering. In others, secondary surgical therapy may be indicated to improve mobility. A tissue defect of the tongue base results in the loss of tongue bulk, and like mobility impairment, may be apparent in poor pharyngeal constriction on the dynamic swallow study. It is important to clinically differentiate problems related to loss of bulk, as opposed to loss of mobility. Tongue bulk defects may improve with surgical replacement of lost tissue with local, regional, or free tissue flaps (Anthony, Singer, & Mathes, 1994; Bodin, Lind, &

Arnander, 1994; Harries, 1996; Pauloski, Logemann, Fox, & Colangelo, 1995; Wolff, Dinemann, & Hoffmeister, 1995).

Defects of glottic valving, such as occur with vocal fold paralyses, result in poor vocal fold closure during deglutition. Aspiration of the bolus during the pharyngeal phase of the swallow, as the bolus passes by the elevated larynx, can typically be detected on the dynamic swallow study. Several surgical alternatives are available for the correction of vocal fold paralyses and other causes of glottic incompetence (Benninger et al., 1994; St. Guily et al., 1994). However, it must be kept in mind that vocal fold medialization may not always be successful in eliminating aspiration (Yip, Kendall, & Leonard, 2005).

Once the bolus has been prepared to be swallowed and has been propelled into the pharynx by the base of the tongue, the upper esophageal sphincter must open to allow passage of the bolus into the upper esophagus. This requires relaxation of the upper esophageal sphincter (the cricopharyngeus muscle). Cricopharyngeal achalasia may result from neuromuscular disease (McKenna & Dedo, 1992; St. Guily, Petrie, Bokowy, Angelard, & Chaussade, 1994) or gastroesophageal reflux (St. Guily, Moine, Perie, Bokowy, Angelard, et al., 1995) and may result in propulsion diverticuli such as a Zenker's diverticulum. Failure of cricopharyngeal relaxation may be identified on the dynamic swallow study by the presence of a "cricopharyngeal bar" or by decreased diameter of the maximum upper esophageal opening (UES). However, neither the dynamic swallow study nor upper esophageal sphincter manometry have consistently pre-dicted patients who will benefit from surgery (McKenna & Dedo, 1992; Shaw et al., 1996). On the other hand, there are studies that have documented that a cricopharyngeal myotomy can cor-rect failure of cricopharyngeal relax-ation as measured with manometry (Ellis, 1995; Schmitz, Bitonti, & Lemke, 1996). A study of 20 patients treated at our center by cricophayrngeal myo-tomy for cricopharyngeal dysfunction used videofluoroscopic swallow stud-ies before and after repair to evaluate patients. Prior to myotomy, the mean UES opening size for a 3-cc bolus was 0.30 cm ± 0.17, which was 57% of the mean of 60 normal controls (0.52 cm ± 0.15) ($p < 0.001$). After repair, the mean UES opening for the same bolus size improved to 0.51 cm ± 0.16 ($p < 0.0001$). The UES opening size in patients who had undergone repair was comparable to that of the normal controls ($p > 0.05$) (Yip, Kendall, & Leonard, 2005).

PES relaxation is no more important to successful swallow than elevation of the hyoid/larynx complex. If these struc-tures are not able to exert pull on the upper esophagus by their superior and anterior displacement, even a relaxed PES may not open. It is often difficult to distinguish patients who fail to relax the PES from those who fail to elevate the hyoid/larynx complex. The under-lying pathology of the dysphagia and the clinical presentation of the patient are currently the best distinguishing features of these two patient groups. Patients with fibrosis of the suprahyoid muscles following head and neck radi-ation, previously removed suprahyoid muscles, or weakened suprahyoid mus-cles following stroke may be unable to elevate the hyoid. The dynamic swal-low study in these cases is likely to demonstrate diminished hyoid bone ele-vation and poor larynx-to-hyoid approx-imation in addition to failure of the PES to open. Surgical therapy to correct this problem has not been performed exten-sively. The largest experience with sur-gery to elevate the hyoid and larynx has been in patients with obstructive sleep apnea in which the surgery is done to permanently enlarge the upper airway (McBride & Ergun, 1994; Riley, Powell, & Guilleminault, 1994; Sher, Schechtman, & Piccirillo, 1996). Anec-dotal experience with surgical cor-rection of poor hyoid and laryngeal elevation in dysphagia has been suc-cessful, however (Kendall, Leonard, & McKenzie, unpublished data).

Esophageal achalasia and strictures are often treated with esophageal dila-tions. The swallow study does not rou-tinely include an evaluation of the entire esophagus but is often helpful in identifying proximal strictures in patients after laryngectomy. The finding of a narrowing that does not change during bolus passage is suggestive of a stricture. The definitive diagnosis is made on endoscopy, which can be immediately followed by dilation.

Dysphagia is often multifactorial. Surgical therapy may be able to correct part of the problem but often other dif-ficulties will persist. Patients need to be counseled about the limitations of sur-gery so that their expectations will be realistic. An immediate return to nor-mal swallow is unusual. Progress after surgery is more likely to be gradual, and a period of postoperative swallow therapy may be required to realize the fullest benefit from surgery.

## TREATMENT IMPLEMENTATION AND FOLLOW-UP

When an appropriate treatment plan has been finalized for a patient, it is the task of the dysphagia team to communicate the plan to the patient and all relevant caregivers. The report accompanying the plan will include summaries of the patient's medical and feeding history, and descriptions of procedures performed as a part of dysphagia assessment. Objective measures from the patient's performance on the dynamic swallow study are compared to available normative data, and summarized in terms of oral, pharyngeal, and laryngeal function. Any pertinent additional observations are noted, and a summary statement of the patient's current capabilities and impairments is offered.

The summary of findings from the clinical and radiographic evaluations should include conclusions that the referring professional may not be able to draw independently, that is, what do the findings suggest about the etiology and severity of the impairment, its impact on nutrition and respiratory health, and prognosis for improvement. For example, research from our own institution indicates that, in post-CVA patients, a pharyngeal transit time between 3 and 5 seconds is associated with a 48% increased risk of developing aspiration pneumonia (Johnson, McKenzie, Rosenquist, Lieberman, & Sievers, 1992). Such information, when available, is included in the summary as an indication of the potential impact of the dysphagia on the patient's respiratory health. In another case, a major feature of the dysphagia might be poor hypopharyngeal clearing. An appropriate summary would categorize the severity of the impairment, suggest its etiology in terms of pharyngeal function (weak pharyngeal constriction, inadequate hyoid/laryngeal elevation, poor PES opening), and remark on the increased risk of aspiration following the swallow. With the summary complete, recommendations from the team are enumerated. Examples of reports generated by our team are included in Figures 18–1, 18–2, 18–3, and 18–4.

It is extremely important that the plan be disseminated not just to caregivers in the patient's immediate environment, but to all those who are likely to be a part of the patient's life until, at least, re-evaluation is planned. If there are timing variables in the plan, that is, it has been recommended that the patient be on a liquid diet for a particular amount of time, then be advanced to a different diet, and so on, it will be critical to note the starting date of the plan in such a way that this information is not lost if the patient is moving from one setting to another. Members of the team who should be contacted in the event of a question regarding the treatment plan also need to be clearly indicated in the written version of the plan. In our setting, copies of the plan will be included in the patient's medical record, but will also be posted at bedside, included in hospital discharge plans, and provided to the patient's primary care and referring physicians. If a final report is not yet available prior to discharge, then oral or handwritten summaries are used. A particularly valuable practice is to encourage the patient, family members, and available caregivers to meet with one or more members of the team to review findings from the evaluation and to discuss the treatment plan at length. This invest-

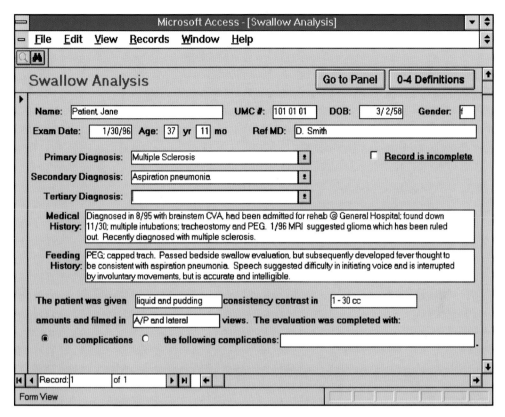

**Figure 18-1.** Information entered into patient information form of database (Microsoft Access).

ment in time and communication is typically educational for all participants and helps to ensure optimal implementation of the plan.

Recommendations for follow-up are included in the report, but it is the responsibility of the patient's referring physician to monitor the patient and determine the need for follow-up visits or re-evaluation. Few generalizations are possible regarding the timing of reevaluation, because this must be tailored to an individual patient. However, it is often dependent on meeting certain objectives or completing other treatments. For example, it may be recommended that a head and neck cancer patient return for re-evaluation

when strategies for airway protection have been learned in therapy and can be consistently performed. Upon demonstration of this capability, changes in diet can be considered. In a patient recovering from stroke, on the other hand, timing of follow-up may be more related to a change in the patient's general condition, in particular, if the patient is more aware, or alert, or cognitively intact, then changes in diet may be appropriate. In other instances, it may be recommended that a patient return for follow-up when other therapies have been completed. For example, a head and neck cancer patient who is undergoing postoperative radiation may need to return at the end of

**A.**

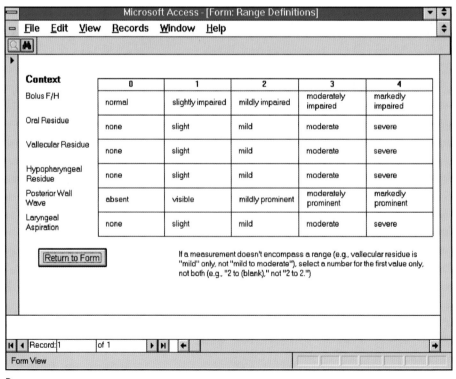

**B.**

**Figure 18–2. A.** Timing and displacement data from DSS entered into objective measures form (database calculates values). **B.** Subjective impressions can also be entered.

A.

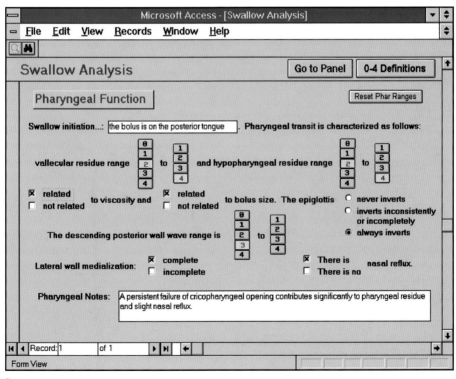

B.

**Figure 18–3.** Observations for oral function (**A**), pharyngeal function (**B**), and laryngeal function (**C**) are included. *(continues)*

C.

**Figure 18-3.** *(continued)*

this treatment. Or a patient with myasthenia gravis may be asked to return when medical therapy for the condition is stabilized. Whatever the individual circumstances, it is important that any changes from the treatment plan in effect be monitored carefully by the patient's caregivers, and that reevaluation be initiated when there is reason to suspect that the patient's capabilities have altered, for better or worse, in a way that raises new questions about the safety and efficiency of swallowing/food management.

In a busy clinical practice, it is easy to be so overwhelmed with the day-to-day problems of individual patients that there may be little provocation for retrospection about groups of patients. However, if we are to benefit from more than just repetition (i.e., performing dysphagia assessments on a large number of patients), it is necessary to build time into the schedule for scrutiny and critical review. One practice that has proved useful to our team is to periodically ask a question of ourselves, for example, how often have we observed a pseudovalleculae in laryngectomized patients, and are there similarities in these patients' surgical reconstructions, or how many of our head and neck cancer patients were swallowing without difficulty within

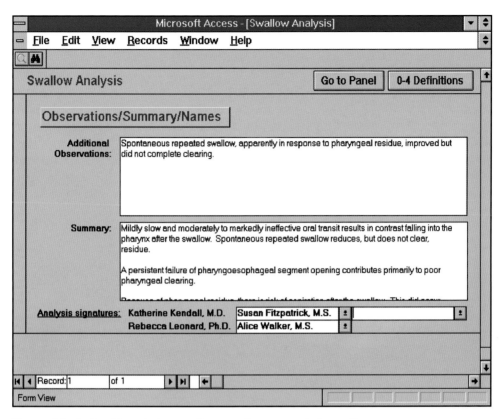

**Figure 18–4.** Additional observations and summary information.

6 months of postoperative radiation therapy, and how many of these underwent dysphagia therapy? One or two team members typically assume responsibility for researching our records for relevant data, which are then presented in preliminary form to the team. The group discussions generated by these exercises have led to a better understanding of swallowing, particular patient populations, and surgical and medical variables that influence swallowing, and have even generated more formal research projects. Our approach to assessment and treatment is subject to continual change as a consequence of such retrospective review, hopefully in ways that advance our care of patients.

## RECORD KEEPING

Our team evaluates and treats several hundred patients each year, and our disordered populations include neurogenic, head and neck cancer, pediatric and adult, and patients who are otherwise healthy with vague complaints of swallowing difficulty. In many cases, we follow patients over time and across multiple treatments. One tool that we have found of great value in managing the amount of "paper work" generated by the team practice is the use of a computerized system that enables us to input patient information data, which can then be used for multiple purposes. The system, based on

Microsoft's "Access" program for PC computers, required some time to learn, set up, and implement. In addition, forms for data input that would be applicable for all patients, allow us to input everything from case history interview information to measures made of dynamic swallow studies, and satisfy the various diverse interests of team members also required repeated efforts. However, as appropriate input parameters and output report forms were finalized, the advantages of a database approach to record-keeping became quite clear. At this point, we are able to enter information about a patient once, use it in multiple reports, and revise only data that need updating when the patient is seen for follow-up. We are also able to query the database to identify patients who meet particular criteria, for example, all patients with vocal-fold paralyses seen from 2004 to 2007 who aspirated liquids but did well on other bolus consistencies. This capability has expedited our clinical work, particularly the time spent away from patients, and has also made the critical review process previously described much more comprehensive and expedient. Our ability to assess treatment outcomes in specific patient groups, or according to specific treatment variables, for example, has benefitted greatly from this approach.

## EVALUATING EFFECTS OF TIME/TREATMENT

As noted, many patients are followed over time and treatments by our team. It is imperative that we have good, that is, valid, reliable, assessment tools not only to diagnose dysphagia, but also to track change in our patients. An excellent way to do this is to examine *biomechanical* measures of swallow before and after treatments, or across time. The dynamic swallow study (DSS) has proven to be an integral part of our repertoire in treatment evaluation, allowing us to quantify changes in bolus transit times, swallow gesture times, and structural displacements associated with our interventions in a standardized manner. We have used this tool to assess effects of behavioral therapies, medical management strategies, and various surgeries. We have also used the DSS to help monitor changes in patients with, for example, degenerative conditions that may eventually require them to consider nonoral methods of eating. Manometry is a related biomechanical tool used to document changes in swallowing pressures associated with time or treatment (discussed in Chapter 13).

Other observations from fluoroscopy studies do not provide quantitative data pertinent to bolus transit timing or swallow gesture displacements, but do provide insights into swallowing function, including, simply, the presence of aspiration or penetration. Aspiration may be seen on an initial study and be absent on a subsequent study. The Penetration-Aspiration Scale is an ordinal scale that provides a more objective rating of these subjective observations, including the extent of bolus entry into the airway, and the patient's ability to respond/clear this stimulus (Rosenbek, Robbins, Roecker, Coyle, & Wood, 1996).

Additional evidence of the effects of time/treatment may be based on other types of *imaging studies*. For example, a chest x-ray that helped document aspiration pneumonia also provides evidence of lung recovery. Endoscopy of the pharynx, larynx (see Chapter 11), and/or the esophagus (see Chapter 13) is another imaging tool that can be used to monitor a patient's progress with behavioral, medical or surgical interventions. *Laboratory studies* are frequently a part of treatment assessment. For example, a CBC (complete blood count) can establish or rule out an infectious or inflammatory disease, and a nutritional evaluation may include the determination of serum protein and albumin levels (see Chapter 10) important to improved nutrition. *Special studies* include pH testing to monitor the effects of medication or surgery on reflux events (see Chapter 6), and scintigraphy, used to determine percent of bolus material aspirated.

Many other criteria can be included in assessing outcomes. *Clinical evidence* of a patient's ability to move from nonoral to oral feeding, reductions in time required for oral feeding, or in restrictions necessary for oral eating, are examples of extremely useful variables to consider in assessment. Stable weight or weight gain, normal temperatures, and improved ability to manage saliva are similarly useful as signs of a patient's improving condition. Measures that incorporate patients' own appraisals of their eating or swallowing abilities are increasingly recognized as important. These might be classified as *self-assessment* tools. The American Speech-Language Hearing Association has developed the NOMS (National Outcomes Measurement System) that includes a section on dysphagia and assesses patients' functional progress and satisfaction with their progress (American Speech-Language-Hearing Association /http://www.asha.org/). Two additional survey tools that have undergone extensive development are the SWAL-QOL (swallowing quality of life) and SWAL-CARE (swallowing quality of care) (McHorney, Bricker, Kramer, Rosenbek, Robbins, et al., Chignell, 2000; McHorney, Bricker, Robbins, Kramer, Rosenbek, et al., 2000; McHorney, Robbins, Lomax, Rosenbek, et al., Chignell, et al., 2002). These instruments are designed for patients with oropharyngeal dysphagia, and involve the completion of a set of questions pertinent to social, psychological, and cultural domains of swallowing/eating function, and to patients' perceptions of the quality of care received for their dysphagia. In a recent study (McHorney, Martin-Harris, Robbins, & Rosenbek, 2006), associations between the two survey tools and results of videofluoroscopy studies were examined in 386 patients. The Pentration Aspiration Scale previously referenced was used to evaluate the fluoroscopy studies. Interestingly, though not surprising to clinicians, relationships between the surveys and the Penetration Aspiration Scale were generally weak. The authors suggest this reflects evidence not only of a generally recognized lack of covariance between patient-based measures of function and clinician-based measures, but also, the need to consider both in evaluating treatment effects. This is a point well-taken, in our opinion. No single test, study, or opinion is likely to adequately and accurately assess changes with time or treatment.

## THE TEAM APPROACH

Nowhere is the advantage of a multidisciplinary approach to dysphagia assessment more obvious than in the team-developed treatment plan. Etiologies of dysphagia cross many disease and disorder categories. The bodily systems that contribute to, or are affected by, dysphagia are extensive in number, and complex. Potential treatments range from medical, to surgical, to behavioral. And the implications of dysphagia for an individual's physical, mental, and social well-being can be enormous. An effective treatment plan must reflect this understanding of the dysphagia gestalt, and this requires, in our opinion, as many relevant and thoughtful specialty resources as we can bring to bear. The likelihood of failing to recognize salient features of either the patient or the disorder is minimized, and the likelihood of developing an appropriate model for treatment is maximized. To some extent, of course, the effectiveness of a team is determined by the relative strengths of each member, and by the interprofessional dynamics that obtain in team activities. But the opportunity to share expertise, to formulate objectives for treatment that reflect each specialist's concerns and knowledge base, and to then collectively prioritize the components of the plan, is well worth the effort required to establish a team and to maintain whatever diligence is necessary to ensure that it functions effectively as a team.

## STUDY QUESTIONS

1. What factors, beyond the results of instrumental evaluations, should be considered in making treatment recommendations for a patient?
2. What are some of the indications for recommending exercises designed to improve strength or mobility of structures?
3. Would respiratory exercises ever be considered appropriate for a patient with dysphagia? Under what circumstances?
4. What is the "IOPI"? The Shaker exercise? What are they designed to do? Is their evidence to support their effectiveness?
5. How might electrical stimulation affect a muscle? What is meant by "selective stimulation"?
6. What characteristics of a bolus might be manipulated to facilitate swallow?
7. What are "postural compensations," and how might they facilitate swallow?
8. Do "facilitative maneuvers" require more from a patient than other strategies? Why? What are some of these maneuvers, and why/when would each be implemented?
9. What behavioral recommendations to patients are typically included in reflux management?
10. What might be useful treatments in managing xerostomia?
11. Which of the following might benefit from a surgical procedure? What kind of procedure(s)?
    a. oral closure defects.
    b. velopharyngeal valve failure.
    c. reduced pharyngoesophageal opening size.
    d. esophageal stricture.
12. What types of assessment tools might be useful in determining the effects of time or treatment?

## REFERENCES

Alexander, R. (1987). Oral-motor treatment for infants and young children with cerebral palsy. In E. Mysak (Ed.), *Semi-*

*nars in speech and language* (pp. 87–100). New York: Thieme.

Ali, G., Laundl, T., Wallace, K., deCarle, D., & Cook, I. (1996). Influence of cold stimulation on the normal pharyngeal swallow response. *Dysphagia, 11,* 2–8.

Anthony, J. P., Singer, M. I., & Mathes, S. J. (1994). Pharyngoesophageal reconstruction using the tubed free radial forearm flap. *Clinics in Plastic Surgery, 21,* 137–147.

Babb, R. R., Notarangelo, J., & Smith, V. W. (1970). Wheezing: A clue to gastroesophageal reflux. *American Journal of Gastroenterology, 53,* 230–233.

Barbay, S., Plautz, E. J., Friel, K. M., Frost, S. B., Dancause, N., Stowe, A. M., et al. (2006). Behavioral and neurophysiological effects of delayed training following a small ischemic infarct in primary motor cortex of squirrel monkeys. *Experimental Brain Research, 169,* 106–116.

Benninger, M. S., Crumley, R. L., Ford, C. N., Gould, W. J., Hanson, D. G., Ossoff, R. H., et al. (1994). Evaluation and treatment of the unilateral paralyzed vocal fold. *Otolaryngology-Head and Neck Surgery, 111,* 497–508.

Bisch, E. M., Logemann, J. A., Rademaker, A. W., Kahrilas, P. J., & Lazarus. C. L. (1994). Pharyngeal effects of bolus volume, viscosity, and temperature in patients with dysphagia resulting from neurologic impairment and in normal subjects. *Journal of Speech and Hearing Research, 37,* 1041–1049.

Blakely, R. W. (1960). Temporary speech prostheses as an aid in speech therapy. *Cleft Palate Bulletin, 10,* 63–65.

Blakely, R. W. (1964). The complementary use of speech prostheses and pharyngeal flaps in palatal insufficiency. *Cleft Palate Journal, 2,* 194–198.

Blakely, R. W. (1969). The rationale for a temporary speech prosthesis in palatal insufficiency. *British Journal of Disorders of Communication, 4,* 134–139.

Blakely, R., & Porter, D. (1971). Unexpected reduction and removal of an obturator in a patient with palate paralysis, *British Journal of Disorders of Communication, 6,* 33–36.

Blumenfeld, L., Hahn, Y., Lepage, A., Leonard, R., & Belafsky, P. C. (2006). Transcutaneous electrical stimulation versus traditional dysphagia therapy: A nonconcurrent cohort study. *Otolaryngology-Head and Neck Surgery, 135,* 754–757.

Bodin, I. K., Lind, M. G., & Arnander, C. (1994). Free radial forearm flap reconstruction in surgery of the oral cavity and pharynx: surgical complications, impairment of speech and swallowing. *Clinics in Otolaryngology, 19,* 28–34.

Bulow, M., Olsson, R., & Ekberg, O. (2003).Videoradiographic analysis of how carbonated thin liquids and thickened liquids affect the physiology of swallowing in subjects with aspiration on thin liquids. *Acta Radiologica, 44,* 366–372.

Burnett, T. A., Mann, E. A., Cornell, S. A., & Ludlow, C. L. (2003). Laryngeal elevation achieved by neuromuscular stimulation at rest. *Journal of Applied Physiology, 94,* 128–134.

Burnett, T. A., Mann, E. A., Stocklosa, J. B., &, Ludlow, C. L. (2005). Self-triggered functional electrical stimulation during swallowing. *Journal of Neurophysiology, 94,* 4011–4018.

Cerny, F., & Burton, H. (2001). *Exercise physiology for health care professionals.* Champaigne, IL: Human Kinetics.

Cook, I. J., Dodds, W. J., Dantas, R.O., Massey, B., Kern, M. K., Lang, I. M., et al. (1989). Opening mechanism of the human upper esophageal sphincter, *American Journal of Physiology, 257,* G748–G759.

Duclone, A., Van Devenne, A., & Jovin, H. (1987). Gastroesophageal reflux in patients with asthma and chronic bronchitis, *American Review of Respiratory Disease, 135,* 327–332.

Easterling, C., Grande, B., Kern, M., Sears, K., & Shaker, R. (2005). Attaining and maintaining sometric and isokinetic goals of the Shaker exercise. *Dysphagia, 20*, 133–138.

Ellis, F. H. (1995). Pharyngoesophageal (Zenker's) diverticulum. *Advances in Surgery, 28*, 171–189.

El Sharkawi, A., Ramig, L., Logemann J. A., Pauloski, B. R., Rademaker, A. W., Smith, C. H., et al. (2002). Swallowing and voice effects of Lee Silverman Voice Treatment: A pilot study. *Journal of Neurology, Neurosurgery and Psychiatry, 72*, 31–36.

Fraser, C., Power, M., Hamdy, S., Rothwell, J., Hobday, D., Hollander, I., et al. (2002). Driving plasticity in human adult motor cortex is associated with improved motor function after brain injury. *Neuron, 30*, 831–840.

Freed, M. L., Freed, L., Chatburn, R. L., & Christian, M. (2001). Electrical stimulation for swallowing disorders caused by stroke. *Respiratory Care, 46*, 466–474.

Fujiu, M., & Logemann, J. A. (1996). Effect of a tongue-holding maneuver on posterior pharyngeal wall movement during deglutition. *American Journal of Speech Language Pathology, 5*, 23–30.

Fujiu, M., Toleikis, R., Logemann, J. A., & Larson, C. R. (1994). Glossopharyngeal evoked potential in normal subjects following mechanical stimulation of the anterior faucial pillar. *Electroencephalography and Clinical Neurophysiology, 92*, 183–195.

Gillis, R., & Leonard, R. (1983). Prosthetic treatment for speech and swallowing in patients with total glossectomy, *Journal of Prosthetic Dentistry, 50*, 808–814.

Gobbo, O. L., & O'Mara, S. M. (2005). Exercise, but not environmental enrichment, improves learning after kainic acid-induced hippocampal neurodegeneration in association with an increase in brain-derived neurotrophic factor. *Behavioural Brain Research, 159*, 21–26.

Gross, R. D., Mahlmann, J., & Grayhack, J. P. (2003). Physiologic effects of open and closed tracheostomy tubes on the pharyngeal swallow. *Annals of Otology, Rhinology and Laryngology, 112*, 143–152.

Hamdy, S., Aziz, Q., Rothwell, J. C., Hobson, A., & Thompson, D. G. (1998). Sensorimotor modulation of human cortical swallowing pathways. *Journal of Physiology, 506*, 857–866.

Harries, M. L. (1996). Unilateral vocal fold paralysis: A review of the current methods of surgical rehabilitation. *Journal of Laryngology and Otology, 110*, 11–16.

Hiss, S. G., & Huckabee, M. L. (2005). Timing of pharyngeal and upper esophageal sphincter pressures as a function of normal and effortful swallowing in young healthy adults. *Dysphagia, 20*, 149–156.

Huckabee, M. L. (2007). Maximizing rehabilitative efforts for dysphagia recovery: SEMG biofeedback monitoring. *Kay Elemetrics: Swallowing application notes.* Pinehurst, NJ: KayPentax.

Humbert, I. A. Poletto, C. J., Saxon, K. G., Kearny, P. R., Crujido, L., Wright-Harp, W., et al. (2006). The effect of surface electrical stimulation on hyolaryngeal movement in normal individuals at rest and during swallowing. *Journal of Applied Physiology, 101*, 1657–1663.

Jacob, P., Kahrilas, P. J., Logemann, J. A., Shah, V., & Ha, T. (1989). Upper esophageal sphincter opening and modulation during swallowing. *Gastroenterology, 97*, 1469–1478.

Johnson, R., McKenzie, S., Rosenquist, J., Lieberman, J., & Sievers, A. (1992). Dysphagia following stroke: Quantitative evaluation of pharyngeal transit times. *Archives of Physical Medicine and Rehabilitation, 73*, 419–423.

Kaatzke-McDonald, M., Post, E., & Davis, P. (1996). The effects of cold, touch, and chemical stimulation of the anterior faucial pillar on human swallowing. *Dysphagia, 11*, 198–206.

Kagel, M., & Leopold, N.A. (1992). Dysphagia in Huntington's disease: A 16 year retrospective, *Dysphagia, 7*, 106–114.

Kleim, K. A., Jones, T. A., & Schallert, T. (2003). Motor enrichment and the induction of plasticity before or after brain injury. *Neurochemical Research, 28,* 1757–1769.

Knauer, C. M., Castell, J. A., Dalton, C. B., Nowak, L., & Castell, D. O. (1990). Pharyngeal/upper esophageal sphincter pressure dynamics in humans. Effects of pharmacologic agents and thermal stimulation. *Digestive Diseases and Sciences, 35,* 774–780.

Koessler, W., Wanke, T., Winkler, G., Nader, A., Toifl, K., Kurz, H., et al. (2001). 2 years' experience with inspiratory muscle training in patients with neuromuscular disorders. *Chest, 120,* 765–769.

Lazarus, C. (2006). Tongue strength and exercise in healthy individuals and in head and neck cancer patients. *Seminars in Speech and Language: New Frontiers in Dysphagia Rehabilitation, 27,* 260–267.

Lazarus, C., Logemann, J. A., & Gibbons, P. (1993). Effects of maneuvers on swallowing function in a dysphagic oral cancer patient. *Head and Neck Surgery, 15,* 419–424.

Lazarus, C., Logemann, J. A., Song, C. W., Rademaker, A. W., & Kahrilas, P. J. (2002). Effects of voluntary maneuvers on tongue base function for swallowing. *Folia Phoniatrica et Logopaedica, 54,* 171–176.

Lazzara, G., Lazarus, C., & Logemann, J. A. (1986). Impact of thermal stimulation on the triggering of the swallow reflex. *Dysphagia, 1,* 73–77.

Logemann, J. A. (1983). *Evaluation and treatment of swallowing disorders.* San Diego, CA: College-Hill Press.

Logemann, J. A. (1997). Therapy for oropharyngeal swallowing disorders. In A. L. Perlman & K. Schulze-Delrieu (Eds.), *Deglutition and its disorders: Anatomy, physiology, clinical diagnosis, and management* (pp. 449–462). San Diego, CA: Singular.

Logemann, J. A., Kahrilas, P. J., Hurst, P., Davis, J., & Krugler, C. (1989). Effects of intraoral prosthetics on swallowing in patients with oral cancer. *Dysphagia, 4,* 118–120.

Logemann, J. A., Kahrilas, P. J., Kobara, M., & Vakil, B. (1989). The benefit of head rotation on pharyngoesophageal dysphagia. *Archives of Physical Medicine and Rehabilitation, 70,* 767–771.

Logemann, J. A., Pauloski, B. R., Colangelo, L., Lazarus, C., Fujiu, M., & Kahrilas, P. J. (1995). Effects of a sour bolus on oropharyngeal swallowing measures in patients with neurogenic dysphagia. *Journal of Speech and Hearing Research, 38,* 556–563.

Ludlow, C., Bielamowicz, S., Daniels Rosenberg, M., Abvalavanar, R., Rossini, K., Gillespie, M., et al. (2000). Chronic intermittent stimulation of the thyroarytenoid muscle maintains dynamic control of glottal adduction. *Muscle and Nerve, 23,* 44–57.

Ludlow, C. L., Humbert, I., Saxon, J., Poletto, C., Sonies, B., & Crujido, L. (2007). Effects of surface electrical stimulation on hylaryngeal movements in normal individuals at rest and during swallowing. *Dysphagia, 101,* 1657–1663.

Martin, B. (1994). Treatment of dysphagia in adults. In L. R. Cherney (Ed.), *Clinical management of dysphagia in adults and children* (Chap. 6). Aspen, MD: Aspen.

McBride, M. A., & Ergun, G. A. (1994).The endoscopic management of esophageal strictures. *Gastrointestinal Endoscopy Clinics of North America, 4,* 595–621.

McKenna, J. A., & Dedo, H. (1992). Cricopharyngeal myotomy. *Annals of Otology, Rhinology and Laryngology, 101,* 216–221.

McHorney, C., Bricker, D., Kramer, A., Rosenbek, J., Robbins, J., Chignell, K., et al. (2000). The SWAL-QOL outcomes tool for oropharyngeal dysphagia in adults: I. Conceptual foundation and item development. *Dysphagia, 15,* 15–121.

McHorney, C., Bricker, D., Robbins, J., Kramer, A., Rosenbek, J., & Chignell, K. (2000). The SWAL-QOL outcomes tool for oropharyngeal dysphagia in adults: II. Item reduction and preliminary scaling. *Dysphagia, 15,* 122–133.

McHorney, C., Martin-Harris, B., Robbins, J., & Rosenbek, J. (2006). Clinical validity of the SWAL-QOL and SWAL-CARE outcome tools with respect to bolus flow measures. *Dysphagia, 21*, 141–148.

McHorney C, Robbins J, Lomax K, Rosenbek J, Chignell K, Kramer, A., et al. (2002). The SWAL-QOL and SWAL-CARE outcomes tool for oropharyngeal dysphagia in adults: III Documentation of reliability and validity. *Dysphagia, 17*, 97–114.

Meyer, G. W., & Castell, D. O. (1983). Anatomy and physiology of the esophageal body. In D. O. Castell & L. F. Johnson (Eds.), *Esophageal function in health and disease* (pp. 1–15). New York: Elsevier Science.

Morris, H. L., Bardach, J., Jones, D., Christiansen, J. L., & Gray, S. D. (1995). Clinical results of pharyngeal flap surgery: The Iowa experience. *Plastic and Reconstructive Surgery, 95*, 652–661.

Morris, S. E., & Klein, M. D. (1987). *Pre-feeding skills: A comprehensive resource for feeding development.* Tuscon, AZ: Therapy Skill Builders.

Nudo, R. (2003). Adaptive plasticity in motor cortex: Implications for rehabilitation after brain injury. *Journal of Rehabilitative Medicine, 41*(Suppl.), 7–10.

Nudo, R. (2005). Neural plasticity and functional recovery following cortical ischemic injury. *Conference Proceedings, IEEE Engineering in Medicine and Biology Society, 4*, 4145–4148.

Nudo, R. (2007). Postinfarct cortical plasticity and behavioral recovery. *Stroke, 38*, 840–845.

Nudo, R., & Friel, K. M. (1999). Cortical plasticity after stroke: implications for rehabilitation. *Revue Neurologique* (Paris), *155*, 713–717.

Palmer, P. M., McCulloch, T. M., Jaffe, D., & Neel, A. T. (2005). Effects of a sour bolus on the intramuscular electromyographic (EMG) activity of muscles in the submental region. *Dysphagia, 20*, 210–217.

Pauloski, B. R., Logemann, J. A., Fox, J. C., & Colangelo, L. A. (1995). Biomechanical analysis of the pharyngeal swallow in postsurgical patients with anterior tongue and floor of mouth resection and distal flap reconstruction. *Journal of Speech and Hearing Research, 38*, 110–123.

Pelletier, C. A., & Lawless, H. T. (2003). Effect of citric acid and citric acid-sucrose mixtures on swallowing in neurogenic oropharyngeal dysphagia. *Dysphagia, 18*, 231–241.

Power, M., Fraser, C., Hobson, A., Rothwell, J. C., Mistry, S., Nicholson, D.A., et al. (2004). Changes in pharyngeal corticobulbar excitability and swallowing behavior after oral stimulation. *American Journal of Physiology—Gastrointestinal and Liver Physiology, 286*, G45–G50.

Riley, R. W., Powell, N. B., & Guilleminault, C. (1994). Obstructive sleep apnea and the hyoid: A revised surgical procedure. *Otolaryngology-Head and Neck Surgery, 111*, 717–721.

Robbins, J., Gangnon, R., Theis, S., Kays, S. A., & Hind, J. (2005). The effects of lingual exercise on swallowing in older adults. *Journal of the American Geriatric Society, 53*, 1483–1489.

Rosenbek, J. C., Robbins, J., Fishback, B., & Levine, R. (1991). Effects of thermal application in dysphagia after stroke. *Journal of Speech and Hearing Research, 34*, 1257–1267.

Rosenbek, J. C., Robbins, J. A., Roecker, E. B., Coyle, J. L., & Wood, J. L. (1996). A penetration-aspiration scale. *Dysphagia, 11*, 93–98.

Rosenthal, S., Sheppard, J. J., & Lotze, M. (1995). *Dysphagia in the child with developmental disabilities: Medical, clinical and family interventions.* San Diego, CA: Singular.

Sapienza, C., & Wheeler, K. (2006) Respiratory muscle strength training: functional outcomes versus plasticity. *Seminars in Speech and Language, 27*, 236–244.

Schmitz, J. P., Bitonti, D. A., & Lemke, R. R. (1996). Hyoid myotomy and suspension for obstructive sleep apnea syndrome. *Journal of Oral and Maxillofacial Surgery, 54*, 1339–1345.

Shaker, R., Easterling, K., Kern, M., Nitschke, T., Massey, D., Daniels, S., et al. (2002). Rehabilitation of swallowing by exercise in tube-fed patients with pharyngeal dysphagia secondary to abnormal UES opening. *Gastroenterology, 122*, 1314–1321.

Shaker, R., Kern, M., Bardan, E., Taylor, A., Stewart, E. T., Hoffmann, R. G., et al. (1997). Augmentation of deglutitive upper esophageal sphincter opening in the elderly by exercise. *American Journal of Physiology, 272*, G1518–G1522.

Shaw, D. W., Cook, I. J., Jamieson, G. G., Gabb, M., Simula, M., & Dent, E. J. (1996). Influence of surgery on deglutitive upper oesophageal sphincter mechanics in Zenker's diverticulum. *Gut, 38*, 806–811.

Shelton, R., Lindquist, A., Arndt, W., Elbert, M., & Youngstrom, K. (1971). Effect of speech bulb reduction on movement of the posterior wall of the pharynx and posture of the tongue. *Cleft Palate Journal, 8*, 10–17.

Sher, A. E., Schechtman, K. B., & Piccirillo, J. F. (1996). The efficacy of surgical modifications of the upper airway in adults with obstructive sleep apnea syndrome. *Sleep, 19*, 156–177.

Silverman, E. P., Sapienza, C. M., Saleem, A., Carmichael, C., Davenport, P. W., Hoffman-Ruddy, B., et al. (2006). Tutorial on maximum inspiratory and expiratory mouth pressures in individuals with idiopathic Parkinson disease (IPD) and the preliminary results of an expiratory muscle strength training program. *NeuroRehabilitation, 21*, 71–79.

Sinclair, W. J. (1970). Initiation of reflex swallowing forms the naso- and oropharynx. *American Journal of Physiology, 218*, 956–959.

St. Guily, J. L., Moine, A., Perie, S., Bokowy, C., Angelard, B., & Chaussade, S. (1995).

Role of pharyngeal propulsion as an indicator for upper esophageal sphincter myotomy. *Laryngoscope, 105*, 723–727.

St. Guily, J. L., Perie, S., Willig, T., Chaussade, S., Eymard, V., & Angelard, B. (1994). Swallowing disorders in muscular diseases: Functional assessment and indications of cricopharyngeal myotomy. *Ear, Nose and Throat Journal, 3*, 34–40.

Stathopoulos, E., & Duchan, J. F. (2006). History and principles of exercise-based therapy: How they inform our current treatment. *Seminars in Speech and Language: New Frontiers in Dysphagia Rehabilitation, 27*, 227–235.

Stepnick, D. W., & Hayden, R. E. (1994). Options for reconstruction of the pharyngoesophageal defect. *Otolaryngology Clinics of North America, 27*, 1151–1158.

Sullivan, P., Hind, J. A., & Roecker, E. B. (2001). Lingual exercise protocol for head and neck cancer: A case study [Abstract]. *Dysphagia, 16*, 154.

Weiss, C. (1971). Success of an obturator reduction program. *Cleft Palate Journal, 6*, 291–297.

Wheeler, K.M., Chiara, T., & Sapeinza, C.M. (2007). Surface electromyographic activity of the submental muscles during swallowing and during expiratory pressure threshold training tasks. *Dysphagia, 22*, 108–116.

Wheeler, R., Logemann, J. A., & Rosen, M. (1980). Maxillary reshaping prostheses: Effectiveness in improving speech and swallowing in post-surgical oral cancer patients. *Journal of Prosthetic Dentistry, 43*, 313–319.

Wolff, K. D., Dienemann, D., & Hoffmeister, B. (1995). Intraoral defect coverage with muscle flaps. *Journal of Oral and Maxillofacial Surgery, 53*, 680–685.

Wong, R., & Johnson, L. F. (1983). Achalasia. In D. O. Castell & L. F. Johnson (Eds.), *Esophageal function in health and disease* (pp. 99–124). New York: Elsevier Science.

Wong, L., & Weiss, C. (1972). A clinical assessment of obturator-wearing cleft palate patients. *Journal of Prosthetic Dentistry, 27,* 632–633.

Yip, H., Kendall, K. A., & Leonard, R. J. (2005). Cricoharyngeal myotomy normalizes the opening size of the upper esophageal sphincter in cricopharyngeal dysfunction. *Laryngoscope, 116,* 93–96.

Zide, B. M. (1990).Deformities of the lips and cheeks. In J. G. McCarthy (Ed.), *Plastic surgery* (Chap. 38). Philadelphia: WB Saunders.

# *Index*